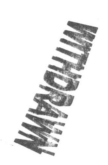

PUBLIC HEALTH POLICIES IN THE EUROPEAN UNION

Public Health Policies in the European Union

Edited by
WALTER HOLLAND, ELIAS MOSSIALOS
with PAUL BELCHER, BERNARD MERKEL

Ashgate

Aldershot • Brookfield USA • Singapore • Sydney

Published by
Ashgate Publishing Limited
Gower House
Croft Road
Aldershot
Hampshire GU11 3HR
England

Ashgate Publishing Company
Old Post Road
Brookfield
Vermont 05036
USA

Ashgate website: http://www.ashgate.com

British Library Cataloguing in Publication Data
Public health policies in the European Union
   1. Medical policy - European Union countries 2. Public health
   - European Union countries
   I. Holland, Walter W. (Walter Werner) II. Mossialos, Elias
   III. Belcher, Paul IV. Merkel, Bernard
   362.1'094

Library of Congress Cataloging-in-Publication Data
Public health policies in the European Union / edited by Walter Holland, Elias Mossialos, with Paul Belcher, Bernard Merkel.
     p. cm.
   Includes index.
   ISBN 0-7546-2072-7
     1. Public health--Europe. 2. Medical policy--Europe. 3. Health planning--Europe. 4. Public health--Political aspects--Europe. I. Holland, Walter W. (Walter Werner)

RA483 .P83 1999
362.1'094 21--dc21   99-043342

ISBN 0 7546 2072 7

Printed and bound in Great Britain by MPG Books Ltd, Bodmin, Cornwall

Contents

Contributors

Arpo Aromaa
Research Professor, Department of Health and Disability, The National Public Health Institute, Helsinki, Finland.

Gerard Breart
Director of Unité 149 (Recherches épidémiologiques sur la santé des femmes et des enfants), Institut National de la Santé et de la Recherche Médicale (INSERM), Paris, France.

Reinhard Busse
Director, Health Care Services and Health Services Unit, Department of Epidemiology and Social Medicine, Medizinische Hochschule Hannover, Germany.

Johan Calltorp
Professor of Public Health Management, Nordic School of Public Health, Gottenberg, Sweden.

Marie-Christine Closon
Professor of Health Economics, Centre d'Etude Interdisciplinaires en Economie de la Santé, Université Catholique de Louvain, Belgium.

David Crainich
Teaching Assistant in Health Economics, Facultés Universitaires Saint-Louis, Brussels, Belgium.

Patricia Fitzpatrick
Senior Lecturer, Department of Public Health Medicine and Epidemiology, University College Dublin, Ireland.

Louise J Gunning-Schepers
Professor of Social Medicine, Vice Dean and Member of the Board of Management of the Academic Medical Centre at the University of Amsterdam, The Netherlands.

Danielle Hansen-Koenig
Director-General, Directorate of Health, Luxembourg.

Bernadette Herity
Professor of Public Health Medicine, University College Dublin, Ireland.

Walter Holland
Former President of the International Epidemiological Association and Visiting
Professor, LSE Health, The London School of Economics and Political Science,
United Kingdom.

Michael Hübel
Principal Administrator, Directorate-General V/F (Employment, Industrial Relations
and Social Affairs – Public Health and Safety at Work), The European Commission,
Luxembourg.

Claudio Macchi
Research Fellow, Dipartimento di Scienze Sanitare Applicate e Psicocomportamentali,
University of Pavia, Italy.

Alessandra Marinoni
Director and Professor, Dipartimento di Scienze Sanitare Applicate e
Psicocomportamentali, University of Pavia, Italy.

Bernard Merkel
Principal Administrator, Directorate-General V/F (Employment, Industrial Relations
and Social Affairs – Public Health and Safety at Work), The European Commission,
Luxembourg.

Johannes Mosbech
Former Consultant and Head of the National Board of Health, Denmark.

Elias Mossialos
Director, LSE Health, The London School of Economics and Political Science, United
Kingdom.

Michael O'Brien
Former President of the FPHM (Faculty of Public Health Medicine, UK) and
Chairman of Northumberland Health Authority, United Kingdom.

George Papoutsakis
Director, Department of Public Health, Ministry of Health, Athens, Greece.

Govin Permanand
Research Assistant, LSE Health, The London School of Economics and Political
Science, United Kingdom.

Eleni Petridou
Associate Professor of Epidemiology, School of Medicine, University of Athens,
Greece.

Victor Ramos
Assistant Professor of Public Health, New School of Public Health, Lisbon, Portugal.

Mady Roulleaux
Principal Advisor, Directorate of Health, Luxembourg.

Claude Rumeau-Rouquette
Former Director of Unité 149 (Recherches épidémiologiques sur la santé des femmes et des enfants), Institut National de la Santé et de la Recherche Médicale (INSERM), Paris, France.

Friedrich Wilhelm Schwartz
Professor of Social Medicine, University of Hannover, Germany.

Andreu Segura Benedicto
Director, Institut Universitari de Salut Publica de Catalunya, Universitat de Barcelona, Spain.

Yannis Skalkidis
Research Associate, School of Medicine, University of Athens, Greece.

Nathalie Swartenbroek
Researcher, Centre d'Etude Interdisciplinaires en Economie de la Santé, Université Catholique de Louvain, Belgium.

Engelbert Theurl
Professor of Health Economics, Institut für Finanzwissenschaft der Leopold Franzens-Universität, Innsbruck, Austria.

Yannis Tountas
Assistant Professor of Public Health, School of Medicine, University of Athens, Greece.

Aphrodite Velonaki
Former Advisor, Ministry of Health, Athens, Greece.

Emmanuel Velonakis
Independent Physician, Athens, Greece.

Acknowledgements

The editors would like to acknowledge the support of the European Commission through grant SOC 95 201 552 05F01 and the research assistance of Kristen Goliber and Anna Maresso. They are also indebted to Sarah Moncrieff for her expert help with the preparation of the manuscript.

1

Public Health Policies and Priorities in Europe

Walter Holland, Elias Mossialos and Govin Permanand

1 Introduction: Health and the European Union

The health of most of the populations of the developed world has never been better. Powles[1] has dealt comprehensively with the historical changes and developments in disease, and attempted to relate these to changes in social and other environmental factors. While recognising that the relationship between disease and economic/social development is complex, he cites several factors as having provided the basis for this change in disease occurrence. Among others, he points to the development of professionally applied public health measures, increasing maternal literacy, and the socialisation of children to now accept as normal the 'historically stringent norms regarding personal cleanliness'. In particular, he concluded that ideological and lifestyle-related changes within society; the cultural incorporation of 'counter-measures' against the negative effects of economic progress; and the crucial role played by modern hygiene in addressing issues pertaining to early life survival, are fundamental reasons for this underlying improvement in the health of the developed world.

In the European Union (EU) specifically, there has been a great diminution in the frequency of infectious disease and a considerable extension of the length of life, with a consequent increase in occurrence in the diseases that are associated with old age – cancer, stroke, and arthritis amongst others. This has serious implications in terms of the measures we must apply for the prevention of disease and improvement in the quality of life. With these changes in disease pattern, new infectious hazards have arisen, including human immunodeficiency virus (HIV), chlamydia and, in some parts of Eastern Europe, a recurrence of conditions such as diphtheria and tuberculosis which we had thought to have eliminated.

All health systems in the EU face the challenges associated with demographic change, most notably the ageing of the population, increasing population mobility, and growing social exclusion. While these place mounting pressures on health service provision at a time when public spending is under tight constraints, there are new opportunities for prevention and treatment, and there is growing interest in prevention and health promotion, and, in improving the quality of life.

In the EU, although the demographic challenges faced by national health care systems may be similar, this is not to say that public perceptions of these systems are therefore also similar. In fact, there are widely differing views on health services in the Community. A 1996 Eurobarometer survey revealed that citizens' satisfaction with their respective national health care systems varies considerably across the EU.[2] For instance, the study reported that approximately 90.0 per cent of respondents in Denmark were 'satisfied' with their health system, as opposed to only 19.9 per cent in Portugal. Perhaps even more noteworthy was that while only 4.7 per cent of Austrians reported being 'dissatisfied' with their health system, the equivalent figure in Italy was 69.4 per cent. In addition to these disparities, the study also pointed to considerable divergencies in per capita expenditure (measured in US$ purchasing power parities), and noted a correlation between higher levels of spending on health and greater levels of satisfaction.

Despite such differences, however, all EU countries face similar problems, including:

- Inequalities in both health status and health service provision between different geographical areas and social groups;

- Variations in the utilisation of services for similar conditions, for example, hysterectomy, immunisation, and family planning;

- Difficulties in the allocation of limited resources to different strategies, for example prevention versus cure, cure versus care or between services, for example, family planning services versus services for abortion; and

- Many of the current health-related problems in European countries are related to lifestyle behaviour and political/economic issues; for example, cigarette smoking and unemployment.

Most countries accept that difficult choices need to be made, and most therefore concentrate on the provision of health care services. However, there is remarkable disparity between the populations' satisfaction ratings with respect to health care services and objective performance measurements thereof.[3] Furthermore, health care services in and of themselves do relatively little to bring about an improvement in the health status of populations. Environmental factors such as housing, traffic and employment, behavioural factors such as smoking, diet and alcohol consumption, and the social factors associated with these, such as poverty, probably make greater contributions. Nonetheless, health care services have an essential role in improving the quality of life and can produce specific and valuable improvements in other aspects of health status.

Bearing these issues in mind, this chapter is divided into three parts. The first part discusses the health-related developments at EU level in terms of the legislative and decision-making frameworks up to the 1997 Treaty of Amsterdam, including an assessment of the roles of the High Level Committee on Health and the Interservice Group on Health. It also considers the changing nature of Community priorities in health, and addresses the complex question of health care in the EU, insofar as the Community has no official competencies in the area. Part two examines public health in the EU, and focuses on the European Commission's current priorities in this field. In doing so, it defines the basis of priority setting in public health generally, and analyses the different methodological approaches in establishing priorities at Member State and European Community levels specifically. And finally, part three draws conclusions from these analyses and offers some concrete recommendations for the future.

1.1 The legislative framework

To date, the lack of progress on the part of the European Union to develop a comprehensive health policy framework is mainly due to the fact that, unlike some other international organisations, it is primarily concerned with economic matters. This may explain why, except in instances where it is specifically related to the needs of the Single Market, health continues to feature towards the bottom of the political agenda. This includes issues related to product safety, health and safety at work, pharmaceuticals and medical devices, and the free movement of professionals.[4]

This lack of attention to health – or failure as some would in fact deem it – is in spite of the fact that the legal framework within which the EU may take action in the field of health policy has evolved considerably since the founding of the European Coal and Steel Community (ECSC) in 1951. At that time, the Community's health concerns were limited only to those related to occupational health in the coal and steel industries. However, a precedent was created by this initiative; a small proportion of the sales of coal and steel was used for research into ways to reduce the hazards in these industries.

The first major Community advance relating to health came in 1986 under the Single European Act (SEA). The SEA amended the earlier European Treaties (Paris, 1951 and Rome, 1957) as, in Article 100A(3), it required the Commission to take, as a base, 'a high level of health protection in its proposals concerning health, safety, and environmental and consumer protection, as they relate to the working of the Single European Market'. Article 118a of the Treaty (also added by the SEA) allowed the Council of Ministers, acting by qualified majority voting, to adopt specific Directives on health and safety issues.

The most significant provision in health was, however, introduced in the 1992 Treaty on European Union (TEU) agreed at the Maastricht Summit. The TEU granted the Commission a new and specific competence in public health through the insertion of Articles 3(o) and 129 in the Treaty establishing the European Community. Article 3(o) stipulated that the Community should contribute to the attainment of a high level of health protection, while Article 129 (Box 1 overleaf) identified two areas for Community action: disease prevention and health protection. Three means through which these objectives were to be achieved were outlined: research, health information

---

Box 1

Article 129 of the Treaty on European Union (Maastricht)

1. The Community shall contribute towards ensuring a high level of human health protection by encouraging cooperation between the Member States and, if necessary, lending support to their action.

   Community action shall be directed towards the prevention of diseases, in particular the major health sources, including drug dependence, by promoting research into their causes and their transmission, as well as health information and education.

   Health protection requirements shall form a constituent part of the Community's other policies.

2. Member States shall, in liaison with the Commission, coordinate among themselves their policies and programmes in the area referred to in paragraph 1. The Commission may, in close contact with other Member States, take any useful initiative to promote such coordination.

3. The Community and the Members shall foster cooperation with third countries and the competent international organisations in the sphere of public health.

4. In order to contribute to the achievement of the objectives referred to in this Article, the Council:

   – acting in accordance with the procedure referred to in Article 189b, after consulting the Economic and Social Committee and the Committee of the Regions, shall adopt incentive measures, excluding any harmonisation of the laws and regulations of the Member States; and

   – acting by a qualified majority on a proposal from the Commission, shall adopt recommendations.

---

and education, and the incorporation of health protection requirements into the Community's other policies. Moreover, there was a requirement that the Member States should coordinate their policies and programmes in these areas, and a guideline that the Commission may take any useful initiative in this respect. However, harmonisation of the laws and regulations of the Member States was specifically excluded.

Nevertheless, Article 129 was criticised as being too vague, especially in defining the specific responsibilities of both the Member States and the Commission in achieving the objectives laid down in the Article, and in policy implementation. This is because the obligation of achieving a high level of human health protection was placed upon the Community as a whole, along with responsibility for directing actions towards the prevention of diseases; in particular, what the Article cited as the 'major health scourges'. Not only does this represent a sharing of responsibility without providing individual competencies, but in relation to the latter point, the Article also failed to make clear what such major health scourges are. The one specifically mentioned, drug dependence, is not necessarily a health matter nor necessarily a major health scourge. Finally, it is not clear what was meant by the 'coordination of activities'. Did it mean the same or similar policy objectives, common programmes, or simply the exchange of information on policy initiatives?

The role of the Council was more specific. Under the Article, the Council could adopt recommendations and, together with the European Parliament, decide on incentive measures for Member States to initiate their own national policies. Still, just what constituted an incentive measure was not defined in the Treaty; was it financial, economic or even political? In addition to this vagueness, it should be noted that a recommendation is not a legally binding instrument for the Member States. Thus, although specific, the Council's role was not made explicitly pro-active in the field of public health.

Box 2

Maastricht Treaty Articles with a health influence

Article(s)	Provision
3 (o)	Stipulates that the Community will contribute to the attainment of a high level of health protection for its citizens.
3 (s)	Defines that one of the objectives of the Community should be to contribute to the strengthening of consumer protection.
36	Permits restrictions on imports and all measures having equivalent effect on grounds of the protection of health and life of humans, animals or plants.
43	Agriculture.
48–51	Free movement of workers.
52–58	Rights of establishment.
59–66	Free movement of services including insurance.
75 (1)	The need to introduce measures to improve transport safety.
100–102	The approximation of laws related to the single market.
118	Prevention of occupational accidents and diseases and occupational hygiene.
129	Public health.
129a	Consumer protection.
130f–130q	Research.
130r (130r–130t of Title XVI)	Environment (and protection of human health).
117–125	Related to social provisions and the setting of a Social Fund.
130a–130e	Economic and social cohesion; the Protocol on social policy; and the Agreement on social policy concluded between the Member States with the exemption of the United Kingdom.
130u	Fostering economic and social development of the developing countries.

Recognising the lack of clarity regarding the nature of 'incentive measures', in Annex 1 (footnote part A) of the Presidency Conclusions of the Edinburgh European Council (11–12 December 1992), it was concluded that:

> 'Where Articles 126, 128 and 129 refer to "incentive measures", the Council considers that this expression refers to Community measures designed to encourage cooperation between Member States or to support or supplement their action in the areas concerned, including where appropriate through financial support for Community programmes or national or cooperative measures designed to achieve the objective of these articles.'

This reference notwithstanding, it remained the case that there was no Treaty-based definition or specification of such so-called 'incentive measures'.

In addition to Articles 129 and 3(o), there were a number of other health-related provisions and requirements in the Treaty – the more relevant ones are summarised in Box 2 (previous page). Beyond the Articles in this list, two Declarations of the Treaty were also related to health: The 'Declaration on assessment of the environmental impact of Community measures', and the 'Declaration on the protection of animals'. But, unlike Treaty provisions, Declarations are not legally binding.

Probably the most important change under the Treaty on European Union was the introduction of the principle of subsidiarity. According to the concept of subsidiarity, as outlined in Article 3(b), the Community is empowered to act either where it has exclusive competence or – in case of mixed competence with the Member States – in instances where it can be more successful than an individual Member State in achieving a particular objective. While perhaps commendable, this concept is rather more political than legal. Thus, the different priorities of the Member States may make it difficult to achieve intergovernmental agreement on when better 'added value' is to be realised at Community level, rather than within national contexts.

1.2 New policy developments: The Treaty of Amsterdam

At the June 1997 Intergovernmental Conference (IGC) in Amsterdam, agreement on the new Treaty resulted in a revision of Article 129 through the introduction of a number of new provisions along with revisions to other parts of the text. In the run up to the 1997 IGC it was not at all clear whether health would in fact even appear on the agenda to discuss a new Treaty, as there had been little interest demonstrated by either the Member States or the European Commission in revising Community activities in the field. This situation changed dramatically with the onset of the Bovine Spongiform Encephalopathy (BSE) crisis, which resulted in a number of proposals put forward both by Member States and the European Commission for the revision of Article 129. Thus, what appeared to be a last minute rush to amend Article 129 – in reaction to the BSE issue – was criticised as a panicky 'knee jerk' reaction rather than the result of a careful review of EU health competencies.[5]

As a result, the revised Article 129 finally agreed in Amsterdam (since changed to

---

Box 3

Article 152 of the Treaty of Amsterdam

1. A high level of human health protection shall be ensured in the definition and implementation of all Community policies and activities.

   Community action, which shall complement national policies, shall be directed towards
   improving public health, preventing human illness and diseases, and obviating sources
   of danger to human health. Such action shall cover the fight against the major health
   scourges, by promoting research into their causes, their transmission and their prevention, as well as health information and education.

   The Community shall complement the Member States' action in reducing drugs-related
   health damage, including information and prevention.

2. The Community shall encourage cooperation between the Member States in the areas
   referred to in this Article and, if necessary, lend support to their action.

   Member States shall, in liaison with the Commission, coordinate among themselves
   their policies and programmes in the areas referred to in paragraph 1. The Commission
   may, in close contact with the Member States, take any useful initiative to promote such
   coordination.

3. The Community and the Member States shall foster cooperation with third countries
   and the competent international organisations in the sphere of public health.

4. The Council, acting in accordance with the procedure referred to in Article 189b, after
   consulting the Social and Economic Committee and the Committee of the Regions shall
   contribute to the achievement of the objectives referred to in this Article through adopting:

   (a) measures setting high standards of quality and safety of organs and substances of
       human origin, blood and blood derivatives; these measures shall not prevent any
       Member States from maintaining or introducing more stringent protective measures;

   (b) by way of derogation from Article 43, measures in the veterinary and phytosanitary
       fields which have as their direct objective the protection of public health;

   (c) incentive measures designed to protect and improve human health, excluding any
       harmonisation of the laws and regulations of the Member States.

   The Council, acting by a qualified majority on a proposal from the Commission, may
   also adopt recommendations for the purposes set out in this Article.

5) Community action in the field of public health shall fully respect the responsibilities of
   the Member States for the reorganisation and delivery of health services and medical
   care. In particular, measures referred to in paragraph 4(a) shall not affect national provisions on the donation or medical use of organs and blood.

Article 152 in the new Treaty) did not represent a comprehensive overhaul of its prede-
cessor (Box 3). It failed to address some of the problems with the earlier version such
as defining what was meant by the 'coordination of activities', 'incentive measures', and
'major health scourges' (as outlined above). Nonetheless, as the ensuing discussion
shows, despite several positive developments, the revised Treaty still fails to recognise

certain fundamental issues and thus represents a missed opportunity for policy-makers to consolidate the EU's competencies in the public health field.

The main feature of the Amsterdam Treaty that has an impact on health was the formulation of the earlier and somewhat ambiguous provision that Community policies ought to contribute to health protection. According to the new text, health protection must now be incorporated into all legislation as an underlying premise. Specifically, health requirements are now to be taken into account in the definition and implementation stages of all Community policy developments. It is hoped that this may ensure a public health input into policies such as tobacco subsidies and agriculture which, while having obvious health implications, had previously been legislated in primarily economic terms. However, despite these good intentions, the new Treaty specifies neither how such an objective is to be implemented, nor who will have responsibility for its enforcement. Thus, it remains unclear as to whether this will actually be accomplished.

On a more positive note, the new Treaty does acknowledge a broader definition of public health in the Community along with a greater Community role; that which had previously been restricted to simply 'the prevention of disease'. That is, it extends this objective to 'improving public health'. But although it reiterates that priority-setting should be based on major diseases, the new Treaty does not consider the broader determinants of health necessary for a comprehensive definition of public health and its consequent role in this. For instance, the World Health Organization (WHO) stresses that 'Health is a state of complete physical, mental and social well-being and not merely the absence of disease or infirmity'. So, by neglecting the questions of the EU's role in poverty alleviation, transport, the environment, education, and housing, etc. the EU has not been able to identify a clear definition (in intersectoral terms such as WHO) as to what public health is.[6] And while skirting issues of welfare policy, inequalities in health and access to health care, along with the more ideological questions related to health might be tacitly embraced by some national governments, it in fact ultimately undermines the nature of the EU's commitment to health under the new Treaty.

Another measure in the new Treaty is the specific recognition of the need for the Community to respect Member States' own responsibilities in health care. The issue of health care and the Community's role in it is taken up more specifically in Section 1.6 of this chapter.

In stipulating that Member States were to respect national competencies in health care, the principle of subsidiarity – which had been introduced earlier at Maastricht – was reinforced by making explicit what was earlier implicit; namely, that 'Community action in the field of public health shall fully respect the responsibilities of the Member States for the organisation and delivery of health services and health care'. As is discussed later in this chapter, this area has been acknowledged as beyond the Community remit and is a carefully protected competence of national governments. It is questionable whether this explicit statement represents a positive development. While it may reflect the EU's willingness and intent to clarify the earlier ambiguity about any Community role with respect to health services, it appears to have not been a well-considered position. For not only does this exclusion of health services from the Treaty contrast with the many current EU policies which affect directly or indirectly the provision of health services, but it may also limit the potential scope for coordinating the European public health activities which are specified in the same text.

For instance, as long as health services are left out of the Treaty, health ministers will not have any real input into other policies affecting their responsibilities. The fact that health services have been excluded may be a point invoked by powerful commercial groups to obstruct moves to develop EU-wide technology assessment activities that conflict with their interests. Equally, by omitting health care systems from the range of Community competencies, some other EU objectives may be compromised. For instance, this exclusion of health services from the Treaty seems to run counter to the goals expressed by the Commission in its 1997 Communication on 'Modernising and Improving Social protection in the European Union' which includes statements on the importance of a 'European dimension' to health services, such as the 'need to improve efficiency, cost-effectiveness and quality of health systems so that they can meet the growing demands arising from the ageing of the population and other factors'.[7] Most importantly, this exclusion of health services may fuel citizens' perceptions that the EU is not dealing with the practical realities of health; namely, that the Community is not undertaking those activities which would appear most necessary.[8] Surely this aim cannot be pursued effectively by the Commission with health services not covered under the Treaty?

Meanwhile, a notable, if not curious, health-related inclusion in the new Treaty is the issue of the health effects of addictive drugs. Although this subject appears in the Maastricht Treaty as well, its inclusion is odd in the sense that drug dependence and its health effects is usually prominent on the agendas of those ministers dealing with social affairs and crime, rather than those with responsibilities for health. Illicit drugs, drug trafficking and trade, and crime are generally considered matters of 'internal affairs' Thus, discussions tend to be undertaken beyond the scope of EU law or the reach of both the European Parliament and the European Court of Justice. Nevertheless, with an eye to expanding the Community's definition of public health, it is a positive development that the Commission has been granted a voice in discussions of the health effects of drugs under the Article on public health.

Equally interesting is the inclusion of a paragraph on the safety of blood, organs, substances and blood derivatives of human origins. It is noteworthy not only for its inclusion but also its detail. The manner in which is has been spelled out in the text goes far beyond the more general language employed in the remainder of the Treaty. While this was intended to serve as a clear indication of the EU's resolve that subjective (national) arguments over the safety of such products should not hinder their free movement within the Single Market, it is undermined by later assertions stating that these measures will not, however, prevent any Member State from maintaining or introducing their own protection measures provided they are more stringent than those laid down by the Commission. The lack of clarity on this position is exacerbated by the fact that those responsible for drafting relevant EU measures will have to do so within the context of not affecting national provisions for the donation or medical use of blood or organs. This runs directly counter to the Treaty's explicit requirement to set agreed standards in this area.

A final health-related aspect of the Amsterdam Treaty is the nature of Article 137. According to the Article:

> '...The Community shall support and supplement the activities of the Member States in the following fields (...including...) social security and social protection of workers;...To this end, the Council may adopt, by means of directives, minimum requirements for gradual implementation, having regard to the conditions and technical rules obtaining in each of the Member States...[and] may adopt measures designed to encourage cooperation between Member States through initiatives aimed at improving knowledge, developing exchanges of information and best practices, promoting innovative approaches and evaluating experiences in order to combat social exclusion.'

Immediately, a potential inconsistency with the provisions of Article 152 becomes apparent. Albeit subject to interpretation, Article 137 would seem to mandate the Community a wider role with respect to health-related competencies. It is not so much that it explicitly lays down the specific powers of the EU, but rather that it does not constrain them to finite areas and issues; perhaps in contradiction to the provisions of Article 152.

For instance, what does the notion of 'supplementing the activities of Member States' mean in practice? Those who would see the Community with a wider role no doubt regard this as indication of the potential for greater EU involvement in abetting the health activities of Member State governments at the national level. Others may adopt a contrary interpretation taking it to mean that the EU is empowered to take action 'only if and in so far as the objectives of the proposed action cannot be sufficiently achieved by the Member States and can therefore, by reason of the scale or effects of the proposed action, be better achieved by the Community'; that is, within the boundaries of subsidiarity (Article 3b, Treaty on European Union). Where does the power of instigation therefore lie? Even if this does represent an endorsement of subsidiarity, what form the 'support' should take is not specified beyond the vague identification of broad fields within which the Community *could* play a role. Should this support manifest itself in financial, policy or consultative terms? Equally ambiguous is the phrase 'social protection'. Leaving aside the fact that this is tied specifically to 'workers' in the text, the question must nevertheless be asked what a Community role in supporting and supplementing the actions of Member States in the field of social protection actually means, if not with at least an implicit relevance for health. For it is undoubtedly the case that 'social protection' carries with it a direct health-related component. And while Article 137 does not pertain to public health *per se*, the areas which it outlines all would seem to have definite and well-established health elements.

Nevertheless, Article 137 represents a changed role for the Council. For not only does it expand the Council's legislative powers, but as it grants the Council the authority to initiate policy in the field of social security – admittedly subject to national level consid-erations – it also represents an extension of its areas of competence. However, the right to initiate in this area is tempered by the fact that in issues relating to social security, the Council is required to act by unanimity and co-decision. What this means in practice is set out in the following section of this chapter. But ultimately, it represents another of the new Treaty's ambiguities with respect to health and related competencies.

In summary, the expectations for a new Treaty with specific and understandable health references promised much in theory, but in practice failed to address the basic issues of institutional reform requisite for the easier development and integration of health poli-cies. As is outlined later in this chapter, there is a compelling case for the establishment of a new Directorate-General for health, one with powers to both initiate and coordinate strategies that could reconcile the multiple, dispersed and often conflicting EU policies relating to health.[9] And although the Amsterdam Treaty negotiations were inevitably preoccupied with topics such as enlargement and common and foreign security policy, health ministers could have done much more to forward their own interests. Particularly, they ought to have at least ensured that all of their concerns were fed into the policy process during the long preparation time leading up to the Amsterdam Intergovernmental Conference.

1.3 The decision-making process at EU level: the roles of the Commission, the Parliament and the Council

Having hinted above at an expansion of the Council of Ministers' powers under Article 137 of the new Treaty, this needs to be put into context. It is necessary to consider the role of the various institutions involved in the EU policy-making dynamic; to appreci-ate not only the formal and structural processes at work in shaping policies at Community level, but also the difficulties in legislating for health policies specifically. The EU decision-making process is complicated, involving several institutions with varying degrees of responsibility and areas of competence. The main three are the European Commission, the European Parliament and the Council of Ministers.

The Commission is responsible for both initiating policies and implementing the provi-sions of the Treaty. It guards this power of initiative quite closely, and thus while it is often encouraged to take action in certain areas by the Member States, the EU Presidencies or the European Parliament, this is not always appreciated, nor necessarily acted upon. The Commission fulfils this role by proposing, and later adopting, propos-als for Regulations, Directives, and Decisions (all which are legislatively binding), as well as providing Recommendations and Opinions (which are not binding). In drafting proposals, the Commission must consult a range of bodies, including the Economic and Social Committee (ECOSOC – which is comprised mainly of representatives of employer and employee organisations from the Member States) and the Committee of Regions (CoR – which brings together regional and local government representatives from the Member States). Once a proposal has been adopted by the Commission, it is then forwarded to both the Council of Ministers and the European Parliament for their consideration. The Council represents the final decision-making authority, but as the

European Parliament may propose amendments to the Council's common position (and since the Maastricht Treaty, may in fact reject a Council proposal), the latter is now directly involved in the legislative process.

The 1986 Single European Act (SEA) and the 1992 Treaty on European Union (TEU) both considerably strengthened the capacities of the European Parliament, so as to ensure it a prominent role in the decision-making process. Prior to these two Treaties, parliamentary power was regarded more as supervisory rather than executive. Although final budgetary approval was within its competence, it had a voice on other future legislation solely under the 'cooperation' and 'assent' procedures. The former allows the Parliament one reading of Council proposals, but Parliament's conclusions are not binding and the Commission could therefore ignore the result. Under the latter, the Parliament may either give or withhold its agreement on the instrument laid before it, but may not amend it. In 1986 the SEA then conferred upon the Parliament the power to veto agreements made between the EU and third countries, as well as instituting a new procedure. This new procedure, the 'cooperation' procedure, granted the Parliament a second reading of Council proposals. Only by unanimity could the Council then overturn a second parliamentary rejection, and as unanimity is always difficult to achieve, the Council would have to seek conciliation (via committee) with the Parliament to ensure that its proposal was approved. The Maastricht Treaty then introduced a fourth procedure, the 'co-decision' procedure, and extended the scope of the cooperation and assent procedures.

The introduction of the co-decision procedure represents the most important change in European Parliament powers under the Maastricht Treaty. The new Treaty of Amsterdam added 23 additional cases of co-decision to the existing 15 and simplified the procedure itself, thereby putting the Parliament and Council on an equal footing in the larger part of normal secondary legislation. Under co-decision, the European Parliament and the Council share decision-making power equally, and adopt legislative proposals by joint agreement. Co-decision grants the Parliament a third reading of proposals, and ultimately, the ability to reject proposed legislation. In cases where, after two readings of a proposal and the invocation of the conciliation procedure (a committee proceeding to resolve the deadlock in a mutually agreeable manner), disagreement between the Council and the Parliament continues, the Parliament is given a third and final opportunity to agree the proposal. Should Parliament, however, continue to reject the proposal – in this case an absolute majority is required – the proposal cannot become a legal instrument. Amongst others, co-decision is used in cases applying to internal market harmonisation, the free movement of workers, consumer protection, public health, the environment, and the framework programme for research and technology. A description of the decision-making process is illustrated in Figure 1.

The co-decision procedure has failed to produce a decision in only two cases to date. The first, on 19 July 1994, saw the Parliament employ the procedure for the first time by vetoing the Council's proposal for an 'Open Network Provision' to voice telephony; whereby the enforcement of the law was to be transferred to a committee comprised of representatives from Member State governments rather than the Commission. The

Figure 1

Passing EU Legislation: the consultation, cooperation and co-decision procedures (under the Maastricht Treaty)

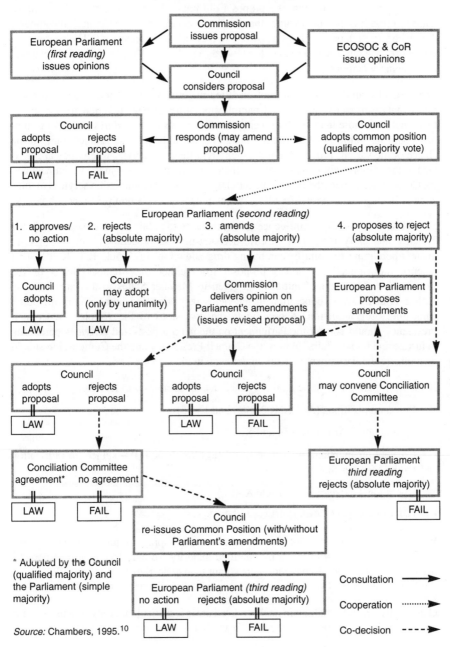

Source: Chambers, 1995.[10]

second instance of co-decision failing took place on 1 March 1995, and was related to biotechnology. While an agreement had been reached in the Conciliation Committee, Parliament nonetheless rejected both the agreement and the original proposal in Plenary session – on the grounds that the proposal did not include a ban on the patenting of human genes. It is also noteworthy that the Parliament is able to introduce amendments during conciliation proceedings, a power that it did not have previously. The co-decision procedure thus represents a major step towards an EU-level system based on bicameral parliamentary democracy.

The TEU also applied the system of qualified majority voting in the Council to many fields of health-related activities. Unanimity is, however, still required for others. In total, there are more than twenty potential combinations of procedures and voting rules that could be followed in legislating health-related policies. The lack of logic in the choice of the various procedures and the different fields of activity where they apply, as well as the complex combination of powers and voting procedures in the Parliament and the Council, along with the involvement of large number of Commission services in initiating policies, makes more difficult the development of a coherent public health policy.

Several other areas with an influence on or relevance to public health are covered in the Treaties, and carry their own specific decision-making procedures. For instance, in matters pertaining to point 6 (combating drug addiction) of Article K.1 (K.3(2), first indent), the Council acts on a proposal from either the Member States or the Commission. The right of initiative is given to Member States in this area because Article K deals with cooperation in the fields of justice and home affairs including combating drug addiction. According to the provisions of the Article, the Council Presidency should consult the Parliament on the main aspects and activities pertaining to justice and home affairs. In turn, the Council Presidency and the Commission should then inform the Parliament of work undertaken in these fields.

In matters relating to Article K, the Council acts unanimously in five cases:

- Common positions (Article K.3(2)(a) and K.4(3))
- Joint actions (Article K.3(b) and K.4(3))
- Conventions pursuant to Article K.3(2)(c) (Article K.4(3) – subject to ratification by the Member States)
- Operational expenditure (Article K.8(2))
- Decisions to apply Article 100c (Article K.9)

With respect to the introduction of measures that apply to joint actions (Article K.3(2)(b)), the Council must act by qualified majority. To introduce measures pertaining to the application of conventions pursuant to Article K.3(2)(c) meanwhile, a two-thirds majority in the Council is necessary unless otherwise indicated.

Community decision-making in health-related areas is difficult not only because there is an overlap in competencies under the Treaty, but also by the fact that eighteen of the twenty-four Directorates-General (DGs) of the Commission – each headed by a different Commissioner with a different mandate – are involved in shaping health-related policies.[11] These include DGV (Employment, Industrial Relations and Social Affairs, with responsibilities for public health), DGIII (Industry, with responsibilities for pharmaceutical policy), DGXII (Science, Research and Development, with responsibilities for health-related research), and DGXIII (Telecommunications, Information Market and Exploitation of Research, with responsibilities for health telematics). In the work of several other Directorates-General health issues can also play an important indirect or direct role (such as the Common Agricultural Policy, and VAT policy). This involvement of numerous DGs in areas that have an impact on health in the Community is part of the problem in forming a comprehensive European public health policy. It should also be emphasised that the EU system is heavily influenced by organised interests precisely because power is so fragmented.

1.4 The roles of the High Level Committee on Health and the Interservice Group on Health

In recognising the need to address the problems caused by the scattered nature of health-related competencies in the Community, two European-level groups have been set up to help integrate these otherwise separated responsibilities. In 1991, with the prospect of a new Community competence in the field of health, the Commissioner for Social Affairs established a High Level Committee on Health. This comprises officials from the Member States, and its function is to advise the Commission on policy developments (Box 4).

Box 4

The role of the High Level Committee on Health

The Committee advises the Commission services on health matters.

Members are designated by the Member States from among senior officials in the Ministries responsible for health.

A Commission's representative chairs the Committee, and the Commission ensures that the Committee is provided with a secretariat that facilitates its work.

The members of the Committee play an important role in advising the Commission services in various policy developments and the Committee acts as a forum for exchanging information and sharing experience between Member States.

However, the Committee has only an informal role, and the members of the Committee do not always represent the same level of responsibility in their respective national Ministries. This creates an imbalance in the degree of importance attributed to the Committee, with some countries treating it with less significance than others; resulting in an often ineffectual arrangement regarding the Committee's mandate. Several Member States have therefore expressed concerns that the potential contribution of the

Committee to shaping policy is not fully exploited, and that the Commission would be more likely to benefit by having advice from the highest possible level of the administration in Member States. In other words, members of the Committee ought to hold fairly high-ranking positions within their national administrations in order for the Committee to shed its informal image and have more of an influence.

This criticism comes despite several later Community initiatives to ensure the appropriate degree of cooperation between the Commission and the Member States in numerous areas including public health. For instance, a Council Resolution of 27 May 1993[12] emphasised that it would be expedient to have a procedure for consultation between Member States and the Commission on questions of public health. A further Council Resolution of 2 June 1994[13] called for further consideration to be given to setting up a mechanism which ensures that Member States are fully involved in the development, implementation and evaluation of Community activities. In its 1994 White Paper on European Social Policy,[14] the Commission indicated its intention to facilitate cooperation between Member States generally, and in particular, to assist Member States in being able to respond to health issues; such as increased access to services and facilities arising from improved mobility within the Union.

In response to the Council's and Member States' request, the Commission has since considered the formalisation of the role of the High Level Committee. This might give more weight to the Committee, although the involvement of the Member States still requires the Committee officials to respect the Commission's right of initiative in proposing policy according to the provisions of the Treaty. Member States will nonetheless be able to advise on, and be informed of, policy developments before the Council of Ministers is given the opportunity to consider them. However, no action has yet been taken towards this end.

A notable recent development has been the Committee's establishment of three working groups to prepare reports on the future of European health policy. One of the working groups has identified a number of objectives for Community action including:

- reducing health inequalities between and within countries and groups in society;

- promoting regard for the health impact of other policies;

- sharing expertise on health promotion, diagnosis and treatment; and

- disseminating research results about best practice.

It is, however, unclear how these recommendations can be translated into specific policies. Reducing inequalities in health will require action beyond the scope of Article 152, and may have implications for the fiscal policies of the Member States, as well as leading to a restructuring of the Community's budgetary priorities. The promotion of awareness of the health impact of other policies would require different Commission structures, since the existing level of coordination between different Directorates-General is in need of improvement. Joint policy developments are rare, and although there are a number of initiatives and programmes, these do not amount to a comprehensive strategy. In some areas of policy development the initiative lies with several Directorates-General which have nothing to do with public health issues and are contradictory (for example, the funding for health education for the prevention of smoking versus subsidies for the growth of better quality tobacco).

A later and separate venture was the establishment of an Interservice Group on Health. It was set up in January 1994 to manage the dispersion of health-related functions throughout the Commission. It was designed to coordinate the activities and programmes initiated by different Directorates-General within the broader field of health. The work of the Group has helped the Commission to better ensure that legislative proposals initiated by different DGs within their own areas of competence do indeed take into account health requirements. In addition, duplication in activities has been reduced, and joint work has been fostered through the coordination activities of the Group.

There is a need for further cooperation between the DGs, for instance between DGV and DGXII on research priorities; between DGV and DGXI on health and the environment; between DGV and DGI on matters relating to Eastern Europe; between DGV and DGVI on agriculture; and between DGV and DGXVI on structural funds. Concerning the latter, contributions from DGV are not currently possible at the design stage of policies and measures, for this remains the prerogative of Member States. The Group needs more support and clout to help ensure that such cooperation is fostered.

One tangible result of the new Interservice Group is the publication of an annual DGV report into the integration of health protection requirements into other Community policies – this Treaty requirement was reinforced in the new Treaty of Amsterdam. Two reports have been produced (for 1995 and 1996), but in their final form, they have been criticised for relying too heavily on policy assessments from the other Directorates-General – assessments which have tended to support the *status quo* (i.e. that which is already being done) rather than to highlight activities which are inconsistent with public health, such as the subsidy of tobacco production by DGVI (Agriculture). It is, however, the case that as the reports have to be 'owned' by the entire College of Commissioners, most critical passages – which, prior to inter-service consultation, are critical of other DGs – are dropped from the final text.

Such 'self-assessment' may be the result of limited resources as much as' politics. The small public health department in DGV is inadequately resourced to effectively undertake such a supervisory function. Nevertheless, the reports are a step forward, and have been welcomed by the Council of Ministers which has supported their continuing annual publication, but without providing additional resources.

The two Committees thus reflect a record of mixed results. While both have served to further the health debate in the Community and put it on the agendas of a diverse range of structures, neither has had a truly tangible effect; at least not in terms of affecting policy in a direct and lasting manner. The advisory function of the High Level Committee on Health requires reform if the body is to fulfil its mandate. The

Interservice Group meanwhile, requires additional support – primarily financial – to improve its ability to safeguard health matters in the formulation of Community policies.

1.5 European Commission priorities

Having outlined the structure and the formal capacities of the EU in the field of health, it is necessary to look at the Community's self-targeted priorities within these formal boundaries. This section, therefore, aims to highlight the health-related actions so far undertaken by the Commission, along with programmes yet to be agreed and future areas still to be dealt with. A more detailed presentation and analysis of the Commission's priorities, programmes and actions in the field of public health is provided by Merkel and Hübel in Chapter 2 of this volume.

General Overview

As a response to the provisions of Articles 3(o) and 129, and following a long process of consultation and negotiation between the various EU institutions, Member States, and other interested groups on proposals made by the Commission, the Commission has defined eight priority areas for European Community action. These areas are:

- drug dependence;
- health promotion;
- cancer;
- AIDS and other communicable diseases;
- monitoring and surveillance of diseases;
- injury prevention;
- pollution-related diseases; and
- rare diseases.

In addition, emphasis is placed on the dissemination of information and evaluation of these policies, especially regarding their effectiveness.[11] It has not been easy to establish these priorities, nor has it been possible to satisfy all the demands for action. But in spite of the criticisms of EU public health policy in some circles,[15] the Community does at least have a list of priorities on which to improve public health policy in the future.

The Commission has also developed specific policies in health promotion, cancer, AIDS and communicable diseases, tobacco, drug dependence, health monitoring, disease surveillance, the environment, and health and safety at work. Proposals have also been put forward for Community action programmes on the prevention of injuries,[16] rare diseases,[17] and pollution-related illnesses,[18] which began in 1998–99. Another area of Community policy is in combating drugs in the EU. Drug addiction has been extensively discussed in many European Councils, including the twice-yearly Meeting of EU Health

Ministers. On this basis, the Commission developed an Action Programme covering the period up to the year 2000.[19] In addition the European Drugs and Drugs Addiction Monitoring Centre (EDDAMC) was established in Lisbon in 1993.[20] The priorities of the EDDAMC include the collection of reliable and comparable data, and the exchange of such information on a large scale.

Community research programmes are already directed at nutrition, cardiovascular diseases, mental illness and the problems associated with ageing. The Commission has prepared draft communications and proposals for European Parliament–Council decisions concerning five-year programmes of action on rare diseases, pollution-related diseases and the prevention of injuries. It has also prepared drafts of communications and proposals for the European Parliament alone, including the recently endorsed proposal on a Community programme for the safety and self-sufficiency of blood and derived products within the Single Market. This is related to the Council recommendation on the suitability of donors of blood and plasma and the testing of donations within the Community.[21] The development of methodologies and capacities for the evaluation of health and health-related programmes and measures is foreseen by the overall health monitoring programme, with preparatory work already carried out.

A further example of Community activity was the May 1996 establishment of a joint US–EU Task Force to develop a global early warning system and response network for communicable disease. This was agreed between the United States government and the European Commission under the Transatlantic Agenda. The Task Force agreed to develop a unified pragmatic and flexible surveillance and response network for communicable diseases, with global geographic coverage, and encompassing a variety of data and communication links employing available and evolving technologies. The Task Force is expected to meet at least once a year to review its progress. To date it has established three working groups on Surveillance and Response, Research and Research Training, and Capacity Review and Strengthening.

Clearly, with existing funding the Community health programmes cannot, and should not, hope to deal with every health problem affecting EU citizens. The real problem is that the current EU approach to public health – that which simply keeps compiling and specifying new diseases to tackle – lacks any coherence. It requires considerably more resources than are currently made available, but this criticism neglects the emphasis that the approach is inappropriate with reality. As it is disease-based and cumulative, it tries to incorporate and fund very specific proposals put forth by both pressure groups and the institutional stakeholders (i.e. European Parliament, Council, etc.). This is not feasible, and may in part account for the widespread criticism of the limited nature of Article 152.

Precisely defined priorities, though difficult to establish, are therefore fundamental for the EU to redress this problem. However, recent decisions in the European Parliament – defined as one of the 'institutional stakeholders' – have emphasised that the search for clearly defined objectives is far from over. In 1996, this lack of a comprehensive strategy of Community objectives was explicitly demonstrated when the European

Parliament (recalling that the Parliament has final budgetary powers) allocated ECU 5 million to a new programme on Alzheimer's disease and a further ECU 4 million for public campaigns aimed at demonstrating to EU citizens the health benefits of the internal market.[22] In identifying two new areas for Community action, simply by the reallocation of resources, the Parliament significantly reduced the Council's proposed total funding of ECU 6.5 million for the broadly-based health promotion programme. This resulted in the already under-resourced Public Health Directorate of DGV having to develop a new Community programme on Alzheimer's disease from scratch.

In light of these two new Parliament-initiated programmes, concern has been raised that by focusing on a single disease, the wider impact of the Health Promotion Programme will be lessened. Moreover, while not disputing the fact that Alzheimer's is an important health problem in the Community, it could be argued that by identifying particular diseases for specific action, the original guidelines laid down in the Treaty for the selection of areas for action no longer apply. This concern has also been heightened by specific references to blood and human organ safety and veterinary and phytosanitary health protection in Article 152 of the Treaty of Amsterdam.

Post-Maastricht

This synopsis of the Commission's priority areas in the field of public health reflects a changing context within which these priorities have been identified and are being pursued. This changing approach is apparent in the Commission's various Communications on public health and other health-related topics since the original 1993 Communication on public health.

Beginning with the 1993 'Communication on the framework for action in the field of public health' (24.11.93),[23] this laid the basis for the development of Community competencies in the area in light of Article 129 of the Treaty on European Union. It outlines a framework for Community action, including a specification of the roles of the individual institutions and Member States. Thereafter it describes and documents the resources available to the Community for the implementation of this framework, along with a detailed listing of the procedures for assessing and evaluating the programmes it establishes. The key areas of action that it identifies are cancer, cardiovascular diseases, accidents, AIDS and communicable diseases, drug dependence and rare diseases. The Commission resisted an all embracing public health policy on the grounds that the coordination of Member State implementation would prove complicated given differing national priorities. It is from this disease-based context with eight priority areas that Community public health policy has since developed.

In its Communication of 07.03.96,[24] the Commission outlined its views on establishing a European Community network for the control and surveillance of communicable diseases; which has since been undertaken. Two years later, in a new Communication (14.04.98) on the 'Development of Public Health Policy',[25] the priority areas pinpointed by the Commission would seem to have evolved. That is, while both the 1993 and 1996 Communications employed a disease-based framework in specifying AIDS and cancer (amongst others) as issues requiring immediate action, the basis of the new Communication espouses a more rational, priority-setting approach. In particular, it concentrates on a three-pronged strategy to developing a Community public health policy. Referred to as the 'three strands for action', they are specified as:

- Improving information for the development of public health

- Reacting rapidly to threats to health

- Tackling health determinants through health promotion and disease prevention

The 1998 Communication begins with an overview of the state of health in the Community as a whole, and then considers individual issues faced by the Member States. With regard to the former, it deals with questions of the longevity/life expectancy of Community citizens, the changing pattern of diseases in Europe and the considerable variations in the health status of Member States and groups. In terms of national issues, the Communication looks at health care costs and social and demographic changes, along with changing health systems and citizens' expectations. The Communication then provides a brief historical overview of the development of Community health policies and competencies before outlining the three strands cited above. The three strands indicate a clear break with the disease monitoring and surveillance strategies of the 1996 Communication – not to mention the rare diseases focus of the 1997 Communication – and a wider interpretation of Community competencies in public health.

It is envisaged that future questions pertaining to the enlargement of the Community and the integration of health requirements in other Community policies will fall within the bounds of this approach. Now that the Treaty of Amsterdam has been ratified, and the revised Article 129 is the new Article 152, the Commission aims to develop specific policies in relation to these strands. In the meantime, the 1998 Communication is expected to at least animate the public health discussion at EU level. Towards this end, the Commission has been widely disseminating the details of its three-strand strategy in order to stimulate debate and gauge response to these plans. This wide dissemination has meant that there have been many responses to the new Communication; two of which are summarised below.

The European Public Health Alliance (EPHA – a non-governmental organisation which 'seeks to protect and promote the public health interests of all people living in Europe' through developing a network of NGOs and other non-profit groups active in the field of public health at all levels) has recently issued a three-part position paper in response to the Commission's plans.[26] Among the thirteen recommendations put forward by the EPHA in its paper are suggestions ranging from the theoretical to the specific. Particular emphasis is placed on the need to dedicate more resources to effective integration of public health priorities at both institutional and policy levels, and on the role to be played by non-governmental organisations given their multi-sectoral status. The EPHA recommendations include:

- Specific public health programmes and research activity which focus on improving the health of those who experience the most severe inequalities in health must be prioritised within this broad policy approach.

- A central focus of the new public health framework should be the development of capacity and effectiveness in the assessment of the impact of all EU policies on human health.

- Responsibility for public health needs to be significantly strengthened within the European Commission – both politically and organisationally. This requires increased resources and the relocation of the public health unit (currently DGV/F) to Brussels in order to bring to an end the geographical and political marginalisation of public health within the European institutions.

- The powers of the European Parliament should be further increased, to ensure that the Parliament has authority over 100 per cent of the EU budget.

- The proportion of the EU budget currently allocated to public health must be increased substantially if the goal of achieving positive health gain for all people living in Europe is to be achieved.

These recommendations do not, however, go far enough, and in part reflect the EPHA's own mandate rather than providing a sound basis for restructuring Community public health competencies. For instance, while it might indeed be administratively easier to coordinate policy should DGV/F be relocated to Brussels, this does not address the real problem of the Unit's lack of power. Equally, while increasing the powers of the European Parliament may indeed help to ensure that public heath priorities receive the attention they are due in creating other Community policies, it remains the case that Members of the European Parliament (MEPs) are not always aware of the most recent developments in the field and may therefore pursue more individualistic agendas than are perhaps required (for example, the Community programme for Alzheimer's disease). Also, an increased budget for public health may be a starting point, but it is not so much the amount of resources as the manner in which they are spent that must be dealt with.

Another notable response came from the Directorate-General for Research of the European Parliament as a Working Document.[27] The report evaluates the cost-effectiveness of the EU's existing public health programmes (specifically those of the 1993 framework: cancer, drug abuse, AIDS and communicable diseases, and health promotion), and considers to what degree the Member States' national interests are adequately represented. It also looks at the issue of subsidiarity and to what extent the programmes take it into account.

In providing a wide range of commentary, recommendation, and criticism, the report highlights the necessity for a more integrated approach to public health at EU level. In so doing, it admits that 'a wider range of disease-based, population-based, risk-based and policy-related studies might also yield value from treatment at international level and that not all possibilities are being exploited'. In this vein, it criticises the existing programmes on several grounds:

- a lack of strategic planning;

- the absence of detailed and operationalised objectives;

- a selection process which lacks the rigour of peer review and is heavily concentrated in the hands of the Commission; and

- uncertain methods of dissemination of project reports.

Another problem mentioned is that the programmes are all too 'rigid', especially in light of 'confusion about the distinction between pure research and action-oriented study'. As well, the report concludes that the Public Health Unit of DGV (DGV/F) is accorded too haphazard a role in these programmes. In light of these, and other criticisms, the report closes with a series of recommendations (Box 5). These recommendations provide a

---

Box 5

Recommendations of the European Parliament Working Paper – *EU health policy on the eve of the millennium*

i The core of the EU's future efforts in public health should be the integration of health impact assessment into health-determining areas of EU policy.

ii This should be supplemented by highly selective funding of projects and research which deliver European value-added and have been assessed for cost-effectiveness.

iii These could include disease-based, population-based and risk-based approaches, as well as comparative analyses of policy and practice. There would be merit in undertaking selective comparative analysis of health-care systems.

iv Projects should have clear, policy-oriented objectives and clearly identified methods of dissemination and take up.

v Direct health education should not be undertaken at EU level.

vi More consideration should be given to the development of a regionally-based health policy, in which priorities would be developed to deal with particular regional problems.

vii Collaboration with other international organisations needs to be improved and extended.

viii A future public health unit should be located in Brussels (or at least should be in the same place as its Directorate-General). Several options exist for organising the health unit in the future, none of them ideal. The most workable option would be to integrate health with social policy and to exploit existing arrangements for inter-service working with other Directorates-General.

ix The key to the future success of health policy lies in visionary leadership and the development of an extensive cadre of well-qualified staff in support. This should include the development of country-specific expertise.

x Administrative budgets need to be increased to support an enlarged cadre of well-qualified staff. Funding programmes need to make better use of existing budgets in the first instance.

good basis for effecting change, though they are in turn dependent on a considerable amount of political will from national and EU policy-makers.

The 1998 Communication's shift away from a disease-specific frame of reference to one which, at least implicitly, endorses a broader application of the determinants of health – and the measures necessary to incorporate them – must be regarded as a positive development. It is perhaps only a pity that this positive (if not natural) evolution to a more multi-sectoral understanding is not in fact echoed in formal terms under the Treaty of Amsterdam.

1.6 The European Community and health care

Before turning to public health itself, the question of health care and services at Community-level needs to be considered. For as stated earlier in this chapter, not only is EU involvement in health care a politically contentious subject but, despite Treaty Articles 59–66 on services, the area of health care delivery has been definitively established as beyond Community competencies.

The Treaty of Amsterdam makes the first explicit reference to medical care and health services as an area of exclusive responsibility for the Member States. It does, however, permit the Community limited involvement in this field, providing that national responsibilities are first taken into account. Political and legal interpretations of this proviso are already giving rise to different opinions as to whether it reinforces subsidiarity and rules out Community action, or if it provides for explicit, albeit limited, scope for Community action in the field of health services for the first time. Indeed, as mentioned earlier, excluding the Community from this field altogether would appear to contradict the European Commission's 1997 Communication which aims to 'improve efficiency, cost effectiveness and quality of health systems' in the EU.[7]

Furthermore, it remains the case that the European Community already acts and legislates in areas which greatly affect health services and the provision of medical care; for instance legislation on private insurance (which includes health care), medical devices, telematics, medical qualifications, the movement and right to establish of medical professionals, and medicines licensing. Accordingly, both despite and because of Article 152, the Community's involvement in these activities is expected to continue in the future; specifically *because,* previously, Article 129 had not been used as the legislative basis for such activities in the health delivery sector.

The lack of explicit EU responsibility in the area of health care delivery contrasts sharply with the large amount of resources and effort spent under the European Commission's PHARE programme in analysing and helping reform health systems in Eastern Europe. There is no current evaluation of the effectiveness (or failure) of the EU-sponsored efforts to reform health systems in Eastern Europe – a number of these countries are experiencing severe problems with the introduction of health insurance systems to replace their formerly centrally planned ones. Therefore – given the Community's lack of competence in its own health care systems – the Member States have never evaluated the work of the EU-sponsored consultants in these countries, and have never questioned why the EU consultants have mostly recommended an insurance-based system (which is not the preferred option in many EU Member States).

The EU's inability to act in the field of health care is contrary to the work and views of other international organisations. The fact that organisations such as the World Bank, the Organization for Economic Cooperation and Development (OECD), WHO and the Council of Europe are all prepared and able to address health care specifically, poses an ironic problem for the EU. The irony is that many EU Member States are also members of these other organisations. Not only that, however, but such organisations also have a much clearer and pro-active role in public health itself. For instance, standing at the other extreme of the Commission's loose commitment to health in Article 152, the Council of Europe states its goal as 'the development of a real European health policy' to be achieved by 'harmonising the health policies of the member states'. However, despite that these international organisations do have explicit competencies in both health care and public health, they do not enjoy any legislative power which would supersede the powers of the national parliaments.

Still, the issue of health care is increasingly discussed on Community agendas. Under an agreement reached in 1996 by the Council of Ministers,[28] the EU has taken the first tentative steps in recognising the 'added value' of collecting and analysing information on health systems. This interim agreement on a Community health monitoring programme defines that amongst the areas for which health indicators may be established in this programme, are the following – which clearly focus on health care:

- sources of financing;

- facilities/manpower (health resource utilisation and health resource personnel); and

- cost/expenditure (in-patient care, out-patient care, and pharmaceutical products).

In addition, in its 1995 Communication on the Future of Social Protection,[29] the Commission identified 'changes in health care systems' as a subject for European analysis and debate.

There are, however, still no Regulations or Directives dealing with health care issues, including coverage for health services provision. The only Community policy document is a 1992 Council Recommendation,[30] which proposed that Member States should:

'Organize the role of social protection in preventing illness and in treating and rehabilitating the persons concerned so as to meet the following objectives:

(a) Under conditions determined by each Member State, to ensure for all persons resident within the territory of the Member State access to necessary health care as well as to facilities seeking to prevent illness;

(b) To maintain and, where necessary, develop a high-quality health care system geared to the evolving needs of the population, and especially those arising from dependence of the elderly, to the development of pathologies and therapies and the need to step up prevention.'

The EU's only involvement with respect to health care is such that the Council simply recommends that Member States provide necessary health care to their populations. The Member States are also expected to decide individually on the manner of doing so most effectively, thus defining on a national basis just what constitutes an issue for them.[4] The Council does emphasise the need for high-quality care and the need for developing therapies to meet the evolving needs of the Community's population, but again it is the responsibility of the Member States to define and develop specific policies.

2 Public health and priority-setting in the European Union

2.1 Contextualising public health – the European dimension

Public health is defined as the science and art of preventing disease, prolonging life and promoting health through the organised efforts of society.[31] It is clear from this albeit terse definition that the scope of potential issues it incorporates is nevertheless considerable. If policy-makers at any level are to legislate adequately for factors and risks affecting citizens' heath and lifespan, they must be prepared to consider and accommodate physical, mental, cultural, social, and economic (including technology-related) issues. These range from the individual to the communal, from one's personal living space to the public domain, and require a broad-based understanding of the manner in which they are inter-related in order to be accounted for in a singular policy or strategy. As the Commission rightly recognised in its 1993 Communication on the framework for action in the field of public health, 'the steps required to protect individuals' health must address both of these environments'.[23] Despite this initial recognition of the wider and more incorporative nature of public health requirements, the content of the Communication still advocated a disease-based framework.

Thus, in spite of this clear definition of the meaning and purpose of public health, and notwithstanding the Commission's own recognition of the approach needed, there has always been confusion in the EU. Although, as we have outlined, and as is further described in Chapter 2 of this book, the EU has had a long involvement with health issues, it was only with the Maastricht Treaty in 1992 that a legal framework was established. The relevant Treaty provisions are linked to 'health protection' and 'promoting public health', but specifically exclude matters pertaining to the provision of clinical services or their financing. Still, the EU does have the authority to identify common problems (and solutions) in these areas, particularly through research. Given that the EU is primarily an economic union, and the cost of provision of clinical services and their financing makes a measurable impact on the social, industrial and economic policies of each of the Member States, it is possible that changes in this area will occur in the future.

This distinction between public health and clinical services is blurred in most of the Member States. In some, public health is equated with the provision of services by the public sector, in contrast to those provided by the private sector. In most, it is recognised that although clinical services can only be a minor contributor to the improvement of health status, the major elements associated with health status are linked to environmental (for example, air pollution), behavioural (for example, tobacco and alcohol consumption), economic (for example, poverty), nutritional, social and genetic factors. Nonetheless, the provision of health services does influence health status. Many preventive, protective and health promoting health services are best delivered with the help of, or through, clinical services. These ambiguities are reflected in the individual chapter descriptions of this book as to how public health priorities are advanced in each of the EU's Member States.

How best to allocate resources to address the needs of public health is complex and difficult since, as explained above, there are many determinants of health and disease. Determining which of the wide range of social factors is to be addressed by the many available social policies is difficult, not least with the decline of the social-democratic welfare state model in Europe. Many of the major public health measures such as water purity, clean air, sanitation and safe food were introduced in the last century. To improve public health now, however, requires a completely different approach since many of the necessary measures require alterations in individual behaviours. This generates debate about the responsibility that individuals have for their own health and the responsibility of society and the state for the health of their populations.[32]

For instance, in the last century, measures to improve sanitation or ensure the purity of the water supply system were introduced by measures such as building a water supply plant or a sewage pipe system. These involved only small, if any, changes in personal/population behaviour. The public health risks were also obvious and common: for example, outbreaks of typhoid and cholera. Although there was some popular resentment to the introduction of these measures at the time,[33] this was sporadic and the benefits so obvious that they were universally introduced, and only opposed in any concerted way by interest groups such as landlords and industrialists.

Nowadays, the major public health hazards are associated with individual behaviours, such as the smoking of cigarettes or the drinking of alcohol. Material deprivation associated with poverty due to such factors as unemployment, long-term illness or disability care also affects health status through a variety of influences, such as poor nutrition and lack of access to health facilities. The effect of these public health hazards are more subtle and take longer to affect individuals. Thus, control measures are far more difficult since they involve changes in individual behaviours (freedoms) and may influence economic/political activity and livelihoods – measures to curb smoking, for example, directly impinge on the rights of tobacco farmers. To change individual behaviours requires far more subtle measures than simply altering the water supply of a town, and are likely to be much more difficult to introduce. It also requires long-term strategies, such as through changes in education.

Choosing between different measures of 'need' to underpin the allocation of resources for public health is also often problematic. Although, for example, the major cause of lung cancer is smoking cigarettes, and the reduction of smoking cigarettes by the population is likely to have a much greater long-term effect on mortality and morbidity from this disease, the immediate service or managerial problem may be palliative treatment or treatment services (radiotherapy or chemotherapy) for patients who already have lung cancer. Information on which national decisions must be made in such competing situations is usually lacking.[34]

A further difficulty arises in that the majority of modern public health issues require inter-sectoral action. For example, the control of cigarette smoking involves agriculture, trade, and communications industries (advertising) as well as the educational system. Bearing these issues in mind, the challenges facing decision-makers with respect to developing appropriate public health measures are obvious. The next section of this chapter addresses these issues, and points to several of the more immediate of these challenges within both a general context, and that of the European Union.

2.2 General requirements for priority-setting in public health

Public health not only influences, but in fact is affected by, all sectors of society; that which includes housing, the environment, the workplace, recreational facilities, tobacco and alcohol policies, and education amongst others. For public health action to be effective, it must be able to mobilise appropriate resources and influence those responsible for executive action to undertake corrective or preventive activities. Public health practitioners cannot act in isolation. They are always dependent on government at central or local level, for the freedom to practise their discipline effectively. Often, public health knowledge and wisdom go counter to belief and to accepted practice.

For example, some politicians believe that cervical cancer screening should be introduced for all women aged between 16 and 64 years, thus (given limited resources) neglecting the fact that the major at risk group are in fact those women over 35 years. Such an over-dilution of effort reduces the overall benefits of the service. This basic misappropriation of resources due to a lack of foresight provides a simple example of how the setting of public health priorities is both a difficult and enormous task.

In order to perform their role, public health practitioners need adequate training and appropriate accreditation to provide quality assurance. The arrangements for this are diverse in the EU and have been described.[35] Essentially, training is required in epidemiological methods to define and describe the health needs of the population, to identify environmental and social hazards to health, and to elucidate the causes and determinants of disease. This knowledge is used to provide advice to those concerned with the setting of priorities and the planning of services. It is essential to evaluate the implementation and outcome of health policies and services provided to populations. Thus, one of the keys to priority-setting is the establishment of a diagnostic surveillance system. This is essential for assessing the current situation and notifying those involved in public health in the event that a problem exists and requires solutions.

2.3 Methods for priority setting in the EU Member States

This book demonstrates the variety of settings in which public health priorities are established and implemented throughout the EU – through central directives, local public health departments, insurance funds and hospital and health service administrations. Member States have a wide variety of consultative and executive mechanisms for the formulation of appropriate public health policies at various levels, ranging from local consultative meetings to inter-ministerial working parties.

Common to most EU Member States is their adoption of the general framework of the World Health Organization 'Health for All' strategy.[36] The following principles underlie this strategy:

• Equity

• Health promotion

• Community participation

• Multi-sectoral cooperation

• Primary health care

• International cooperation

It is important to recognise that by using targets one can highlight important areas of strategy, and that they are also of help in the process of converting policy into programmes. They provide a tangible means of monitoring progress and can act as a stimulus for the collection of good quality data. There are disadvantages however. Firstly, they can lead to spurious priority being given to that which is measurable – as the earlier example on cervical cancer would indicate – and, if taken in isolation, can present an over-simplistic description of policy. Equally, they can appear unrealistic and as a result be dismissed as unattainable.

Public health action that could have a significant impact on important causes of morbidity and mortality can be subdivided into the following categories:

• Improvement of health status

• Risk factor reduction

• Improvement in services and protection

• Surveillance and data needs

Criteria for indicators and targets should be:

Credible: They should address important public health issues that are likely to remain current.

Clear: They should be easily appraised by, and relevant to, a wide general audience.

Selective: The choice of topic should be used to highlight areas that are a high priority for action.

Compatible: They should be compatible with current public health strategies.

Achievable: Interventions should be available or potentially available. The target must take account of evidence of effectiveness and the delay between intervention and effect.

Balanced: They should monitor progress through a mixture of process and outcome measures.

Quantifiable: Data are required. If necessary, proxy indicators should be used or specific recommendations made for the collection of data.

Ethical: They should respect the autonomy of individuals and avoid unnecessary value judgements.

Examples of priority areas in the EU are:

- Alcohol-related harm
- Drug and other substance abuse
- Healthy physical and social environment
- Physical and sensory disability
- Maternal and infant health
- Surveillance and control of infectious disease
- Blood pressure control
- Occupational safety and health
- Mental health
- Exercise
- Nutrition
- Dental health
- Screening for cancer
- Smoking
- Accidental injuries
- Birth control

It is important to understand what is involved with priority-setting in public health. Only when proper understanding has been achieved is it possible to set priorities for action, let alone determine whether innovations have reached their objective. Ideally, public health priorities are based on knowledge of the occurrence, socioeconomic consequences and preventability of health problems, taking into account prediction of future trends and the expected costs and benefits of the public health measures. In this vein, two specific and separate elements must be considered. These are the 'burden of disease' and 'preventability and accountability', and are outlined as follows.

1. Burden of disease:
This is measured by mortality statistics, hospital admission rates, general practitioners' consultation rates and the presence of morbidity in the community. The use of surveys is the main tool by which to gather and compare such data. These figures allow one to examine the burden by, for example, age, sex, geographical area, potential years of life lost, and degree of disability. Analysis of burden of disease enables an assessment of the impact of a disease (or of diseases in general) to be made because of the loss of duration and quality of life due to the effects of diseases and disorders. It also provides an estimate of the cost of health, social care and other services concerned with the prevention and treatment of disease, and assisting people with diseases and disorders. Loss of duration and/or quality of life represents a burden to individuals and their families and thus a burden to society. The cost of health and social services also represents a burden

on society, as part of national income is used to meet the costs.

Although most EU countries have data on mortality and usually morbidity, comprehensive data on quality of life is not available. Thus, most estimates of disease burden tend to be limited.

2. Preventability and availability:
Epidemiological knowledge is required to understand the causes of the major conditions in a country or area. This knowledge involves research into the natural history of the disease, and the suitable age and/or stage for effective intervention. For example, it is now known that about 90 per cent of lung cancer cases in Europe are due to the smoking of cigarettes. Thus to prevent the occurrence of the disease one must either stop children from starting to smoke or persuade those that already do, to stop. It is known that if one stops, the risk of lung cancer reverts to that of a non-smoker within 3–5 years. It is furthermore known that screening for lung cancer in order to identify individuals at an early reversible stage, by X-ray or sputum cytology for example, is ineffective.[37] Treatment of lung cancer is also not very effective, and few patients survive for more than 1–3 years. Thus, if one wishes to reduce the burden of cancer of the lung, one needs to influence the smoking habits of the population.

For ischaemic heart disease the problem is more complex. There are a variety of risk factors for this disease, with smoking, high blood pressure, diet, and exercise as the most important. Early treatment, such as with thrombolytics, is effective in reducing case fatality after a myocardial infarct. Long-term treatment and rehabilitation are effective in prolonging survival and improving the quality of life following an infarct. Thus, the development of a public health strategy for this disease will involve (advocating) the reduction of smoking habits, identification and treatment of those with raised blood pressure, an increase in the amount of exercise taken, reduction of fatty diet, as well as the improvement and speed of access to facilities that enable individuals to receive early treatment with thrombolytics. It will also involve ensuring the appropriate long-term rehabilitative treatment.

The appearance of the HIV virus in Europe in 1982–83 highlighted the need for public health to be concerned with the prediction of future trends; for example the proportion of individuals likely to become infected (and then to require treatment), as well as methods of identifying high risk groups – in this case, those with particular sexual habits. It also showed the need to plan methods of prevention (in the absence of an effective immunising agent or therapy) such as the use of condoms.

The precise ranking of priorities in any area will be largely determined by local circumstances, including the availability of facilities, ability to mobilise effective inter-agency activity, as well as the feelings/wishes of the population. Thus, for example, in an area with few elderly and many young, priorities are likely to be focused on the needs of children and young people rather than those of the elderly. Areas targeted for activity will therefore embrace immunisation, the prevention of road accidents, and reproductive health, rather than disability and care in the home. In setting priorities it is, however, important to bear in mind that there are often local variations which can only be determined through consultation with local people. An excellent example of this was provided in Watts, a very poor area of Los Angeles, and the site of major riots in the late 1960s.[38]

Following these riots the local resident population was asked what they felt their major health-related problem was. This was a relatively young, black neighbourhood, and to the surprise of the officials, disability in young adults was identified as a major cause of concern. An in-depth analysis discovered that the frequency of young disabled, partly as a result of a very high rate of congenital malformations and partly through road accidents, had a profound effect on the economic status of the community. In households with a disabled youngster only one of the adults could go out to work – in contrast to many other communities with community care facilities or less youth disability, and where both parents were employed. Thus, the main priority areas lay in the identification and prevention of congenital malformations, the prevention of road accidents, and the provision of community care facilities.

The precise ways in which communities can, and are, consulted for the determination of priorities is described in the following chapters. The ways in which EU countries list their priorities are also provided. It is obviously important to identify risks that are associated with particular causes of diseases. Identification of the risk rather than the disease does help, in that some risks including cigarette smoking, alcohol consumption, blood pressure, and exercise are associated with more than one disease. It is thus administratively easier and has a greater impact on public health to convince people to tackle, for example, smoking, as this will have an effect on cancer of the lung, chronic respiratory disease and ischaemic heart disease. Use of the disease as a priority may hide the importance of attacking the risk factors of relevance. Further, by identifying risk factors it is clear that the action taken to implement a public health policy should involve more than just the health service. It necessarily also involves education, agriculture, transport and housing.

An example of how this can be tackled according to a simplistic four-part strategy is provided by looking at two separate cases. The first is the smoking of cigarettes (Box 6), and the second, mental health (Box 7), provides a contrasting model.

Box 6

Smoking

1. Background information

In all EU countries smoking is the most preventable cause of death. To demonstrate this, it is important for health officials to research and then make available some of the following basic information:

- The number of deaths from smoking-related diseases, i.e. cancer of the lung, chronic respiratory disease, ischaemic heart disease; and their representation by age and sex. (In the UK it is estimated there are approximately 100,000 smoking-related deaths per annum.)[39]

- The (increasing) concern over passive smoking. (In the UK, it is considered that there are several hundred deaths from lung cancer each year due to environmental tobacco smoking.)
- The proportion of smokers by age and sex, and if possible by socioeconomic status.
- Changes in smoking habit by age and sex over a specified time-period.
- Type of cigarettes smoked, for example, high, medium, or low tar.

2. Target-setting:

Having obtained this information it is then possible to formulate reasonable targets for action. For example:

Improved health status

(a) Reduction in ischaemic heart disease (ICD 410–414) death rates by 30% over a 12 year time-period.

(b) Reduction in lung cancer death rates (ICD 162) by 10% over a 12 year time-period.

Reduced Risk Factors

(c) Reduction in the proportion of adults who smoke by 35% over a 12 year time-period.

(d) A 50% reduction in smoking by pregnant women over a 12 year time-period.

(e) The proportion of children aged 11–15 and adolescents aged 16–19 years who smoke should be reduced to a half of present levels in 12 years time.

3. Improved services and protection

Smoking prevalence is influenced by price, availability of tobacco, and advertising as well as knowledge of the risks of smoking. Thus, in setting such targets, the next step is to devise and set in place the appropriate structures and programmes by which to meet them. For example:

(a) The European directive on tobacco product labelling should be fully implemented and tobacco products labelled with health warnings and tar and nicotine content. These warnings should cover at least 10% of the printed surface.

(b) In 2 years time no smoking should be permitted in any public place.

(c) Over the next 2 years there should be a complete ban on cigarette advertising except at the point of sale.

(d) Over the next 10 years major life and health insurers should offer differential premiums to smokers and non-smokers.

(e) Within 3 years all schools should provide a non smoking environment and high-quality no smoking education.

(f) Within 3 years all health records of those aged 18 years and over should include information on smoking status and this should be updated annually.

(g) Within 3 years all general practitioners should offer no-smoking advice to those of their patients who are regular smokers, and they should also offer practical support in stopping smoking to these patients.

4. Data and surveillance needs

In ordor to undertake these measures and meet the set targets, health officials will have practical certain requirements, including:

(a) Annual mortality data by age and sex for ischaemic heart disease and cancer of the lung.

(b) Annual (if possible) or at least periodic data to track the targets 2(c), 2(e).

(c) Periodic surveys to track the target 2(d), 3(a), 3(b), 3(c), 3(d), 3(e), 3(f), 3(g).

Box 7

Mental Health

1. Background information

There is no good measure of mental health, nor even a good instrument for measuring mental ill health in the Community. Most of the available questionnaires have been designed to detect mental illnesses, or more precisely, to classify subjects as meeting criteria for being a case of a defined mental disorder. Mild degrees of mental ill health or disease are common, and cross-sectional surveys in the UK using such instruments as the Nottingham Health Profile (NHP) or the General Health Questionnaire (GHQ) typically show that up to 30% of an adult population have one or more mental ill health symptoms.

There is a reasonable amount of information on the prevalence of specific mental disorders (for example, schizophrenia), but it is doubtful that purposeful activity will affect the prevalence.

There is a reasonable amount of information on the incidence of suicide and para-suicide. As the rate, particularly among young adults, has been rising and since some effective programmes of prevention have been introduced (for example, those that address drug over-dose and poisoning by coal gas), it would seem sensible to set targets for reduction in the suicide rate to ensure that this continues to be monitored.

People with severe mental illness are a small but significant segment of the population, whose health and functioning deserves special attention. Monitoring mental health policy calls for at least a network of sentinel case registers.

Stress is considered commonly to be a major problem of modern society. The concept is poorly-defined; however, there are certain circumstances which are commonly considered to 'cause' or increase stress, for example, inadequate housing, child abuse, unemployment, and violence. It thus seems reasonable to include some of these as risk factors.

2. Target-setting

Improved Health Services

   (a) Reduce the rate of suicide over the next 10 years in young people aged 15–34 by 10%.

   (b) Reduce the hospital admission rate for drug overdoses by 10% over the next 5 years.

Reduced Risk Factors

   (c) Within three years reduce the number of households in temporary accommodation by 30% and no one should be 'sleeping rough'.

   (d) The incidence of child abuse should be reduced by 25% in the next 3 years.

3. Improved services and protection

   (a) Within 3 years 95% of the population should have someone with whom they can talk over worries or problems.

   (b) Within 3 years 95% of the medical records of those aged 75 or more should document routine enquiry about the presence or absence of depression.

   (c) Within 3 years each area of the country should have an annual first contact rate for community psychiatric nurses as good as that of the top 10% of the country.

4. Data and surveillance needs

   (a) Data to track targets 2(a), 2(b), 2(c), 2(d), 3(a), 3(b), 3(c).

   (b) In addition it would be helpful to have:
       – Data on unemployment by area, age and sex.
       – Data on homicide rates.
       – An instrument to measure mental health in the community.

These two disparate examples attempt to show some of the steps that need to be taken when decisions have been made about appropriate public health activity in specific cases. Formulating the problem in this way also demonstrates the necessary actions that must be taken, and how the implementation of the policies can be monitored.

The separation of the commissioning and provision of services in many EU countries theoretically enables better decisions to be made within a given budget. In theory, there-fore, it should be possible to balance preventive, curative and rehabilitative services. For this to be effective, an adequate knowledge of the natural history of a condition and its epidemiology is essential. It is of course not always available, but for some common conditions we do have the necessary knowledge, for example, ischaemic heart disease and cancer of the lung. An example of how such knowledge can be applied is with respect to ischaemic heart disease. The frequency of the condition (incidence and preva-lence) can either be determined by appropriate surveys or estimated from nationally available figures. Thus the burden of disease can be estimated.

Many of the factors responsible for ischaemic heart disease are known: cigarette smok-ing, blood pressure, diet, and so on. The effectiveness and cost of introducing preven-tive measures such as anti-smoking education in schools, banning tobacco advertising, screening for and treating those with raised blood pressure, providing dietary advice, and labelling foodstuffs, are either known or can be estimated. Evidence of the effec-tiveness of various treatment strategies such as thrombolytic treatment for myocardial infarction, treatment of early angina, and coronary artery bypass grafts, is available. It is thus possible to develop an appropriate local (or national) model of the requirements for different strategies – preventive use of thrombolytics, ambulance services, aspirin, coro-nary care beds, and operating theatres, for example. From this complex model it is thus possible to consider the balance of resources to be devoted to, or invested in, the devel-opment of effective methods to both reduce the burden of ischaemic heart disease and improve the outcome of those who develop the condition. That said, implementation of course poses another set of problems. And while this section has shown the complexi-ties in working out and setting in motion the priorities for two diseases, the following section outlines to what extent this becomes even more difficult at European level.

2.4 Establishing priorities at EU level

Under the principle of subsidiarity and given the limitations of Article 152 in the Amsterdam Treaty and the general character of Article 3(o) of the Treaty of the European Union, the development of all-embracing health policies is the responsibility of each EU Member State. Each Member State is faced with a unique pattern of chal-lenges to the health of its population. This diversity is partly a result of differences in the complex interplay of government policies and consumer preferences as they affect factors such as tobacco, alcohol, diet, and transport, as well as biological and environ-mental factors. Consequently, there is significant scope for Member States to learn from the experience of others as they develop their own policies. However, there are many areas in the field of health promotion and disease prevention where European Community policies have an important role, ranging from agricultural policy and tax harmonisation to safety legislation. Some of these problems, as well as efforts to integrate health into other Community policies, are considered in two reports already published by the Commission.[40,41] The integration of public health into other Community policies was also raised in the Commission's Green Paper on 'Commercial Communications in the Internal Market'.[42] It looks at reducing barriers to the free movement of goods and services between Member States in order to promote more efficient marketing of commodities, and thereby making more goods available at a lesser cost to EU citizens.

Nevertheless, there is an urgent need to define where the European Community can act in public health matters, and which areas should remain the preserve of Member States – the present lack of clarity has already led to disputes over the Community's role. Amongst other reasons, a clear framework for setting priorities is needed with respect to defining the criteria for Community actions (Box 8); where they can be performed more cost-effectively for the Community as a whole; where there is a need for the coordination of activities at European level; where other Community policies have health implications; and where there are issues that cross national boundaries.

Box 8

Criteria for defining European Community functions in the field of public health

- Where there is a clear need for the coordination of activity or to learn from the experiences of other Member States.

- Where functions can be performed more cost-efficiently for the Community as a whole (for example, economies of scale).

- Where there are issues which cross country boundaries such as epidemics, environmental issues and the consequences of the free movement of persons and goods, including pharmaceuticals.

- Where action is needed to standardise definitions so as to make the exchange of information reliable.

- Where the actions and policies of the Community have important health implications.

Priorities for European public health policy could therefore be determined on four criteria:

- the extent and seriousness of the problem;

- whether effective preventive or curative methods are available;

- whether rehabilitation is possible; and

- whether such methods can be used appropriately and efficiently.

This general format of the basis on which priorities are set is helpful in providing those involved in policy formulation with a framework. However, as the individual chapters of this book will illustrate, it is an idealistic scenario because of several problems.

A fundamental issue in every country is the lack of information whether at a national or local level. Although all countries have a comprehensive system for mortality statistics – enabling estimates to be made according to age, sex, area, etc. – this does not necessarily give a complete picture of the diseases in a population. For instance, almost every country analyses mortality by 'underlying cause of death'. But with the majority of deaths being amongst the elderly, and therefore in fact the product of several 'causes' of death – such as coronary heart disease coupled with diabetes – this framework is often inappropriate and generates incomplete results. This example of a manner of death in fact caused by a secondary factor would (according to the 'rules') be classified as due to 'coronary heart disease'. Within this framework it would therefore be difficult, except by special inquiry, to identify that the underlying factor was in fact diabetes, and not a coronary condition.

Furthermore, mortality is only one expression of the burden of disease. Many people are ill, disabled or handicapped, reflecting different expressions. Although most countries have morbidity statistics relating to numbers (or rates) of hospital admission or sickness absence, few if any, have comprehensive systems of recording morbidity in the community, and outside institutions. In addition, there are differences between countries in the manner of collecting or recording such data. Only a few EU Member States (i.e. Sweden, Denmark and Finland) operate a system whereby individuals are identified by personal numbers. The majority of others instead employ 'events' as the basis for collating statistics. Thus, under the latter system, for example, persons with tuberculosis who may be admitted several times in a year for one episode of illness, will appear as more frequent than a person with pneumonia admitted on only one occasion. It is also important to recognise that there is variation in the diagnostic terms used both within, as well as between, specific hospitals, practices, areas and countries. There are many other problems in trying to estimate both the extent and severity of a problem that may influence decision-makers. These include age, sex, ethnic group, and the definition of severity. Thus, it is important to recognise that such figures can only give a very rough idea of the size of a problem in any area or country. And, there are similar difficulties with the other three criteria. For although it is known that effective policies exist for a number of conditions, such knowledge is lacking for many others. The ability to measure such factors as efficiency are also dubious; they may save money to the provider, but may cost a great deal to the individual sufferer or their family.

With these caveats in mind, it is important to recognise that the setting of public health priorities remains an inexact procedure. It is dependent on a large variety of factors, of which the national ones outlined above are only one part. Perceptions and political factors also play an important role. There can be no doubt that the most important factor predisposing to ill health in Europe is poverty, and thus inequality in the provision of services. This, however, presumes that those who pay the taxes and who are the most vocal (certainly not the poor) are willing to accept that poverty alleviation is the first priority – an unlikely scenario. It is thus important to recognise the utility of a framework which underlies the concept, but equally to recognise that methods of priority-setting and resource allocation in Member States will differ greatly.

Another fundamental definition that needs clarification is that of 'added value'. This is supposed to guide Community action, but there is little understanding of what it actually means in practice. Given the differences between Member States in the development of their public health policies, health systems and socioeconomic status, what constitutes 'added value' is not necessarily the same for all Member States. Within this context, knowledge transfer based on best practice available between Member States and adapted to the local environment should be a priority. Human resources development ought to be another. Current initiatives under the Fourth Framework Programme for Research support the mobility of doctoral, post-doctoral and experienced researchers between Member States. But it is important that the Commission also supports local developments and centres of excellence in training and research in the Member States.

3. Conclusions and recommendations

The Community's current role in the field of health is based on a limited definition of public health, and one restricted to specific areas such as 'prevention', 'major health scourges', and 'drug dependence'. This disease-based approach was outlined immediately after Maastricht in the Commission's framework document.[23] While it may have proved politically successful, such an approach has reduced the Community's ability to make a substantial contribution to the health of European citizens. As this chapter has argued, instead of a disease-based strategy, a greater focus on risk factors associated with diseases and the determinants of health is needed. This calls for a multi-sectoral approach that incorporates subjects such as poverty, unemployment, agriculture, transport, housing, and education. The reason being, that many other areas of European Community policy (such as agriculture and industry) can and do impact on health. Accordingly, there is great potential for an integrated approach to health at Community level. This was recognised under the Maastricht Treaty in that it stipulated that health protection must be integrated into other areas of Community policy. However, this has not happened effectively to date. And while a longer term, risk-based approach may be less politically appealing, it is likely to be more effective in health terms.[5]

Implementing a new framework for setting priorities must go hand in hand with reforms of European Community institutions. So too is a reorganisation of the decision-making process necessary in order to redress the relative weakness of those responsible for health, particularly in the Commission. As discussed above, health-related activities are currently scattered throughout the Commission without any effective central focus. This was obvious during the height of the BSE crisis when agriculture and not health officials took the lead in both the Commission and the Council of Ministers, leading one analyst to ask: 'where is the public health community in all this?'[43] Health-related policies are also discussed by ministers of transport and industry at European level, for example, but are omitted from the agendas of health ministers' meetings. This is not altogether a bad practice as it does enhance a multi-sectoral approach, but there remains a pressing need for an effective mechanism to bring together all health-related discussions. The structural portrait of EU policy-making is therefore consistent with current political realities – there is a lack of long-term strategies and incremental measures, and short-term policies do not always address new challenges.

This need for an effective coordination mechanism was recognised in the findings of the European Parliament's Temporary Committee of Inquiry on BSE. The Committee's report influenced developments at the 1997 Intergovernmental Conference, and prompted a rearrangement of health-related responsibilities at Community level, especially within the Commission. Amongst the reforms, DGXXIV was mandated responsibility for 'Consumer Health' as complementary to its continuing role in Consumer Policy. This reshuffling of competencies – it must be reiterated, in the wake of the BSE crisis – has meant that DGV (and the Public Health Unit specifically) has been, to a certain extent, marginalised (or at least relieved of some of its duties) with respect to its role in public health. Nevertheless, the extension of DGXXIV's portfolio to take up consumer and food health issues does not address what many perceive as the fundamental issue; namely, the need for a new Commission portfolio to focus exclusively on public health. The creation of a new Directorate-General or even separate department dedicated solely to health (and with functional, executive powers), could play a significant role in coordinating (or even initiating) policies, programmes, and activities in the area of health. This would, however, only represent one component of the wider task to redefine, in an appropriate manner, the nature of public health in the EU context.

3.1 Piecing together the puzzle: institutions, structures, individuals and agendas

Reorganising the basis of EU health competencies from a disease-based to a priority-setting framework will require a four-part process. The first step, as in putting together a jigsaw puzzle, is to establish the institutional framework, that is, to build the borders. With respect to a new EU public health setting, this will involve developing the necessary institutional capacity within which all plans and programmes can be effectively undertaken. In this vein, the idea of establishing a new portfolio or Directorate General to focus exclusively on public health would be a positive, if not necessary, first step. As with a puzzle, however, a border alone does not provide a complete picture, and is not able to convey any real meaning – the creation of a new DG therefore is not sufficient for the development of a comprehensive EU public health strategy. Also imperative is the establishment of formal structures and networks to enable and underpin the pursuit of specific health-related aims – there is little point in continuing a jigsaw puzzle in the centre of the void created by the borders, that is, in isolation. Rather, it is necessary to build on those pieces already in place, as they provide a firm and accountable starting point. The one step therefore leads to the other in an interdependent manner. In this regard, the tasks of a new DG should involve the grounding of specific structures which, *inter alia*, could include:

- The development of a Europe-wide system of surveillance and control of the incidence of communicable disease (including a system for the quick dissemination of information across frontiers).

- The development of cooperative arrangements for the evaluation of methods of treatment and technology assessment.

- The development of a European Health Services Information Facility to:
  - develop a set of indicators appropriate for the Community as a whole, taking account of the data which is available or can be made available or developed. (Data would be gathered from Europe as a whole, in order to provide comparable data for other countries);
  - in collaboration with other international agencies, work out common standards and definitions so that comparative studies can be undertaken to assess possible variations in health needs, utilisation, health expenditure and outcome;
  - compare the incidence and prevalence of various diseases in different environments, taking advantage of the heterogeneity of the populations, services and customs in the EU;
  - make use of the existing wide variation in the incidence of many diseases to investigate the aetiology of major causes of mortality and morbidity so as to identify possible preventive strategies;
  - sponsor appropriate experiments in the control of diseases for which preventive measures are known, including building on the successful experience of 'Europe against Cancer'; and
  - identify the health consequences of migration and develop ways of abating its harmful effects.

- Assistance in the development of appropriate educational programmes in health (services) research.

- Help in the grounding of safety legislation which emphasises safety and is not diluted by unjustified arguments about competitiveness.

- Aid in the development of a system for learning from experience of health promotion and disease prevention in different Member States.

- The development of medical purchasing guidelines in order to assist Member States to reduce unnecessary services.

- The development of systems of information dissemination to promote research in defining effective health care and how best to give patients an informed choice.

- The establishment of a Community programme for coordinating technology assessment.

- The development of a European-level system of coordination activities to eliminate, through immunisation, those diseases for which this is technically possible.

- The establishment of a programme for the promotion of greater awareness of rare diseases affecting migrants amongst health care professionals who may be called upon to treat them but have little experience of them.

- The development of a network for the pooling of the experience of different Member States to acquire better knowledge of the causes of health inequalities and develop remedial policies.

- The establishment of a Community-level programme to support efforts to enable people to make health choices about their diet through:
  - strategies aimed at relieving poverty;
  - improved food labelling;
  - ensuring that agricultural policies are consistent with health; and
  - improving understanding of the effect of nutrition on health.

- A leading role in establishing a system of common standards for training in public health and promote public health education (the Community should also find the extra finance for such promotion through the reduction of subsidies on those agricultural commodities which can be damaging to health).

- The establishment of a monitoring capacity to:
  - monitor developments in cost containment policies;
  - assess the success of different policies; and
  - communicate the findings to the Member States.

  (of particular importance is to study the effects of the major reforms which have been recently introduced or planned in increasing the efficiency with which resources are used);

- Ensuring that the intelligence network upon which public health is dependent is made responsible at all levels for the design and implementation of appropriate information systems; in order to be able to react rapidly to any threats to health, be comparable, comprehensive and flexible.

These structures must be based on solid methodologies and be applicable across the EU in its entirety. They must also be flexible and accommodating enough to evolve in tandem with further enlargement of the Community. In this view, Berlin and Hunter regard the next round of accession countries from Central and Eastern Europe as facing the challenge of hitting a 'moving target' with respect to meeting the changing public health criteria of the EU.[44] Cooperation between Member States is of course critical, and planning and implementation must be taken together. Thus, the establishment of relevant institutions and structures – or setting and building upon borders in a puzzle – is vital to a new Community public health role based on priority-setting measures.

Nevertheless, institutions and structures are still not in and of themselves sufficient to produce a new Community public health understanding. The third step therefore is to fill in the detail, to try and complete the picture. This will involve matching like with like;

distinguishing between possibility and certainty; deciding on the constitution of Community programmes; and making use of the more formalised structures already created. Here, the emphasis in creating a new and more contemporary (relevant) EU public health context is on individuals and agendas. A new entity with a host of comprehensive and valid structures is of little use without specific programmes and the persons to implement them.

In order to run such a new Directorate with its various systems and structures, the EU must have at least a professionally qualified Director-General for Public Health. As well, the staff of this new DG must be trained in public health and have sufficient strength in numbers and quality to be able to participate in and guide the EU policies that have an impact on public health. As mentioned, there are many such EU activities which impinge on the health of the population. It is thus crucial that those responsible for the formulation of EU policies are informed of their health consequences and that the staff of a new EU Public Health Directorate is capable of coping with the problems and solutions that have been outlined earlier. The Directorate must have access to adequate resources, both to promote public health policies, as well as to mount the necessary research in order to formulate effective policies. Thus, for the DG to be able to carry out its new mandate effectively, it is in turn reliant on the quality of the individuals who will run it.

The fourth and final step in completing the jigsaw puzzle is to ensure that the health-related programmes run the by the new DG are valid and relevant. That is, to ensure that the new institution has the proper agenda(s) to make appropriate use of its structures and fulfil its role. The underlying mandate for any such body should therefore be the development of a singular and coherent health strategy, along with an operational policy to meet the Treaty stipulations for the proper integration of health requirements into other Community policies.

Should the role of the High Level Committee on Health be formalised, this will – when combined with the significant powers of the European Parliament and Council – ensure that the elected representatives of the peoples of the Community and the Member States' authorities play an important role in policy formation and implementation. In order to fulfil this overarching agenda, two primary tasks of the new public health body must also be:

- the development of common standards and definitions (in collaboration with WHO and other international organisations) to ensure that comparative studies to assess possible variations in health needs, utilisation, health expenditure and outcome can be undertaken; and

- since the major causes of morbidity and mortality have been identified, to evaluate, as a priority, appropriate preventive strategies for their control.

In terms of the 'how?' with respect to setting up such a body, it could be achieved through an amalgamation of those individual units with a health-related function or influence from various DGs in the existing Commission structure. For instance, aspects

---

Box 9

Proposed regrouping of the European Commission's health and health related dossiers

Public Health

[Environmental health and chemical substances, radiation protection, disease prevention, health promotion, health monitoring and health telematics, research and G7 health projects, epidemiology and surveillance of diseases, actions on specific risks, combating drug dependence, programmes for the disabled, medical ethics]

Medical Care and the Internal Market

[Medicinal products (orphan drugs, vaccines, consumption, pricing and reimbursement), technology assessment, effects of other Community policies on health systems, health professions, health economics and policy analysis, priority setting and policy evaluation]

Safety and Standards Regulation and Consumer Protection

[Occupational safety and health, medical devices, veterinary and phytosanitary regulations and controls, nutrition and food safety, biotechnology, relations with and information to consumers, pricing, marketing and liability issues]

Health Developments in Other Countries and Humanitarian Aid

[PHARE, ACE and TACIS programmes on health, Euro-Mediterranean projects, health planning in developing countries, humanitarian aid]

---

of DGV's role (Social Affairs, specifically the Public Health Unit) could be combined with those of DGVI (Agriculture), DGXI (Environment), and DGXXIV (Consumer Policy). A tentative regrouping of responsibilities is outlined in Box 9, and is based on current needs and potential future developments and requirements.[45]

3.2 Recommendations – the way forward

As was originally pointed out in Section 1.5 of this chapter regarding the European Parliament's recommendations in response to the Commission's 1998 Communication, political will is crucial to all reform of Community public health competencies. Thus, here too must it be reiterated that the completion of this four-part process – the establishment of institutions and structures, and the securing of qualified personnel assigned relevant agendas – is still not enough to develop a priority-setting based framework for public health in the Community. For as with the jigsaw puzzle, while the pieces may all have been put together, the picture remains incomplete without it being interpreted. That is, in order for this four-part process to have the desired effect, it depends most crucially on the political will to change things. This political interest must, therefore, be forthcoming not only from the Community but so too from other institutions, bodies, and individuals, and of course the Member States themselves.

Accordingly, to develop such a comprehensive EU-level public health strategy, several recommendations are here offered. In addition to those tasks and structures mandated a new DG, these recommendations also represent a potential first step. For them to be successful, however, they must be recognised and taken into account by policy-makers:

- The provision of much greater support for public health research in Europe. We do not exploit sufficiently the wide variability in populations, the migration of individuals and communities through the 'free movement' Directive nor the wide variation in environments, culture and work that exists to determine some of the causes of ill health and better policies for health improvement.

- Public health must be forthright in the advocacy of programmes that improve health and be able to state clearly and openly the dangers and consequences of some actions – whether clinical, environmental or political.

- Public health, at all levels, must have the ability to influence the budget for its activities. Usually short-term clinical or 'outbreaks' or 'scandals' take precedence and overwhelm public health resources. If public health is to play the required role, it must ensure that long-term issues are not omitted in favour of short-term demands.

- At all levels within the EU and its Member States, public health must have a clear role to guide not only the policies of health authorities or bodies, but also of schools, welfare agencies, housing departments, environmental agencies, agriculture, industry, etc.; as well those of practising clinicians in hospitals and in general practice and the community.

- For the effective monitoring of health needs and the outcome of services, data needs to be linked to individuals, as is done in only three Member States (Denmark, Sweden and Finland), rather than only recording 'events'. For this to be implemented, not only do we require appropriate information systems, but we also need to integrate these needs into the EU Data Protection policies.

- In all EU countries there is a need to improve the education in public health for a variety of disciplines, for example, doctors, nurses, statisticians, psychologists and health educators. This implies the recognition of the multi-disciplinary nature of the subject and the different needs of the individual disciplinary groups. In addition to education, a structured, supervised training programme must be established in those EU countries that have no such programme, and in all countries for all the disciplines involved, in order that the EU can call upon a cadre of trained persons to tackle public health problems and provide public health expertise at all levels: local, regional, national and supranational.

- Many public health problems depend upon the assessment of risk and their communication to both the public and those responsible for the formulation of policy. Examples range from the transport of nuclear materials on public highways, to contaminated food or water, to the smoking of cigarettes. Unfortunately, such assessments and their communication have not, in the past, been tackled in a sufficiently satisfactory, systematic manner. This problem needs to be tackled by research, education and discussion (with, for example, the media) if we are to improve our present practice.

• It is a *sine qua non* that EU public health policies should be based on evidence, rather than only beliefs. It is unfortunate that this needs to be stated, as it is so obvious, but there are several examples of current policies which do not meet this criterion.

• As stated, public health has a difficult role to fulfil – and its practitioners require not only scientific, professional but also diplomatic skills. For it to be effective it has to act as a 'change agent'. Within the EU and its Member States there is a great need for the development and application of public health policies. For the formulation and implementation of such policies, properly trained people are needed. Thus it is essential that we have policies that encourage, sustain and promote individuals who show the appropriate leadership qualities.

The amount of political will to achieve this cannot be understated. For until a political consensus over all potential areas for action emerges, policies may continue to develop merely as a series of individual responses or reactions to new ideas, problems and requests as they arise, and not as a coherent strategy with clear objectives. The earlier-mentioned 'knee-jerk political reaction' to the BSE crisis resulting in the hasty revision of Article 129 of the Maastricht Treaty is a prime example of this. At present, the institutional and legal conditions are unfortunately not the most appropriate for the development of a coherent EU public health framework.

The various chapters which follow describe public health policies and the methods of priority setting in EU countries, and demonstrate the enormous variability both in the methods used and in the amount of care taken to consult the population and consumers of health services. These ensuing chapters cover policies and developments in the Member States up to late 1998. There is also wide variation in the contribution, training and competence of those whose major task is the promotion of public health. Only if there is greater appreciation of the need for a well-trained group of public health practitioners capable of undertaking the types of study outlined, are we likely to see a community-wide improvement in health. The ability to undertake such work will enable the EU to develop a rational public health policy supported by those who will benefit from it. And while this cannot be simply imposed from above, the Community does have a role to play in setting down guidelines and principles which Member States can then implement of their own accord. Rather than straight-out harmonisation, therefore, the emphasis ought to be on the gradual realisation of wider Community objectives through national-level implementation. For as has already been mentioned in this chapter, the reform process is predominantly a political one.

References

1. Powles J. Changes in disease patterns and related social trends. *Social Science and Medicine* 1993;35:337–87.

2.   Mossialos, E. *Citizens and Health Systems: Main Results from a Eurobarometer Survey.* (Based on Eurobarometer 49 (1996). International Research Associates (Europe). This summary was undertaken by LSE Health, London School of Economics.) Luxembourg: Office for Official Publications of the European Communities, 1998.

3.   Holland WW. (ed.) *Atlas of Avoidable Deaths.* 3rd edition. Oxford; Oxford University Press, 1997.

4.   McKee M, Mossialos E, Belcher P. The influence of European Community law on national health policy. *Journal of European Social Policy* 1996;6(4):263–86.

5.   Belcher P, Mossialos E. Health priorities for the European intergovernmental conference. *British Medical Journal* 1997;314:1637–38.

6.   Mossialos E, McKee M. The Amsterdam treaty and the future of European health services. *Journal of Health Serv Res Policy* 1998;3(2):65–66.

7.   Commission of the European Communities. *Modernising and Improving Social Protection in the European Union.* COM (97) 102 final 12.03.97.

8.   Bury J. A future for an EU public health policy? *Eurohealth* 1998;4(4):5–6.

9.   Mossialos E, Permanand G. A new European Commission: Wendezeit or déjà vu for public health? *Eurohealth* 1998;4(5):1.

10. Chambers, G. Inside the labyrinth: how the EU works. *Eurohealth* 1996;2(3):7–11.

11. Merkel B, Hübel M. Public health policy in the European Community. In this volume. pp. 49–67.

12. European Commission. Resolution of the Council and the Ministers for Health, meeting within the Council of 27 May 1993 on future action in the field of public health. *Official Journal of the European Communities* 1993;C174(36):1–3.

13. European Commission. Council Resolution of 2 June 1994 on the framework for Community action in the field of health. *Official Journal of the European Communities* 1994;C165(37):1–2.

14. European Commission. *European Social Policy – A Way Forward for the Union: A White Paper.* COM (94) 333 final/2, Brussels, 1994.

15. Coghlan T. Commission report on the integration of health protection requirements – a response. *Eurohealth* 1996;2(4):6–8.

16. *Communication from the Commission Concerning a Community Action Programme on Iinjury Prevention in the Context of the Framework for Action in the Field of Public Health.* COM(97)178 final of 14.5.97.

17. *Communication from the Commission Concerning a Programme of Community Action on Rare Diseases within the Framework for Action in the Field of Public Health.* COM(97) 225 final of 26.5.97.

18. *Communication from the Commission Concerning a Programme of Community Action on Pollution-related Diseases in the Context of the Framework for Action in the Field of Public Health.* COM (97) 266 final of 4.6.97.

19. *Communication from the Commission to the Council and the European Parliament on a European Union Action Plan to Combat Drugs (1995–1999).* COM (94) 234 final of 23.6.1994.

20. Council, Council Regulation (EEC) No 302/93 establishing a European Monitoring Centre on Drugs and Drugs Addiction. *Official Journal of the European Communities* 1993;L36/1.

21. *Proposal for a Council Recommendation on the Suitability of Blood and Plasma Donors and the Screening of Donated Blood in the European Community.* COM (97) 605 final of 17.11.97.

22. Belcher P, Mossialos E. Editorial. *Eurohealth* 1996;2(1):1.

23. *Commission Communication on the Framework for Action in the Field of Public Health.* COM (93) 559 final of 24.11.93.

24. *Commission Communication Concerning Communicable Disease Surveillance Networks in the European Community.* COM (96) 78 final of 07.03.96.

25. *Communication from the Commission to the Council, the European Parliament, the Economic and Social Committee and the Committee of the Regions on the Development of Public Health Policy in the European Community.* COM (98) 230 final of 15.04.98.

26. European Public Health Alliance. *Position Paper in Response to the Commission Communication on the Development of Public Health Policy in the European Community COM (1998) 230 final.* Brussels: EPHA, 1998.

27. Mountford L. *European Union Health Policy on the Eve of the Millennium.* Public Health and Consumer Protection Series, Working Document (SACO 102 EN), DG for Research – European Parliament: Luxembourg, 1998.

28. European Commission, Common Position (EC) No 35/96 of 18 June 1996 adopted by the Council, acting in accordance with the procedure referred to in Article 189b of the Treaty establishing the European Community, with a view to adopting a European Community and Council Directive adopting a programme of Community action on health monitoring within the framework for action in the field of public health. *Official Journal of the European Communities* 1996;C220(39):36.

29. European Commission, Communication from the Commission. *The Future of Social Protection: A Framework for a European Debate.* COM (95) 466 final, Brussels, 1995.

30. Council. Recommendation on the convergence of social protection objectives and policies (92-442). *Official Journal of the European Communities* 1992;L245/49.

31. Acheson ED. *Public Health in England. Report of the Committee of Inquiry into the Future Development of the Public Health Function.* London: HMSO, 1988.

32. Green DG. (ed.) *Acceptable Inequalities. Essays on the Pursuit of Equality in Health Care.* London: Institute of Economic Affairs Health Unit, 1988.

33. Porter D. Public health and centralization the Victorian British state. In: Detels R, Holland WW, McEwen J, Omenn G (eds). *Oxford Textbook of Public Health.* 3rd edition Vol. 1. Oxford: Oxford Medical Publications, 1997. pp. 19–34.

34. McCarthy M, Rees S. *Health Systems and Public Health Medicine in the European*

Community. London: Faculty of Public Health Medicine and Royal College of Physicians, 1992.

35. Holland WW. Achieving an ethical health service, the need for information. *J. Royal College of Physicians* 1995;29:325–34.

36. World Health Organization Regional Office for Europe. *Targets for Health for All: Targets in Support of the European Regional Strategy for Health for All*. Copenhagen: WHO, 1985.

37. Holland WW, Stewart S. *Screening in Health Care*. London: Nuffield Provincial Hospitals Trust, 1990.

38. Breslow L. *Personal Communication*, 1969. (Dr L. Breslow was Commissioner of Health in California.)

39. Royal College of Physicians. *Health or Smoking*. London: Pitman Medical, 1983.

40. European Commission. *Report from the Commission to the Council, the European Parliament and the Economic and Social Committee on the Integration of Health Protection Requirements in Community Policies*. Luxembourg: European Commission, COM (95) 196 final of 29.05.95.

41. European Commission. *Second Report from the Commission to the Council, the European Parliament and the Economic and Social Committee on the Integration of Health Protection Requirements in Community Policies*. Luxembourg: European Commission, COM (96) 407 final of 04.09.96.

42. European Commission. *Commercial Communications in the Internal Market*. Luxembourg: European Commission, COM (96) 192 final of 08.05.96.

43. Palmer S. The BSE crisis – an assessment. *Eurohealth* 1996;2(2):10–12.

44. Berlin A, Hunter W. EU enlargement – the health agenda: public health challenges and opportunities. *Eurohealth* 1999;4(6 Special Issue):5–7.

45. Mossialos E, McKee M. The European Union and health: past, present and future. In: Harrison A. *Health Care UK 1997/98*, London: King's Fund, 1997.

2

Public Health Policy in the European Community

Bernard Merkel and Michael Hübel

Introduction

Responsibility for financing and operating health systems has traditionally been the prerogative of each individual country in the European Community. This is largely still the case today; both the provision of health services and the organisation of health systems remain in essence the responsibility of Member States, although rules and conditions governing health services and attaching to certain components of health systems have been laid down at Community level. Right from the outset of the European Community, it has had an involvement in the area of health, and for a number of years its legislation and activities have had important consequences both for the health status of European citizens and for the functioning of the health sector.

This chapter gives an overview of a number of Community policies and priorities with an impact in the health field. It focuses particularly on the Community's activities in the field of public health, which are based on Article 129 of the Treaty establishing the European Community.*

Before looking at the development of health-related policy at Community level and at the specific activities and priorities in the field of public health, it is necessary to give a short description of the decision-making process in the Community and of the structures at Community level relating to health.

---

* The Amsterdam Treaty has modified this Article which, in the consolidated version of the Amsterdam Treaty, has become Article 152. The new Treaty came into force on May 1st 1999.

Decision-making

All of the European Community Institutions play an important role in preparing, adopting and implementing health-related Community legislation. The Treaty contains provisions for a number of different decision-making procedures, which cannot be presented here in detail. With regard to public health in particular, legislative measures and other actions are taken on the basis of Article 129 of the Treaty which specifies that, apart from non-binding recommendations to be issued by the Council on a proposal by the Commission, the so-called co-decision procedure should be used. This procedure is set out in Article 189b. It means in essence that agreements have to be on the basis of a joint co-decision between the Council and the European Parliament.

The steps leading to this decision are broadly as follows.

The European Commission puts forward a proposal for a decision by the Council and the European Parliament. This proposal will originate with a draft prepared by one of the Commission services. For public health this would normally be the public health and safety at work Directorate within the Commission's Directorate-General V (DGV/F).* Before a proposal is put on the agenda of the Commission for agreement (that is to say the College of 20 Commissioners), it will have gone through several stages. First, discussions with experts and national representatives. Second, the development of a draft proposal, comprising a draft legal instrument: a decision together with an explanatory document. Third, consultation with all relevant services of the Commission. This last is not by any means a formality. All Directorates-General (DGs) concerned have to agree to a proposal, or if they cannot agree, they must set out clearly their positions and reasons for disagreement before it is put to the College of Commissioners for a decision on its adoption, modification or postponement. Every effort is made to ensure that proposals before the College have the backing of all the DGs concerned, and that the concerns of all its Members are fully addressed.

The proposal would be presented to the Commission by the particular Commissioner(s) responsible for that area of activity.

After the proposal has been adopted by the Commission, it is presented to the Council and the Parliament for co-decision. It is also presented to the Economic and Social Committee (representing employers organisations, trade unions and consumer interests) and the Committee on Regions (representing regional and area authorities) which can give an opinion on the proposal.

Once the Council receives a proposal it decides which Council working group should deal with the topic. All working groups consist of officials representing Member States' governments. The groups are chaired by an official of the Member State holding the Presidency of the Community which rotates every six months. For public health issues,

---

* *See below for the Commission's structure and services dealing with health.*

the normal working group is the 'Health Group'. However, a particular issue may be dealt with instead by another group. This could happen, for example, in respect of a proposal that involved psychotropic substances, health and environmental policy issues, or health and safety at work issues.

The Council Group concerned will have a series of meetings at which they will aim to prepare a decision on the Commission's proposal which takes the form of a 'Common position'. Commission representatives attend these meetings to explain the proposals and provide input into the debate. When a common position has been arrived at, it has to be agreed formally at a meeting of the Council: this could be the Council devoted to health issues in which Health Ministers take part (the so-called Health Council) which generally takes place at the end of each Presidency i.e. twice a year. Alternatively another Council can formally adopt the common position, if political agreement has already been obtained at the Health Council.

While the Council has been discussing the proposal, Parliament will have started its own consideration of the Commission's proposal. In accordance with the Treaty, Council has to await the results of Parliament's deliberations before agreeing the common position.

Parliament attributes the proposals it receives to the relevant committee; for public health matters this is normally the Committee on the Environment, Public Health and Consumer Protection. Other Comittees may be associated with the preparation of the opinion. The Committee appoints a rapporteur who draws up a draft report and a reso-lution on the proposal. Once the Committee has agreed to this report (taking into account also the opinions of associated Committees, for example, social affairs, women's rights) this is then sent to the whole Parliament for debate and decision. The Commission services will be present during these discussions to provide clarifications and supplementary information when required.

On the basis of the Parliament's opinion, the Commission may put forward an amended proposal to Council. Following the adoption of the common position, the Commission forwards to the Parliament its observations and reasons for its reserves, if any, on the common position. This is the basis for the second reading in Parliament and of Council's further consideration. The Parliament may table amendments to the Council's common position, following which the Commission may again present a revised proposal to the Council. If both Institutions' positions are then in accord, the decision will be adopted by the Council. However, given that the two Institutions have rather different philoso-phies about what the Community should be doing in the public health field – the Parliament usually wanting it to be more proactive and the Council usually trying to place restraints on Community actions, especially in their budget and modes of manage-ment – it is not surprising that they tend to arrive at rather different views of the merits of the Commission's proposals and how far and what changes might be desirable.

The position is not helped by the fact that the two bodies normally conduct separate and parallel examinations of the Commission's proposal and usually do not formally confer while doing so.

Thus, to date, in order to secure the agreement of the Council and the Parliament to the various proposals, it has been necessary to use in the end the conciliation procedure provided for in the Treaty to resolve their differences. This involves a conciliation committee being convened which comprises the Members of the Council or their representatives and an equal number of representatives of the European Parliament. The Commission also takes part in the discussions. The aim of this process is to try to find a compromise between the positions of the two Institutions. It has been used for all the proposed decisions for public health programmes. So far agreement has always been reached at the end of this procedure. However, it has to be said that the whole co-decision procedure is both time-consuming and complex. In the case of the public health programmes put forward, the complete procedure from the date of presenting the Commission's proposal to the date of the programme coming into force has generally taken about two years. To this must be added the period of the development of the proposal and its adoption by the Commission.

Health policy within the Commission

Within the Commission, health-related matters are attributed to different services and departments. Many Community policies have clear implications for health (e.g. agriculture, food policy, research, trade and transport policy), but legislation in these fields would not normally be dealt with by the services in charge of public health matters. There is, however, a procedure of internal consultation to ensure that all services associated with a particular matter agree to the proposal (see above).

The European Commission is structured as a number of Directorates-General, roughly corresponding to Ministries in national administrations. Matters of public health are dealt with primarily by Directorate-General V (Employment and Social Affairs), which has a Directorate on Public Health and Safety (V/F; based in Luxembourg)*. An overview of other Commission DGs with policy responsibility in areas with a potential impact on health is provided in the annex.

Within the DG V Directorate in charge of public health, a number of public health programmes are administered which support activities in Member States. These are intended to provide a certain European Community 'added value' and are of direct relevance to Member countries and more generally to the Community as a whole. In implementing the programmes, the Commission is assisted by programme committees consisting of representatives of Member States. These Committees, which are chaired by the Commission, give their opinion on the programme's priorities, project selection and evaluation procedures, and annual work programmes, and on individual project applications. The Commission regularly evaluates the programmes and presents reports on their implementation to the Council and the European Parliament.

---

* *European Commission, DG V/F, L-2920 Luxembourg.*

Background

The European Community has had an involvement with health issues for four decades. The Treaty of Rome of 1957 contained provisions, for example, relating to restricting free movement of goods on health grounds. The Single European Act of 1987 introduced further areas of health-related work such as a large-scale research programme and the development of health and safety at work legislation.

The first action programme specifically on public health (Europe Against Cancer) began in 1987, and was followed by a second action programme on the same subject which began in 1990. These initial programmes, which aimed at supporting collaboration activities across the Community in the field of cancer, provided a model for two further initiatives. These were the Europe Against AIDS programme, which began in 1991, and a drug dependency prevention programme, which formed part of the European action plan against drugs (which also covered drug trafficking etc).

These were very limited funding activities, without a specific legal basis. It was only with the 1993 Treaty on European Union (the Maastricht Treaty), with its new public health provisions, that the Community had the opportunity to create a broad and coherent strategy in the field of public health.

The Maastricht Treaty on European Union

The Treaty of Maastricht, ratified on 1 November 1993, provided the Community for the first time with a specific legal competence in the field of public health. In Article 3(o), the Community is given a new objective of making 'a contribution to the attainment of a high level of health protection'. This general objective is, of course, applicable to all Community policies.

Article 129 of the Treaty then sets out a framework for Community action to be undertaken in pursuit of this objective.

The Article's main provisions are as follows:

- Member States shall coordinate programmes and policies in collaboration with the Commission. The Commission can take initiatives to promote such coordination.
- Community action on health protection should be focused on the prevention of diseases. This has the (implicit) implication that they should not deal with the provision of health services and the organisation of health systems. Member States' responsibilities in these areas should not be touched.
- Community activities in the field of public health should concentrate particularly on the major health 'scourges', including drug dependence, which is mentioned specifically,
- in these areas, the Community is to cooperate with other organisations active in the field.

In addition, the Treaty stipulates that health protection requirements shall form a

---

The Maastricht Treaty

Article 3

... the activities of the Community shall include, as provided in this Treaty and in accordance with the timetable set out therein:

Article 3(o). A contribution to the attainment of a high level of health protection.

Article 129, Public Health

1. The Community shall contribute towards ensuring a high level of human health protection by encouraging cooperation between the Member States and, if necessary, lending support to their action.

Community action shall be directed towards the prevention of diseases, in particular the major health scourges, including drug dependence, by promoting research into their causes and their transmission, as well as health information and education.

Health protection requirements shall form a constituent part of the Community's other policies.

2. Member States shall, in liaison with the Commission, coordinate among themselves their policies and programmes in the areas referred to in paragraph 1. The Commission may, in close contact with the Member States, take any useful initiative to promote such coordination.

3. The Community and the Member States shall foster cooperation with third countries and the competent international organizations in the sphere of public health.

4. In order to contribute to the achievement of the objectives referred to in this Article, the Council: acting in accordance with the procedure referred to in Article 189b, after consulting the Economic and Social Committee and the Committee of the Regions, shall adopt incentive measures, excluding any harmonization of the laws and regulations of the Member States; acting by a qualified majority on a proposal from the Commission, shall adopt recommendations.

---

constituent part of other Community policies. This means in effect that when other policies and measures are being developed attention should be paid to their potential consequences for health.

Commission communication on the framework of action in the field of public health

Directly after the coming into effect of the Treaty in November 1993, the Commission published a communication on 'the framework for action in the field of public health'.[1]

This document, which gained the support of Council and Parliament, set out how the Commission intended to implement the new public health powers included in the Treaty.

The first part of the communication deals with the context in which Community public health strategy has to be developed. This discusses the background to health-related activities in the Community and the principles governing Community action, such as subsidiarity. It also considers the major causes of mortality and morbidity in the Community today – cancer, cardio-vascular diseases, accidents, mental illness, respiratory conditions and musculo-skeletal conditions, and the main trends in Community health status, such as lengthening life expectancy.

The communication then looks at the major problems faced by the Member States in the field of health.

The first of these is that resulting from the falling birth rate and lengthening life expectancy, the population is ageing. Progressively there will be larger numbers of elderly people who have different health needs and are disproportionate users of health services to provide for. It also means that the burden of paying for these services will fall on a relatively smaller working population.

Second, the development of powerful technologies for diagnosis and treatment, including new and costly pharmaceutical products, has contributed to continually rising health care costs.

Third, and linked to the improvements in therapy, there are rising expectations among the public about what health services can provide – and rising demands about what they should provide. The increasing awareness of differences in levels and standards of provision within countries and between them tends to accentuate this.

Fourth, population mobility is increasing, both within and into the Community, which can spread communicable diseases and can produce migrant communities with special health needs.

Finally, there are diseases arising from changes in the natural and working environments, such as rising levels of asthma and certain forms of cancer and stress and musculo-skeletal problems.

As a result of these developments health spending has risen rapidly in Member States over the last two decades.

This has been happening at a time when Member States are facing serious economic difficulties, notably slow growth and persistent high levels of unemployment. These put pressure on public finances and have lead Member States to place constraints on public expenditure on health services and social assistance.

In recent years Member States have made strenuous efforts to control the rise in health expenditure and in certain cases have stabilised or even reduced health care spending as a proportion of GDP. States have tried to control health spending by for example limiting the numbers of doctors being trained, limiting the range of drugs they can prescribe or imposing charges on patients.

Criteria for Community priority actions

The Community programmes cannot attempt to address every health problem and every kind of disease. To be effective Community actions must be properly focused. The

Communication therefore sets out various criteria to be followed in determining priorities. The criteria are:

- a disease's impact on mortality and morbidity
- a disease's socio-economic impact
- how far a disease is amenable to effective preventive action, and, of particular importance
- how far there is scope for Community actions to complement and add value to what is being done by the Member States

Priority areas for Community action programmes

On the basis of this analysis, the Communication proposed eight priority areas for which multi-annual programmes would be developed:

- cancer
- health promotion, education and training
- AIDS and other communicable diseases
- drug dependence
- health monitoring
- rare diseases
- pollution-related disease
- accidents and injuries

The situation today is that five of these programmes have been adopted and are underway.

A set of three programmes was adopted in April 1996:

First, there is the Community action plan to combat cancer, which covers cancer prevention, screening and early detection, training of health professionals and support to research.[2]

Second, the programme on AIDS and other communicable diseases.[3] The aim of this programme is to help contain the spread of HIV and AIDS and reduce morbidity and mortality from other communicable diseases by improving information on the incidence and development of these diseases, identification of situations and behaviour putting people at risk, early detection, and appropriate social and health support.

Third, there is the programme on health promotion, education and training.[4] This covers health promotion strategies and structures, prevention and promotion measures, health information, health education, and training in public health and health promotion.

Early in 1997, Council and Parliament reached agreement on the programme on drug dependence,[5] which includes actions in the area of data collection, studies and evaluation, and on information, health education and training.

A fifth programme, on health monitoring, was agreed by the Council and the European Parliament in June 1997.[6] The aim of this programme is to develop a Community monitoring system in which common health-related indicators can be defined, data can be collected and rapidly exchanged using electronic communications, and a capability for undertaking surveys and examinations can be built up. This will provide a more comprehensive and better validated data basis for both the Community and Member States, and an improved analytical capacity to inform and target policy development and establish priorities in the field of public health at Community level. It will include building up a telematics network between Member States' administrations dealing with health and health-related data.

Proposals for the remaining three programmes, on pollution-related diseases,[7] injury prevention[8] and on rare diseases,[9] have been adopted by the Commission. The proposed programme on pollution-related diseases focuses on prevention of asthma, allergies and other diseases where air pollution may be a causal or precipitating factor. That on injuries includes both accident prevention and prevention of self-inflicted injuries and suicide; and the programme on rare diseases aims inter alia at bringing together knowledge and expertise in the different Member States on particular diseases of low prevalence requiring special joint efforts, improving the information available and supporting patient groups. These proposals are currently being considered by Council and Parliament in the co-decision procedure.

In the context both of the preparations for the enlargement of the Community and the European Economic Area (EEA) agreement, provisions have been put in place to open the public health programmes to allow the participation of EEA and Central and Eastern European countries associated with the Community, as well as Cyprus.

Other public health activities

In addition, a large amount of work has been carried out in areas not directly linked to the specific action programmes proposed in the framework for action.

Communicable diseases

A decision creating a network for the epidemiological surveillance and control of communicable diseases in the European Community was adopted by the European Parliament and Council in July 1998.[10]

Communicable diseases caused by various microbial agents tend to spread through populations and through space, essentially as a result of environmental changes, the movements of people, the movement of goods, and the distribution of drinking water and foodstuffs. The more and faster that people travel, the greater the risk of these diseases spreading in the form of epidemics and, as a corollary, the greater the health risk to populations.

In order to take the measures necessary to block the progression of these diseases or prevent their appearance, national health authorities clearly need to have as precise a picture as possible of the epidemiological situation. This requires effective epidemiological surveillance, with the results being used in order to control and prevent these diseases. Consequently, the networks's aim is to establish a system of close cooperation and effective coordination of routine and emergency surveillance between Member States.

Blood safety and self-sufficiency

The Commission's strategy on blood, first presented in its Communication on Blood Safety and Self-sufficiency in the European Community,[11] aims to improve consumer confidence in the safety of the blood transfusion chain and to promote Community self-sufficiency. It includes the following main activities:

- Development of policies and agreed procedures in the donor selection process.
- Implementation of efficient validated and reliable screening tests.
- Development of quality assessment criteria and good manufacturing practices.
- Development of a haemovigilance system.
- Development of educational programmes on optimal use of blood and blood products.
- Dissemination of information on the blood transfusion system.
- Establishment of basic criteria for inspection and training of inspectors.

Following up its Communication to Council on Blood Safety and Self-sufficiency as well as a number of Council Resolutions on the topic, work has begun on a series of recommendations in this field. The Council has already adopted a recommendation on donor selection and testing of donations, based on a survey to collect information about the current regulations and practices in the Member States.[12]

In addition, a feasibility study for a haemovigilance network has been completed as has a project supported by the Commission on the inspection and accreditation of blood collection establishments.

With regard to self-sufficiency, the objective is directly linked to voluntary unpaid blood and plasma donations which are considered to be safer than those coming from remunerated donors. In an effort to assess the progress being made towards this goal, the Commission, with the cooperation of the Member States, prepares reports on this subject.

Health status

In order to inform and support policy makers, the Commission has decided to publish annual reports on the state of health in the Community. Two reports have so far been published. The first of these presented a general overview of trends in demography, morbidity and mortality in all Member States.[13] Similar general reports will be produced at regular intervals. In between these, the reports will focus on the health status of specific population groups, or on specific health determinants. The second report, published in May 1997, focused on the state of women's health in the Community.[14] The next report is intended to be on health and migration, followed by a report on the state of health of youth in the Community.

Reporting instruments, such as the reports on the state of health, will be developed further and will both feed into the health monitoring programme (see above) and draw on its results and experiences. Further reports, for example providing overviews of trends in health systems, could be developed as complementary tools. In this context, it is important also to draw on Member States' experiences with health reporting.

Integration of health requirements in Community policies

In order to carry out the Treaty obligation that health protection requirements should be part of other Community policies the Commission has taken several initiatives.

First, it has introduced measures to ensure that the Commission services in charge of public health are consulted on all health-related proposals before they are presented to the College of Commissioners.

Second, an Inter-service Group on Health was created which provides a forum to exchange information and discuss major health-related issues among Commission DGs. In addition, this group provides contact persons for health-related questions in all Commission services.

Third, the Commission has prepared annual reports on the integration of health requirements in Community policies which describe how health considerations have been taken account in different areas of Community policy. Three reports have already been presented to the Community Institutions.[15] The Fourth report, covering activities in 1997, is currently under preparation.

Although the Commission has thus taken several measures in this area, the development of a comprehensive strategy for the implementation of this Treaty obligation has not proved easy. For one thing defining health protection requirements and determining what constitutes a high level of health protection is not straightforward. Nor is it obvious what is the best methodology to use. The programme on health monitoring will provide an opportunity to refine the methodologies further.

Through its involvement with proposals and policies originating in other Commission services, the Commission services in charge of public health are following and contributing to policy areas as diverse as food law, research, transport policy, pharmaceuticals, and development aid, without of course being able to follow all possibly relevant policy proposals in depth.

Additional activities

A number of projects relating to the development of health systems have been undertaken, and others are under preparation. They serve to support cooperation with Member States and inform policy development. They concern areas such as:

- common problems and choices faced by Member States,
- cost containment measures taken by Member States,
- public health priorities and priority-making systems,
- public attitudes to health, their concerns and priorities and views of the effectiveness of health systems, and
- health technology assessment.

A further area of activity is non-ionising radiation, where a comprehensive review and a feasibility study have been presented and proposals for Council recommendations are being prepared.

Future possibilities

Public health has recently become a very high profile political issue in the EU, not least because of the BSE/CJD crisis. This part of the chapter gives an overview of the main political issues of relevance for future developments.

Current issues and new challenges

New challenges are constantly emerging and indeed it was already envisaged in 1993 that the framework for action in the field of public health and the action programmes proposed would need to be reviewed in the light of experience.

Since the communication was adopted a number of issues have been growing in importance and these are likely to have major consequences for health policy at the Community level. These include :

- changes to the legal basis for public health
- enlargement of the EU
- the growing recognition that socio-economic inequality is an important factor in differences in health
- emergence of new communicable diseases (Ebola, BSE/CJD) and resurgence of old ones (TB) and development of microbial resistance to existing drugs
- pressures on health systems from, for example, socio-economic and demographic factors, such as ageing populations, and the costs of introducing new technology
- similar responses being made by Member States to their problems (cost containment, health reforms and signs of greater willingness to work together in tackling

common problems e.g. the recent agreement on tobacco advertising which had previously been stalled for a long time).

These factors have been accompanied by rising public interest, deep concern over the impact of technology (GMOs, etc.) and about the effects of other policies on health and heightened expectations about Community actions on health.

In view of these developments and of the fact that the existing public health programmes will come to an end soon after the turn of the century, it will be necessary for the Community to formulate a Community strategy for public health beyond 2000.

This requires developing a policy with clear priorities and concrete actions which takes full account of

- the new challenges to be met, as outlined briefly above
- the changes to the legal base introduced at Amsterdam, (see below) and
- an evaluation of the effectiveness of the existing framework and the action programmes that have been undertaken.

New legal basis

The Amsterdam Treaty includes a substantial revision of Article 129 (Article 152 in the new Treaty) which sets out the Community's public health competence (see Box over leaf). This revision will have a major impact on the scope and content of future public health activities and priorities. The consequences of the new wording therefore need to be very carefully considered. The following paragraphs describe the most important changes introduced.

The provisions regarding health in other policies have been widened. A high level of human health protection is to be ensured in the definition and implementation of all Community policies and activities. This amounts to a strengthening of the original wording particularly since it implies that Community policies and activities should aim at achieving a high level of health protection, rather than saying that health protection requirements should be a constituent part of other Community policies, which may well be interpreted as requiring merely that policies should not have a negative effect on health. Moreover the new wording refers not only to legislation, but also to proposals for policy and to their implementation (which is, of course, largely an obligation on Member States).

Another significant change is to broaden the aim of Community action so that it now includes not just preventing human illness and diseases, but also improving public health, and obviating sources of danger to human health. Moreover, action against 'the major health scourges' ceases to be the main focus of Community activities in this field, as now. It is simply to be 'covered' by actions.

Paragraph 4 of the new Article refers to actions the Community can undertake on the basis of this Article. Two additions are made:

AMENDED VERSION OF Article 129 (ARTICLE 152)

1. A high level of human health protection shall be ensured in the definition and implementation of all Community policies and activities.

Community action, which shall complement national policies, shall be directed towards improving public health, preventing human illness and diseases, and obviating sources of danger to human health. Such action shall cover the fight against the major health scourges, by promoting research into their causes, their transmission and their prevention, as well as health information and education.

The Community shall complement the Member States' action in reducing drugs related health damage, including information and prevention.

2. The Community shall encourage cooperation between the Member States in the areas referred to in this Article and, if necessary, lend support to their action.

Member States shall, in liaison with the Commission, coordinate among themselves their policies and programmes in the areas referred to in paragraph 1. The Commission may, in close contact with the Member States, take any useful initiative to promote such coordination.

3. The Community and the Member States shall foster cooperation with third countries and the competent international organisations in the sphere of public health.

4. The Council, acting in accordance with the procedure referred to in Article 189b and after consulting the Economic and Social Committee and the Committee of the Regions, shall contribute to the achievement of the objectives referred to in this Article through adopting:

(a) measures setting high standards of quality and safety of organs and substances of human origin, blood and blood derivatives; these measures shall not prevent any Member State from maintaining or introducing more stringent protective measures;

(b) by way of derogation from Article 43, measures in the veterinary and phytosanitary fields which have as their direct objective the protection of public health;

(c) incentive measures designed to protect and improve human health, excluding any harmonisation of the laws and regulations of the Member States.

The Council, acting by a qualified majority on a proposal from the Commission, may also adopt recommendations for the purposes set out in this Article.

5. Community action in the field of public health shall fully respect the responsibilities of the Member States for the organisation and delivery of health services and medical care. In particular, measures referred to in paragraph 4(a) shall not affect national provisions on the donation or medical use of organs and blood.

4(a) says the Community can adopt 'measures setting high standards of quality and safety of organs and substances of human origin, blood and blood derivatives'. The following paragraph clarifies that this excludes 'measures...(which) affect national provisions on the donation or medical use of organs and blood'. Subparagraph 4(b) brings into the scope of this Article (and therefore the co-decision procedure) 'measures in the veterinary and phytosanitary fields which have as their direct objective the protection of public health'. This follows the Parliament's wish, which originated in the context of the BSE crisis, to be involved in these fields.

The revised Article 129 has introduced a number of specific and potentially important changes which should enable the Community to make some progress on a number of public health issues, such as forging closer links between health and other areas of policy.

The development of the Community's public health policy

In response to these developments and the challenges the Community and Member States have to face in the health field, the Commission has recently put forward a Communication on the development of public health policy in the European Community.[16] The communication does not present any formal proposals for implementing the Community's public health policy since this would not have been possible before the Amsterdam Treaty came into force. It nevertheless represents a significant step towards a reorientation of the Community's activities in this field. Indeed the communication's main conclusion is that 'in order to build on what has been achieved, while taking proper account of the trends in health and the changing situation in the Community, a new public health policy is required'.

The Commission intends to develop public health policy based on three strands of action, and two horizontal tasks:

- **Improving information for the development of public health,** through the development of a comprehensive Community system for collecting, analysing and disseminating information, focusing on trends in health status and health determinants and on developments in health systems. The rationale behind this proposed activity is that while health systems of the Member States are distinct, they all face common problems, in particular how to contain costs while ensuring high quality health services. There is a huge potential to exchange ideas about how to address these problems and pass on information about those approaches that have worked. Activities would be developed largely on the basis of experiences gained in the health monitoring programme and related activities.

- **Reacting rapidly to threats to health,** by means of a Community surveillance, early warning and rapid reaction capability. At present, there is no effective Community mechanism to deal comprehensively with emerging health threats. Work would build on the European Community network for the epidemiological surveillance and control of communicable diseases, and the proposed programme on rare diseases. In addition it would also link up with, and take into account, those Community early warning and rapid reaction systems which are already in place.

- **Tackling health determinants** through health promotion and disease prevention. The Commission has acquired a great deal of experience from the existing Community programmes in these fields. The intention is to build upon this experience. About 600,000 deaths in the EU each year are premature and a large number of these are avoidable. Some are due to unhealthy environments, and thus issues such as pollution, living conditions and inequalities have to be tackled. In addition, people sometimes contribute to their own ill health through poor diet and unhealthy lifestyles. Actions will be developed on the basis of the existing disease prevention and health promotion programmes, but the future approach will try to bring together disease prevention and health promotion. The Commission also intends to give more weight to large-scale sustainable initiatives that support the development and implementation of policy.

Moreover, in all three strands proposed, it is intended to undertake work on two horizontal areas of activity:

- Integrating health requirements in other Community policies, as the new Treaty Article stresses this provision, it will be necessary to review whether more needs to be done to ensure that all Community policies contribute to ensuring a high level of health protection. Although, as outlined above, there are serious methodological questions to be overcome, it should not be forgotten that this kind of activity also raises sensitive political issues which will need to be addressed.

- The health impact of enlargement, which will be important both for health status and health systems, in existing Member States as well as in accession countries. There are a number of challenges in this context. These include issues related to communicable diseases, food safety, medicinal products and blood, and the free movement of health professionals. The opening of the Community towards Central and Eastern Europe will thus force the Community to adapt its public health strategy in response to new needs and requirements.

All in all, the Commission communication represents a significant step in the short history of public health activities in the Community. It is an attempt to set out the elements of a new 'public health policy' which amounts in effect to a movement away from an approach based on a series of separate action programmes, largely disease-oriented, to a more structured approach linked to clearer policy objectives and considerations. The Commission's intention is to present concrete proposals and the necessary legal instrument(s) once the Treaty of Amsterdam has been ratified. These will take into account the response to the communication.

Conclusion

This is a particularly significant period in the development of public health activities and policy by the European Community. The Community has always had an involvement in this field and in a range of policy areas with implications for health. But it was only with the coming into effect of the Maastricht Treaty that it had the necessary legal base to develop a coherent public health policy. Now with the increasing emphasis being put on public health issues in the Community, arising in part from the BSE crisis, and the widened provisions set out in the new Treaty, there is a good opportunity for the Community to develop its work in this field and to improve its effectiveness. But progress will be made only if the Community shows itself willing to be proactive, to set the most relevant goals and objectives, to identify priorities, to evaluate activities objectively and to strengthen existing capabilities, methods and information systems.

The Commission's communication on the development of public health policy has launched a debate on how the Community could move forward in this area which is of great concern to citizens and policymakers. The next years will be crucial and it remains to be seen how the Community will respond to this challenge.

References

1. COM (Official Commission document) (93) 559 final of 24.11.1993.
2. *OJ (Official Journal of the European Communities)* L 95,16.4.1996, p. 9.
3. *OJ* L 95, 16.4.1996, p. 16.
4. *OJ* L 95, 16.4.1996, p. 1.
5. *OJ* L 19, 22.1.1997, 25.
6. *OJ* L 193, 22.7.1997, p. 1.
7. COM (97) 266 final of 4.6.1997.
8. COM (97) 178 final of 14.5.1997.
9. COM (97) 225 final of 26.5.1997.
10. *OJ* L 268, 3.10.98, p.1.
11. COM(94) 652 final of 21.12.1994.
12. *OJ* L 203/14 of 21.7.1998.
13. COM (95) 357 final of 19.7.1995.
14. COM (97) 224 final of 22.5.1997.
15. COM (95) 196 final of 29.5.1995, COM (96) 407 final of 4.9.1996 and COM (98) 34 final of 27.1.1998, COM (98) 34 final of 27.1.1998.
16. COM (98) 230 final of 15.4.1998.

ANNEX

Health policy involvement of Commission Directorates-General

DGs I, IA, IB
External relations   Cooperation with third countries in the field of health (many health-related projects are covered in the context of the Community's development aid, and its support for Central and Eastern European countries)

DG III
Industry   Free movement of products: e.g. Pharmaceuticals (including responsibility for the European Medicines Evaluation Agency, London), Medical devices, Food law, cosmetics, etc.

DG V
Social policy   European social funds: actions to combat unemployment, social security/health insurance, disability, poverty, etc. – Health and safety at work, public health

DG VI
Agriculture   Veterinary public health, plant health, specific products: fruit and vegetables, tobacco, milk, alcohol

DG VII
Transport   Transport of dangerous goods, safety of cars, planes and ferries, access to public transport

DG VIII
Development   Cooperation with ACP countries in the field of health (many health-related projects are covered in the context of the Community's development aid)

DG IX
Personnel   Health of Commission staff

DG X
Information   General information activities of the Community, responsibility for sports

DG XI
Environment   Radiation protection, water safety, safety of chemicals, environmental impact assessments

DG XII
Research   Fourth Framework programme: Programmes including BIOMED
                         (Biology and Medicine, including public health), BIOTECH
                         (Biotechnology), Agricultural research (including food safety),
                         Environment and climate research. A new Framework
                         programme is being prepared for 1999 onwards

DG XIII
Telematics   Telematics in the health sector, e.g. telemedicine, electronic
application   health data networks, etc.

DG XIV
Fisheries   Community fisheries policy, including safety issues

DG XV
Internal market   Free movement of professions and services: recognition of diplo-
                         mas, advertising, etc.

DG XVI
Regional policy   Regional funds and cohesion funds, which can also support
                         health-related projects

DG XVII
Energy policy   Environmental and health effects of production and use of energy

DG XXI
Taxation   Taxes on certain products relevant to health (e.g. tobacco,
                         alcohol)

DG XXII
Education,   Programmes in this field include a specific focus on health
training and youth   (e.g. AIDS, drugs, etc.)

XXIV
Consumer   Consumer policy, Scientific committees related to health
protection   protection, Veterinary inspection services

Eurostat
Statistical offices   Health statistics, Community household surveys, etc.

ECHO
Emergency aid   Emergency aid in disasters

Notes: names of Directorates-General (DGs) have been abbreviated. The table shows
examples, and not necessarily all, health-related activities of the respective DGs.

Further details are given in the Commission's reports on the integration of health protection requirements in Community policies.

3

Public Health and Health Policy in Belgium

Marie-Christine Closon, David Crainich and
Nathalie Swartenbroek

Introduction

The state of health of the Belgian population can be considered to be relatively good if one refers to common public health indicators. However, life expectancy and infant mortality rates, though better than those of many countries, are not among the best in the European Community.

In 1996 life expectancy for men at birth was 73.1 years (which is lower than Italy, Spain, Netherlands and United Kingdom but higher than France, Germany and Ireland). Life expectancy of women at birth was 79.8 years (which is higher than Germany, Ireland, and the UK, but lower than France, Italy, Netherlands and Spain), see Table 1 overleaf. The infant mortality rates per 100,000 live births were 993.1 and 796.6 for males and females respectively. These are largely below those of the United Kingdom (737.9 for males and 574.5 for females), Germany (769.5 for males and 602.1 for females) of France (832.9 for males and 603.5 for females) and Ireland (854.7 for males and 657.4 for females).[1]

The funds allocated to the health sector have been increasing in Belgium. According to Poullier, health expenditure amounted to 3.4 per cent of total domestic expenditure in 1960, 5.9 per cent in 1975 and 8.0 per cent in 1996.[2]

However, the strict cost containment measures within the compulsory health insurance scheme, combined with the Belgian government's difficulties in managing its public deficit, make it difficult to allocate more funds to the health sector. Moreover, the ageing of the population may be 'the most important single cause of increasing need for health care'.[3]

Table 1
Life expectancy at birth in eight countries of the European Union

Country	All	Men	Women
Belgium	77.9	73.1	79.8
France	78.8	73.0	80.8
Germany	76.7	72.7	79.0
Ireland	76.6	72.6	78.1
Italy	78.3	74.2	80.6
Netherlands	77.9	74.4	80.4
Spain	78.0	74.6	80.5
United Kingdom	77.1	73.6	78.7

Source: WHO. World Health Statistics Annual,1996.[1]

To tackle these issues, decision-makers have introduced progressive but profound reforms in the Belgian health care system since the 1980s.[4] Overall, stakeholders are required to assume a growing financial responsibility as mechanisms based more on diseases, case-mix and share of risks replace the old financial mechanisms based on the simple reimbursement of costs or medical treatment. The new orientation in the financing of hospitals, the increase of patient cost-sharing and the financial responsibility of the sickness funds* reflect some of the recent changes. Another trend is a reduction in health care supply (such as decreases in the numbers of beds and doctors). The aim is to reduce supplier-induced demand for health care. In all cases there are attempts to match health care supply with the needs of the population. The evaluation of health policy and medical practice within the context of cost control and with the aim of reinforcing efficiency and quality of care, but without prejudicial effect, has now been given greater priority. Thus, with increasing budgetary restrictions, priority setting is ever more essential in public health and health policy. However, the management and the structure of the Belgian health system have not been formally organised around a precise definition of priorities. This may be a challenge for the future.

The framework of public health policy

The distribution of competencies

The way in which policies in prevention and health promotion are established is related closely to the political structure of the country. The structure is very decentralised and as a consequence health policy decisions are made at various levels. Figure 1 outlines

---

* *The sickness insurance funds are called 'Mutualities'. These private, not-for-profit societies have a special function in Belgium as they act – for historical reasons – as defenders of the patients' rights.*

the framework for responsibility in public health and decision-making. There are three levels of political responsibility that are organised between various institutions around two concepts: territory and language.

The three regions (Flanders, Wallonia and Brussels) are responsible for matters related to citizens living in those areas (mainly housing and the environment including water,

Figure 1
Public health related responsibilities and decision-making

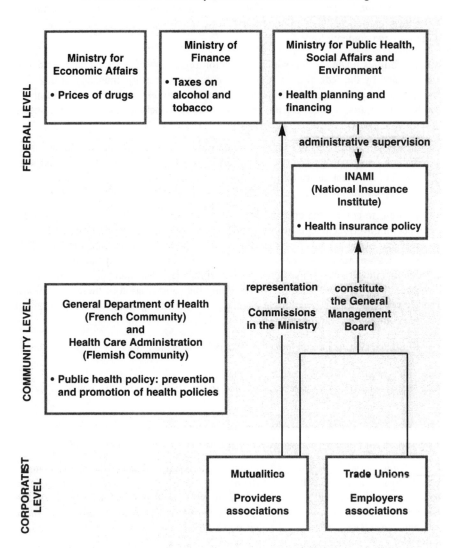

energy, pollution and forests). 'Regional' health is mainly focused on environmental policies (pollution, noise, treatment of waste material).* Regions are also responsible for health institutions, such as centres for mental care, family planning, medical centres, and elderly rest homes.

The three communities (the French-speaking community, the Dutch-speaking community and the German-speaking community) are responsible for matters related to citizens speaking the same language (including cultural affairs, education, and public health). The communities have all the competencies in health matters except those specified in the *'Loi Spéciale'*. They are responsible for developing prevention, health promotion and education policies (excluding tertiary prevention: physical readjustment and rehabilitation) and epidemiology.

Responsibilities related to the whole population regardless of language and residence are assumed by the federal government (justice, social security, monetary policy, and national defence). Federal health matters, which are the responsibility of the Ministry for Social Affairs, Public Health and Environment, include all the competencies described in the *'Loi Spéciale'*. These are:

- Supervision of financing (which is organised by trade unions and employers associations) and management (which is left to sickness funds and providers associations) of the compulsory health insurance which covers almost all the curative care and represents the major part of the funds allocated to the health care system;

- In order to control the cost of health care insurance, the *'Loi Spéciale'* gives the Federal government legislative power concerning hospitals, psychiatric care homes, rest and nursing homes, centres for mental health and home care services. This includes – as far as they have an impact on health insurance expenditure – criteria for planning (for example, university hospital beds and number of institutions), price fixing and the basic rules concerning the subsidisation of these institutions. However, the execution of these planning criteria is delegated to the regions (and to the communities for the university hospitals);

- Compulsory vaccination policies (the polio vaccination is the only one designated).**

Moreover, some fields that are not included in the *'Loi Spéciale'* are managed by the

---

* *Excluding radioactivity monitoring which is dealt with at the federal level.*

** *It should be noted that a draft agreement has been reached between the Federal government and the Communities concerning the hepatitis B vaccination. It specifies that this programme will be implemented by the Communities and financed by the federal government, despite the fact that vaccination against hepatitis B is not defined as compulsory. The Federal government expects future savings for the health care insurance. However, the legality of such an agreement may be questioned.*

Federal government, both in terms of policy-making and implementation. These include:

- Product standards (for example, food and pharmaceutical products)
- Radioactivity
- Professional norms and standards for those working in the health care sector
- Pharmaceutical policy
- Emergency services policy
- Blood policy

Developing a health policy

The difficulty in establishing a comprehensive health policy framework in Belgium stems from the fact that any proposal must be unanimously accepted by the various Ministers involved.*

Health policy developments in Belgium are initiated by the Ministry for Social Affairs, Public Health and Environment while the insurance policy is administered by the National Insurance Institute for Sickness and Work Disability (INAMI). This body is composed of representatives of employers, trade unions, sickness funds and health care providers. It is responsible for the management and financial administration of health care insurance. The INAMI is the most direct way through which these various stakeholders exercise their influence on the Belgian health care system. Moreover, they also use the consultative function of the INAMI within various Committees of the Ministry for Social Affairs, Public Health and Environment. The INAMI cannot, however, take the lead in any policy, including health policy, outside the area of financing as its power is restricted to defining which services or interventions are to be reimbursed. The Ministry for Social Affairs, Public Health and the Environment has the legal power to propose measures in order to protect the rights of patients.**

The power of the INAMI within the Belgian health care organisation is significant in terms of the resources it manages in health care insurance. That is why INAMI has tried to play a greater role beyond its field of competence.

---

* *A recent example concerns the new emergency services policy. The administration of the Ministry for Social Affairs, Public Health and the Environment had to notify policy proposals to three Ministries. A veto by one of them would have blocked policy developments.*

** *The Ministry for Social Affairs, Public Health and the Environment makes, for example, strict rules concerning access to the profession for health providers. This is the case for specialised physicians whose access to the profession is restricted by the fact that the number of places available annually is determined by the Ministry for Social Affairs, Public Health and the Environment.*

The following new policies have been introduced recently to reinforce the role of the Ministry of Public Health in health policy:

- New orientation of financing based more on real needs rather than on the existing structures.

- Promotion of alternatives to in-patient care.

- Creation of a more defined status for emergency services, intensive care, neonatal care, units for terminally ill, pharmaceutical policy etc.

- Reinforcing the importance of evaluation and quality of care.

- Control of medical supply.

- Possibility of establishing criteria for good medical practice.

In addition, the Ministry for Social Affairs, Public Health and Environment will present a report with its health policy priorities.

Better integration between insurance policies and health policies is necessary. This integration is expected to be achieved through the creation of the so-called 'multipartite' which brings together all the actors (including sickness funds, trade unions and doctors) involved in the sector to define policy priorities. Financing and priority setting will be considered simultaneously. This also facilitates a more global approach to the problems and favours consultation and exchange of data between the Ministry for Social Affairs, Public Health and Environment, and the INAMI. Although this 'multipartite' is only an intermediate body in the policy-making process, it may play an important role in the future. The most recent proposals concern hospital policy, emergency services policy and blood policy. The 1998 report on health policy of the Ministry for Social Affairs, Public Health and Environment defines the general orientation of health policy in Belgium. It outlines clearly the public health priorities:

- *Health protection:* greater control regarding food production and sale, veterinary checks (in order to better detect the presence of growth stimulants in meat) and the production of pharmaceuticals.

- *Environment:* concrete measures have been/will be implemented regarding:

  Ozone (measures to reduce emissions of fumes in petrol, promotion of railway transport and public transportation and an information campaign to increase people's awareness of the issue).

  Dioxins (stronger policy regarding the incineration of household waste which is the main source of dioxins in the environment, and fixing the maximum level in food).

  Benzene in fuel (limits on lead content in petrol).

- *Tobacco:* reducing advertising, protecting non-smokers, banning misleading presentations ('light' cigarettes, for example), banning sales of packs which are mainly bought by the young i.e. those with less than 20 cigarettes.

- *Drugs:* a legal basis to efficiently organise the exchange of syringes has been approved.

- *Specific policies:* Important financial support for scientific research into diabetes, specific training for medical staff dealing with babies to prevent cot death, promotion of feeding, and an action plan against flu to improve detection and prevent transmission.

The section of the 1998 report concerning social integration takes stock of the policy situation concerning disabled persons, needy persons and refugees. Measures have been implemented to improve these groups' social situation, including their health.

Public health in Belgium

Characteristics of the Belgian health care system

The main features of the Belgian health care system are the following:

Health system funding: Total health care expenditure in Belgium in 1994 is estimated at BEF 630 billion, slightly more than 8 per cent of GNP.[5] Social security contributions make up 36 per cent of the finance for these expenditures whereas 38 per cent of the expenditure is met out of general taxation. Out-of-pocket expenditure (co-payments) accounts for 17 per cent and a further 9 per cent is raised from other sources (mainly complementary health insurance and indirect taxes). This system ensures a high level of solidarity between different socioeconomic classes and between the sick and the healthy.

Coverage and cost sharing: Compulsory health insurance covers almost the entire Belgian population (although the self-employed who represent 15 per cent of this population are only covered for major risks). Patients have to share the cost of the service through co-insurance ('ticket moderateur'). For a typical home visit they pay a co-payment of 35 per cent (the co-payment for widows, disabled, old-age pensioners and orphans with an annual gross income below a certain threshold is 8 per cent). The co-payment rates were substantially increased in October 1993 and January 1994 and social and fiscal exemptions were also introduced. Patients are exempt from co-payments once the sum of the latter exceeds a certain annual amount that is related to income.

About 2,500 medicines (of a total of between 5,500 and 6,000 available in Belgium) are reimbursed by the health insurance. The proportion of the cost reimbursed depends on the therapeutic value of the medicines, which are divided into six categories. A patient who utilises health services but who does not belong to the health insurance scheme can appeal to the Public Centres for Social Help ('Centre Public d'aide sociale' CPAS) for financial assistance.

Availability of health care services: Belgian health care delivery is mainly private and based on independent medical practice or 'medecine liberale'.[6] Ambulatory care is dominated by sole practitioners working as self-employed physicians, dentists and pharmacists. Patients can choose their providers freely (general practitioners, specialists and hospitals). Access to secondary care is direct. Belgium has one the highest physician/population ratio in the industrialised world (the average number of patients was 555 per general practitioner and 598 per specialist in 1997).[7]

Partly because the physician/population ratio is high, ambulatory medical care is highly competitive and doctors seem to be very responsive to patients.[8] There are no waiting lists. In Belgium 60 per cent of beds belong to private not-for-profit hospitals while the remaining 40 per cent belong to public hospitals often serving towns or districts ('inter-communales'). Hospitals are usually required to accept every patient and to recover the reimbursement bill for patients not possessing health care insurance from the CPAS of the town where they reside.[9]

Quality of care: WHO Europe's Health for All targets have been endorsed by succes-sive Ministers of Health. In practice, the Law on hospitals requires the evaluation of quality of care and makes the medical director responsible for its implementation. It gives the Council of Doctors overall responsibility to see that it is carried out. In addi-tion, in general practice a medical record scheme has been developed, with targets for improved quality of care. The financing system provides incentives for efficiency in health care as it is based on the function of the hospital, its needs and its performance rather than – as it was before – financing based only on medical treatment provided and costs incurred. The difficulty of assessing medical care made necessary the creation of evaluation committees to consider the medical care provided within each hospital while taking into account the quality of care, in order to remove negative effects on the patient's health that may be induced by the financing system. The committees are charged with evaluating new technologies and the process of care according to the objectives of quality and efficiency.*

The accreditation formula also has better quality of care as a target. The basic idea behind the accreditation system (proposed in 1994 and implemented from 1st July 1995) is the selection of the best health care at the lowest cost, by encouraging doctors to prescribe cost effectively. Accreditation is granted to doctors satisfying certain quality requirements. In practice, doctors seeking accreditation must establish good communi-cation with other health care providers, prepare a medical brief for each patient treated, participate in an adult continuing education course (20 hours/year including health economics and ethics courses), not abuse prescribing and therapeutic responsibilities, and see a sufficient number of patients.** Both fee-for-services and the patient reim-bursement rates are higher for a consultation with an accredited doctor so that financial incentives are given to prescribe (for the physician) and to use (for the patient) better quality health care services.

---

* *The location and membership of these committees have not yet been established.*

** *The Ministry for Public Health has defined a minimum target of 1250 contacts with patients as being sufficient. An exception has been made for new doctors (i.e. who have practised for less than three years).*

Health knowledge of patients: There is no health education in primary school programmes and although some associations deal with this issue, it seems that the level of knowledge of the population in health matters is still quite poor.

Prevention and health promotion policies

Public health research

The collection of data related to health and epidemiological research is the starting point for developing a public health policy. According to Detels and Breslow,[10] 'Effective intervention in factors affecting community health depends upon reliable knowledge concerning the occurrence and distribution of these factors, as well as health, in the community'. Thus the backbone of public health strategy is the development and the maintenance of accurate and reliable health information systems upon which rational action can be based. In Belgium, medical data related to stays in acute hospitals must be submitted to the Ministry for Social Affairs, Public Health and Environment. Thus, the Ministry has access to data to develop further policies in this sector. The communities are also obliged to collect data in order to develop a database related to demographic statistics and communicable diseases. Once this information is gathered and classified, it is subject to statistical analysis at two levels:

- at the Federal level the National Institute of statistics INS ('Institut National Statistiques') analyses data collected by the communities.

- at the Community level the data is analysed by the Institute of Hygiene and Epidemiology (IHE).

The main scientific activities in public health are conducted through the IHE, which has the status of 'State Scientific Establishment'. The IHE facilitates the public authorities in terms of scientific research or technical analysis and the decision-making centres define their priorities in term of public health on the basis of research conducted by this institution. The financing and administration of the Institute is carried out by the federal state, the regions and the communities. A co-management Committee (composed of representatives of the federal, community and regional ministries dealing with health and environment) selects the programmes which are to be financed. The main activities of the IHE are:

- The monitoring of the changing effects of some determinants of health. The IHE deals with the monitoring of air pollution and the monitoring of radioactivity in the air, the water and the food chain, etc.

- The epidemiological monitoring, which includes the control of general morbidity.

- Regulating the composition of foodstuffs, vaccines, and some consumer goods such as toys, cosmetics, glues, cleaning products, etc.

- The evaluation of the quality of results obtained by laboratories and application of 'good laboratory practice' (GLP) within the framework of international legislation (OECD and European Union).

The role of research-based evidence is important. There has been an increase in research projects dealing with development strategies in the last 10 years in Belgium. Research projects are carefully allocated to Universities of each political tendency (catholic/non-catholic) and of each language (French/Dutch speaking). In this way, the government can have a broad perception of possible issues and of possible measures to deal with them. National projects are funded by:

(i) the SPPS ('Service de Programmation de la Politique Scientifique') finances projects dealing with incentive programmes in health informatics, health economics and social indicators;

(ii) the Ministry for Social Affairs, Public Health and Environment is currently developing standards in processing information (minimum data set for clinical and nursing procedures, input controls, feed back, classification systems) and to deal with a number of specific issues (expensive medicines, quality of care indicators, role of financial incentives on providers practices).

Public health intervention

Effective intervention is the heart of public health efforts to protect communities from health hazards. These efforts include reducing the numbers of individuals susceptible to infectious and chronic diseases, treating people early in the course of disease, modifying the environment and promoting healthy behaviour of both communities and individuals.[10]

A number of decisions directly related to public health are made by the federal government, which controls most resources devoted to health care. This is the case with the price of medical services (ambulatory care, in-patient care etc.) and with medicines that are established after negotiation between sickness funds and representatives of medical associations (for medical services) and between sickness funds and the pharmaceutical industry (for medicines). However, in both cases these decisions have to be approved by the government.

Taxes on alcohol and cigarettes (which aim to reduce their consumption) are also decided at federal level. In theory the revenue from these taxes should be devoted to some aspects of preventive care. In practice, it goes into the budget of the INAMI and finances the reimbursement of curative health services.

As it is known that there is a risk of lung cancer from passive smoking, legislation in this area is important for public health but the Royal Decree of 26 May 1993 is vague. It states only that employers have to take the necessary measures in order to establish the right conditions for tobacco use, while taking into account the expectations of both smokers and non-smokers. These measures are required to be based on reciprocal tolerance respecting individual freedom and on courtesy. In January 1997 the Belgian parliament passed a new law to introduce a total ban on tobacco advertising and sponsorship. This decision followed concern over the increasing number of young smokers. As well as banning tobacco advertising the new law will also cover the use of tobacco brand names to sell non-tobacco products.

As public health concerns all citizens, the communities are given the responsibility of dealing with public health policy in Belgium. The following section briefly deals with the implementation of public health policies in the French-speaking and Dutch-speaking communities.

The French-speaking community of Belgium and the Walloon region The competencies of the Walloon region are related to housing and the environment. Currently, these include public health activities such as the financing and regulation of detoxification centres, family planning clinics, mental health centres, and geriatric centres. The region is responsible for regulating hospitals. The Walloon region is also in charge of defining and implementing policies for disabled people.

The responsibilities of the French region are as follows:

All the competencies in Public Health are administered by the General Department of Health (Direction Generale de la Santé) within the Ministry of Culture and Social Affairs. The only exceptions are matters dealt with by the National Office for Childbirth and Infancy ('Office de la Naissance et de l'Enfance', ONE), the Agency for the Prevention of Aids ('Agence de prevention du SIDA') and by the Royal Academy of Medicine.

* The General Department of Health has competence in the schools of medicine, the prevention of communicable diseases and health education.

* The National Office for Childbirth and Infancy* is responsible of the child policy. This institution is a public interest which is supervised by the Ministry of Culture and Social Affairs of the French Community of Belgium.

* The Agency for the Prevention of AIDS is required to set up an action plan to fight against AIDS and has to submit proposals on budget provisions for actions it will undertake itself or through numerous associations – some of them having been created and managed by patient groups.

* The Royal Belgian Academy of Medicine** promotes scientific and medical research by funding awards, organising scientific conferences and other related activities.

---

* The National Office for Childbirth and Infancy is an inter-community organisation. Child policy is organised by the 'Office de la Naissance et de l'Enfance' in the French-speaking Community and by the 'Kind en Gezin' in the Flemish Community.

** The Royal Belgian Academy of Medicine is a National institution and collaborates with each Community.

The French-speaking Community implements its policy in various ways including:

- Sponsorship of local coordination centres that centralise every project submitted by non-profit organisations. There are ten local coordination centres in the French Community. They are charged with gathering information from the population particularly about needs. Non-profit organisations working in the area can contact these centres to get information for their particular project.

- Funding particular projects.

- Management of several institutions including the schools' medical check-up centres where the compulsory medical examinations of pupils are made.

- Vaccination programmes in collaboration with the ONE (an independent institution funded by the Community).

- Introduction of decrees on subjects such as non-smoking areas, etc.

The priorities are set on the basis of epidemiological studies conducted by the IHE. In particular, the Centre for Operational Research in Public Health ('Centre de Recherche Operationnelle en Sante Publique', CROSP) processes public health information and may suggest policy recommendations.

Priorities are also based on surveys conducted to evaluate the overall health status of the population. The interviews cover all aspects related to the health status of the population including the general quality of life. A new project with the participation of the population was introduced in January 1997. Five thousand families will be interviewed about their health, their way of life, their socioeconomic environment, their consumption of medical services, etc. The objective of this research is to use the information collected to find the relationship between way of life, health determinants, and welfare and health care consumption. Federal government and the Communities will work together on this project.

In terms of prevention policy, cancer and cardiovascular diseases are the main focus. Health education among young people is a main priority of the Community since it is one of the most effective ways of promoting health among the population.

The main preventive services and educational programmes that have been organised concern:

- Immunisation services. Mandatory childhood immunisation (controlled by ONE) including poliomyelitis (compulsory) and diphtheria, pertussis, tetanus (highly recommended). 92.8 per cent of the population was vaccinated against poliomyelitis in 1991 (whilst 98.1 per cent was vaccinated in 1989). 94.2 per cent of the population received three doses against Diphtheria Pertussis Tetanus in 1991 and 68.4 per cent received four doses. This mandatory immunisation is provided free of charge by the ONE and given by paediatricians or General Practitioners. They receive no positive financial incentives to undertake these vaccinations but are assessed financial penalties (fines) in cases of non-immunisation. A vaccination programme (PROVAC) is conducted in collaboration with the ONE. This programme covers non-compulsory vaccinations for measles, rubella and mumps and is also starting to promote hepatitis B and meningitis vaccinations.

- The fight against respiratory infections. The Community is strongly involved in the prevention of tuberculosis through the Foundation for Respiratory Conditions and Health Education ('Fondation pour les Affections Respiratoires et l'Éducation a la Santé', FARES) Programme. Radiological examinations are focused on high-risk individuals. Statistical data concerning the evolution of the disease is collected by the FARES.

- Childhood policy. This is conducted by the ONE, which is allocated a large part of the Community health budget. ONE provides antenatal services and consultations for children. It regulates and finances day nurseries. It is also involved in preventing child abuse.

- School health programmes. The French-speaking community funds the authorities which organise medical inspection teams for schools. The Schools Medical Inspection comprises the following:[11]

  (i) For pupils, the detection of psychological or mental problems, the detection of communicable diseases, and the supervision of the vaccination programme,

  (ii) For members of staff, the detection of sources of infection,

  (iii) For pupils and members of staff, preventive measures which are necessary to avoid the spread of contagious diseases.

- Screening programmes: The early detection of cancer is organised by the university anti-cancer centres and the provincial anti-cancer centres which are sponsored by the community in order to undertake their primary prevention activity. The screening programmes undertaken in Belgium are those whose usefulness is proven and recognised. That is why the anti-cancer centres deal with breast cancer in the French-speaking community.

- School health services: The community organises a school health programme, in collaboration with the ONE. It includes screening (detection of physical or mental deficiencies, transmissible diseases etc.), collection of morbidity statistics and health education programmes (on a trial basis).

- AIDS: AIDS prevention is coordinated by the agency for the prevention of AIDS (discussed earlier).

- Cigarette consumption: The community has introduced decrees on non smoking areas. The cigarette consumption policy is partly conducted by the FARES, but local initiatives are not coordinated.

- Health needs of ethnic minority populations: Health education programmes for ethnic minority populations are generally local initiatives. They are partly coordinated by the community.

The Flemish-speaking community   The Flemish community comprises the Flanders region and the Dutch-speaking community and these two communities are merged to constitute one single administrative body. The health care administration which is included within the Ministry for Health Care, Welfare and Culture is responsible for the preparation, evaluation and the implementation of the policies. Two sub-sectors of the health care administration of the Flemish community are particularly concerned with public health.

- The Royal Medical Academy of Belgium ('Konninklijke Academie voor Geneeskunde van Belgie') promotes medical progress, publishes scientific works, grants awards for scientific research, and publishes reports on administrative and medical problems regarding medical practice or public health.

- The Preventive and Social Health Care Division is involved in public health and its responsibilities include the following:[12]

  (i) payment of the share of kidney dialysis and haemophilia costs which are not refunded by the INAMI;

  (ii) covering treatment costs for cancer and tuberculosis patients whose revenue is beyond a certain threshold;

  (iii) informing the Minister about the vaccination policy and the fight against communicable diseases; and

  (iv) registering, coding and processing birth and death data statistics.

  The Preventive and Social Health Care Division can also intervene in public health matters through its local services, which monitor drinking water quality and work to prevent the spread of communicable diseases.

Until the 1980s, public health problems were dealt with by organisations such as the sickness funds, the Red Cross, doctors' associations, and anti-alcohol groups whose actions were dispersed. Coordination was introduced in 1991 through a decision of the Flemish government to create a formal structure. The decision included three important issues:

- the establishment of criteria to be met by the associations in order to be recognised (and therefore subsidised),

- the establishment of criteria for the approval of projects (in order to assess the value of subsidies to be allocated to each project),

- the creation of the Flemish Institute for Health Promotion ('Vlaamse Instituut voor Gezondheidspromotie', VIG) which coordinates the allocation of resources to different programmes.

The Flemish Community intervenes in public health matters through an administration (the 'Preventive and Social Health Care Division') which evaluates and funds projects in the field of health promotion and scientific research related to preventive health interventions. This administration works in collaboration with the VIG as they both make recommendations to the Ministry which develops the public health strategy. The Minister finally decides which projects may be implemented. These projects are financed for a period of one year since the budget is fixed annually.

The starting point for setting priorities is the Flemish government's declaration on the broad outlines of its policy. The health associations are also asked to set out their plans of action (which include the way the plans will be administered).

Mortality statistics classified according to several criteria – such as age, sex and region – are also used to formulate policy. This makes it possible to detect at-risk groups and enables the targeting of prevention policies. This information is also used to evaluate the development of health problems in the medium term (five to ten years) which is useful in policy formulation. According to the Head of the Preventive and Social Health Care Division, projects are selected according to four criteria:

- the importance of the issue involved, assessed according to the number of persons concerned and according to the threat to life;

- the potential benefit of the action to undertaken. This means that an action will only be undertaken if the causes of the problem are known* and if the action is likely to result in improvement in the population's health;**

- the budget necessary to implement the project; and

- the way the problem is perceived by the population and the media. Of course, this is not an official criterion but it is, for obvious political reasons, important in the final decision-making. Media perception is evaluated subjectively.***

The importance given to child policy is reflected in the Communities' allocation of resources in 1994. About 55 per cent of the budget dedicated to medicosocial activities was granted to fund health activities in schools and about 10 per cent of the budget was allocated to health education. These activities are mainly organised by the association

---

For example, as it is known with certainty that smoking causes throat cancer, actions aiming at the prevention of throat cancer aim to reduce smoking. Action will not be taken where the causes of a public health problem are unproven.

**The action must have a positive consequence on public health. For example, an anti-tobacco campaign will be undertaken if the population is sensitive to this kind of campaign and is therefore likely to reduce its cigarette consumption.*

***For example a large action to combat AIDS is considered to be 'normal' as AIDS is seen as one of the big issues at the end of this century (this may, however, seem irrational when compared to risks associated with other illnesses). In contrast, large funds dedicated to combating issues for which there is less awareness will be called into question by the population.*

'Child and Family' ('Kind en Gezin') which is responsible for child policy in Flanders. The importance given to the fight against cancer by the Flemish Community is also reflected in the fact that more than 5 per cent of the budget dedicated to medicosocial activities is allocated to two activities (screening; 4.8 per cent and research; 0.3 per cent) related to these areas. It constitutes the third section of the budget (classified in decreasing order).

The main services related to prevention concern the following areas:

(i) Health inspection. There are several policies developed including:

- the distribution of free vaccines;

- the reduction of communicable diseases;

- the prevention of infectious diseases;

- the promotion of a healthy environment.

(ii) Cancer prevention. The Flemish Advisory Committee for cancer prevention ('Vlaamse Adviescommissie voor Kankerpreventie') makes recommendations and proposals regarding cancer prevention. These include:

- advice on early cancer detection and coordination of initiatives in this field;

- policy suggestions regarding cancer in the field of applied research, early detection and diagnosis, prevention, health education and information; and

- sociomedical supervision, longitudinal statistics, research and epidemiology.[12]

(iii) Perinatal care. The Flemish Advisory Committee on perinatal care ('Vlaamse Adviescommissie vor the Perinatal Zorg') makes proposals in the field of perinatal health care regarding:

- perinatal counselling aiming at a better insight into and a further decrease in perinatal mortality;

- the possible establishment and specific funding of perinatal centres;

- setting priorities concerning scientific research in perinatal care and perinatal epidemiology.[12]

(iv) Health protection. A team based within the Community is charged with improving all the factors that have an impact on health such as lifestyle. It collaborates with the VIG in funding projects and participates in research groups specialising in health education.

(v) Sports practice. The Council which advises on the medical aspects of sport ('Raad voor Medisch Verantwoorde Sportbeoefening') offers advice with the help of:

- the Committee for Medical Examination in Sport (dealing with all medical aspects of sport) which offers advice on recognising medical examiners for sports;

- the Committee for Top Level Sports and Promising Athletes: which offers advice on medically justified sports practice; and

- the Anti-doping Committee: offers advice on doping, more particularly on the list of substances enhancing the performance of athletes in an artificial manner, and on the approach to the doping problem generally.[12]

Collaboration between authorities with a competence in health   In total there are eight ministers dealing with public health in Belgium. Other ministers are also involved in health related policy questions. The Ministry for Economic Affairs sets the price of medicines, the Ministry of Interior deals with disasters, the Ministry of Justice reviews the legitimacy of all laws dealing with public health, and the Ministry of Finances can raise taxes on alcohol and tobacco.

As the various competencies are divided between the different authorities, collaboration is strongly encouraged. For example, the French community deals with health education relating to drugs but it is the Walloon region which runs the detoxification centres. Without collaboration, it is difficult to develop a consistent health policy. However, a formal framework for this collaboration between the community and the region does not really exist at present.

Collaboration between the community and the federal state is difficult as well. Formal inter-ministerial meetings exist but are generally used to resolve conflicts related to competencies and not for improving collaboration. In addition, although the health policies of the French and the Flemish communities are similar, there is no real collaboration between the communities.

Collaboration is required to lead an efficient policy in these areas where each level has a role to play and where the efficiency of prevention depends on the simultaneous application of sanitary measures. The main field of cooperation between the communities, the regions and the federal government concerns the prevention of communicable diseases. Collaboration is necessary in this area because:

- the communities are responsible for prevention;

- the federal state is responsible for sanitary control of airports, the vaccination of travellers, the application of compulsory vaccinations inside the country, and, above all, for the coordination at federal level of emergency sanitary measures which is a requirement of the World Health Organisation; and

- the regions have competencies in areas such as water, pollution, housing, etc.

Conclusion

The Belgian political landscape is characterised by a great decentralisation of its institutions. Thus, there are three different decision-making centres (the federal government, the communities and the regions) which deal with policies of health prevention and promotion. One may pose the question of the desirability of such a structure when the health problems seem to be similar in Flanders and in the Walloon area. Altogether, there are eight Ministers of Health and Environment in Belgium. This situation may create a number of problems:

- As three decision centres (the Federal government, the Communities and the Regions) deal with policies of health promotions, the competencies of these three centres must be defined clearly to avoid conflicts. Since the definition of the prevention in the matter of health is not clearly established, these conflicts based on the competencies happens between the communities, the regions and the federal government.

- Secondly, it is difficult to define a single health policy. This could be possible in a decentralised system where there is also coordination between the various decision-making centres. But since this is not really the case in Belgium, health policy seems to be reduced to dispersed actions.

At the moment there is no real government plan concerning health objectives and priorities. A number of health policy priorities are defined implicitly through budgetary decisions (negotiations within the INAMI on the price of various treatments and on the reimbursement rates of these treatments). These decisions may favour some sub-groups of the population (through the choice of categories of care to be reimbursed) in access to care. The problem lies in the way in which these decisions are made by the various stakeholders involved in the negotiations (sickness funds, health providers, government etc.). As such decision-making mostly tends to take into account the financial imperatives, it seems that the Belgian health system still lacks a comprehensive framework of public health priorities. The new obligation for the Ministry for Public Health to present its health policy priorities is definitely a step in the right direction within the current context of budgetary restrictions implemented at each level of the health care system and for each category of social expenses.

References

1. WHO. *World Health Statistics Annual.* Copenhagen: WHO, 1996.

2. Poullier JP. Public health strategies in Europe: doing better and feeling worse. In: Detels R, Holland WW, McEwen J, Omenn GS (eds). *Oxford Textbook of Public Health, 3rd Edition.* Vol. 1, pp. 275–96. Oxford: OU Press, 1996.

3. Muir Gray JA. Lesson and challenges. In: Detels R, Holland WW, McEwen J, Omenn GS (eds). *Oxford Textbook of Public Health, 3rd Edition.* Vol. 1, pp. 343–8. Oxford: OU Press, 1996.

4. Crainich D, Closon M. Cost containment and health care reform in Belgium. In: Mossialos E, Le Grand J (eds.) *Health Care and Cost Containment in the European Union.* Aldershot: Ashgate, 1999, pp. 219–66.

5. Kesenne J. *Health Care Reform and Risk Structure Compensation: The Case of Belgium.* AIM seminal proceedings, Maastricht, October 11, 1995.

6. Nonneman W. Van Doorslaer E. The role of the sickness funds in the Belgian health

care market. *Social Science and Medicine* 1994;39(10):1483–95.

7. Ministry for Social Affairs, Public Health and the Environment. Personal communication, 1998.

8. Hurst J. The reform of health care. A comparative analysis of seven OECD countries. *Health Policy Studies No.2.* Paris: OECD, 1992.

9. Closon M-C. *The Health Care System in Belgium.* Université Catholique de Louvain. Unpublished paper, 1995.

10. Detels R, Breslow L. Current scope and concerns in public health. In: Detels R, Holland WW, McEwen J, Omenn GS (eds). *Oxford Textbook of Public Health, 3rd Edition.* Vol. 1, pp. 3–18. Oxford: OU Press, 1996.

11. Anon. The French Community of Belgium. In: La Santé en Belgique-De Gezondheid in Belgie – Health in Belgium. SA Media Belgium International NV, 1996. pp. 348–52.

12. Anon. The Flemish Community of Belgium. In: La Santé en Belgique-De Gezondheid in Belgie – Health in Belgium. SA Media Belgium International NV, 1996. pp. 341–6.

Further Reading

Longfils R. L'éducation pour la santé, l'affaire de qui? *Education Santé* 1994;93:2–3.

Ministry for Social Affairs, Public Health and Environment. *Krachtlijnen voor het Toekomstig Gezondheidsbeleid – Lignes de Force de la Politique Future en Matiere de Santé.* Brussels, 1995.

Ministry for Social Affairs, Public Health and Environment. *Note de Politique Generale du Ministre des Affaires Sociales, de la Santé Publique et de l'Environnement pour L'anne Budgetaire 1997 – Beleidsnota van het Ministerie van Sociale Zaken, van Volksgezondheid en Leefmilieu voor het Begrotingsjaar 1997.* Brussells, 14 November 1996.

4

Public Health Policy and Priority Setting in Denmark

Johannes Mosbech

Country and population

The population of Denmark is 5.2 million with a density of 123 inhabitants per square kilometre. The country is divided into 14 counties and 275 municipalities.

Mean life expectancy at birth is 73 for males and 78 for females with 15 per cent of the population aged 65 years or over.[1] In 1996 there were 67,600 births and 61,000 deaths in Denmark.

Annual immigration into Denmark is approximately 45,000. On average 3,500 people leave the country each year. In 1994 there were 197,000 foreign nationals in the country (comprising 4 per cent of the population) with 115,000 of these from countries outside Europe.

Public health care expenditure accounts for 9 per cent of total public spending, 4.8 per cent of Danish GDP and 6.7 percent of total expenditure. In 1997 there were 2.9 doctors per 1,000 inhabitants.[1,2]

Basic principles of the health care system

In Denmark health care is considered a public responsibility. Virtually all health care services are financed, planned and operated by public authorities. Financing derives mainly from general taxation. All residents in Denmark have equal access, free of charge to almost all health care services, regardless of employment, financial and social status.

The system is characterised by a far-reaching devolution of responsibility for health care to politically elected regional and local councils. Thus, responsibility for health care services is distributed among the three administrative levels in Denmark: national, regional and local. The authorities of these three levels cooperate closely to ensure a coherent health care system.[3]

Over the last decade, a general trend in Danish health policy has been the transfer of tasks from the hospital sector to the primary health sector. More services have been made available at community level and the services of the primary health sector have been expanded. This trend reflects the idea that citizens should be offered treatment at the local level.[3]

In recent years, it has been widely recognised that existing health problems cannot be solved by treatment alone. Consequently, efforts to prevent disease have been strengthened. Much weight has been attached to lifestyle factors such as nutrition, tobacco, alcohol, etc.[4-6]

Health promotion is not only the responsibility of the health care system. It comprises a wide range of tasks in many sectors, for example improving the work environment, increasing road safety, improving housing and the community environment and strengthening social services at community level. Consequently, health care policy is developed through cooperation among a wide range of authorities and organisations. One result of this cooperation is a comprehensive programme on health promotion. Twelve ministries have been involved in the creation of this programme which has been coordinated by the Ministry of Health.[7]

Administrative organisation

The Danish health care sector comprises two subsectors: hospital services and primary health care services. Responsibility for these services is distributed among the national, regional and local levels, and is illustrated in Figure 1.[8]

I. National level

At the national level, the task is essentially to define, coordinate and supervise the health care system. One of the main tasks is to set the goals for the national health policy. The Ministry of Health is the principal health authority and is responsible for legislation on health. This includes legislation on health care, personnel, hospitals and pharmacies, pharmaceutical products, nutrition, vaccinations, maternal and child care, patients' rights, etc.

The Ministry controls the health care system mainly by issuing general rules and guidelines. It runs a number of central agencies with various executive, advisory and supervisory functions.[3,8] These are as follows:

The National Board of Health

The main functions of the National Board of Health are:

- executive tasks for the administration of health services
- advisory functions with respect to national government

Figure 1
Responsibility for health care services in Denmark

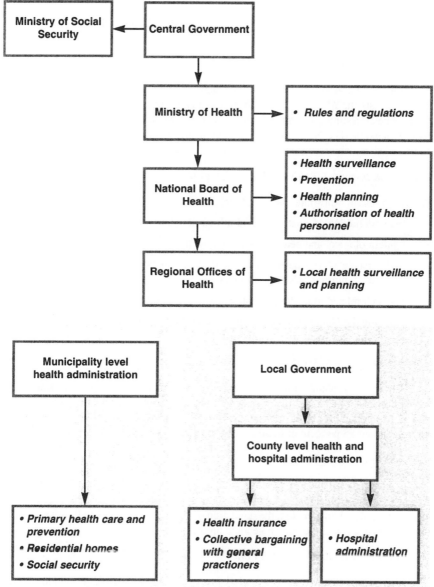

Other parties: Medical associations, private patient organisations

- advisory functions with respect to local authorities and health professionals
- supervisory functions with respect to health professionals
- regulation and planning of the education of health professionals.

At regional level, the tasks of the Board are carried out by state-employed public health officers.

The National Food Agency

The National Food Agency oversees the legislation on foodstuffs in Denmark. The agency assists the Ministry of Health in law-making and acts as adviser on food and food-related questions. The municipalities are responsible for ensuring compliance with food legislation. The National Food Agency operates and supervises the Danish food control system, which consists of 38 municipal food control units.

The Danish Institute for Clinical Epidemiology (DICE)

DICE is a research institute. Its main functions are:

- the undertaking of a national Health Interview Survey Programme
- epidemiological and health services research
- maintenance of computerised registers, e.g. a national mortality register and a register of multiple sclerosis sufferers
- research related to health promotion and disease prevention
- assisting the National Board of Health and other public authorities in carrying out epidemiological and statistical investigation.[9]

The Patients' Complaints Board

The Patients' Complaints Board is an independent body composed of lawyers and non-professionals as well as health personnel. The Board considers complaints about professional errors made by health personnel. One thousand cases are put before the Board each year, and 85 per cent of these concern doctors.

The Danish Council of Ethics

The Council has an advisory function and has issued several reports and recommendations on various ethical matters. Amongst these are reports on brain deaths, patients' self determination and information, the regulation of research conducted on fertilised human ova and foetuses, and the human genome project.

The Council on Health Promotion Policy

The Minister for Health has set up an independent Council on Health Promotion Policy which consists of 24 members. The main functions of the Council are:

- to follow developments in health promotion

- to survey and evaluate public health promotion efforts
- to make proposals for new health promotion initiatives
- to make health promotion the subject of public debate.

Under the Council on Health Promotion Policy, the Minister for Health has set up an independent Council on Alcohol, which consists of nine members. This Council has the same functions as the Council on Health Promotion Policy, but restricted to alcohol issues.[3]

The Danish Council on Smoking and Health

The Council is an independent council of experts under the Ministry of Health and consists of nine members appointed by the Minister for Health.

The main functions of the Council are:

- to reduce the health damage from smoking
- to reduce the number of new smokers, particularly among children and adolescents
- to secure smoke-free environments
- to reduce rates of tobacco consumption amongst existing smokers.

The State Serum Institute

With a staff of about 900, the State Serum Institute is the central public health institute for Danish hospitals and general practitioners in the field of medical microbiology, immunology and related disciplines, and a national and international research centre. In addition, the institute produces vaccines and blood products.

II. Regional level

Denmark's 15 counties are general administrative entities at regional level. They are headed by politically elected county councils. One of the counties' major tasks is the provision of health care services. The counties are responsible for hospital care and primary, curative care (except home nursing) as well as for health promotion initiatives.

These activities are mainly financed through county income taxes. The level of the county income tax being a crucial political issue, planning the health care services requires a balance between good services and taxes. Differences in income and demography are compensated for by government block grants. The Association of County Councils in Denmark coordinates matters that are common to all county councils.[7]

III. Local level

Denmark's 275 municipalities are the general administrative entities at local level. Like the counties they are headed by elected councils. They finance their activities in much the same way as the counties.

The municipalities have a wide range of responsibilities of which health care tasks constitute only a minor part. They are responsible for home nursing services and a number of preventive programmes, including public health nurses, school health and child dental services. Municipalities are also responsible for planning and running most of the social welfare system, including services related to health care, such as nursing homes for the elderly.

Primary health care

Today, primary health care constitutes the backbone of the Danish health care system. Over the past decade much has been done to redistribute services from the hospital sector to the primary health sector. The idea is that health care tasks should be conducted as near to the citizen as is appropriate in a given situation.

Primary health care services comprise general practitioners and practising specialists, practising dentists, physiotherapists and home nurses employed by the municipalities.

General practitioners

Every citizen in Denmark has the right to register with a general practitioner of which there are about 3,200 throughout the country. On average 1,600 citizens are enlisted with each general practitioner.

The pillar of the health care system is the so-called 'family doctor system'. Anyone aged 16 or over may choose his or her own general practitioner. Families often keep the same family doctor for a number of years which gives the doctor a thorough knowledge of the family's social and medical condition.

The general practitioner acts as a 'gatekeeper'. When a person falls ill or has a health problem, he or she contacts the general practitioner. In cases where the doctor considers it necessary, the patient will be referred for further examination or treatment either to a practising specialist or to a hospital. The doctor may also call on the services of health visitors, home nurses and the community social services.

This system functions round the clock and all facilities are available to the patient free of charge. The only deviation from the 'gatekeeper' system occurs in the case of sudden, serious injury or disease. In this case the patient may be treated at the hospital without referral to the general practitioner.

In principle, the general practitioner either runs a private practice on his or her own or in collaboration with other general practitioners. The main part of the general practitioner's income, however, derives from the Health Care Reimbursement Scheme.

Practising specialists

Generally, the practising specialists examine and treat patients referred to them by general practitioners. There are about 800 full-time practising specialists in Denmark.

Practising dentists

The majority of dentists have private practices. There are 3,400 practising dentists in Denmark. According to an agreement with the Health Care Reimbursement Scheme the patients are reimbursed part of their expenses for dental treatment. The population has a free choice of dentist.[10]

Physiotherapists

General practitioners can refer patients for treatment to physiotherapists, who themselves are permitted to establish private clinics. They work under an agreement with the Health Care Reimbursement Scheme which partly reimburses the fees paid by their patients. Many municipalities also employ physiotherapists, for instance in nursing homes.

Home nurses

A home nursing service is compulsory for all municipalities. The general practitioner or the hospital can refer patients to home nursing care, which is free of charge and often integrated locally with the home help services.[11]

Nursing homes

Nursing homes receive elderly people who are not in need of hospital treatment, but who require sheltered housing with some degree of care. The municipalities pay for the main expenses of the nursing homes.

Hospital services

Denmark has about 30,000 hospital beds with an average occupancy rate of 81 per cent. There are about 1.1 million admissions to hospitals per year and approximately 4 million out-patient visits annually. The average length of stay is approximately 7 days.

The counties are responsible for the supply of hospital services to their citizens free of charge. Virtually all hospitals are owned and run by the counties. For specialised hospital services that cater to catchment populations larger than one county, an inter-county market has been established.

Since January 1st 1993, Danish citizens requiring hospital treatment can choose between all public hospitals and a number of private clinics which cooperate with the public hospital services. This means that a patient, who has been referred for hospital treatment by their general practitioner has the choice of hospital without regard to geographical considerations. The county of residence will be under obligation to pay for the treatment. Admission to highly specialised wards, however, is granted only when this is considered necessary on medical grounds.

During the last decade there have been major changes in the way hospitals function. The total number of hospital beds has decreased by 25 per cent from more than 40,000 in

1980 to some 30,000 in 1992, corresponding to 6 beds per 1,000 inhabitants. However, the number of admissions has increased by about 15 per cent in the same period from about 950,000 admissions to about 1,100,000. This has been possible through a rapid decline in the average length of stay, which is now less than 7 days (excluding psychiatry), and a correspondingly rapid expansion of out-patient services. Thus the hospitals have been increasingly directed at out-patient treatment, which relieves the pressure on in-patient facilities.[2,3]

Hospital structure

Danish hospital physicians are full-time, salaried staff members. Hospital treatment is free of charge to people resident in Denmark. Patients are only admitted to hospital after referral from a general practitioner or via the hospital emergency units, which are available to everyone.

General social situation

The Danish welfare model is based on the principle that all population groups should enjoy acceptable living conditions and all citizens be guaranteed certain fundamental rights in the event of unemployment, sickness or old age.[8] The main elements are:

Universalism: Every citizen is entitled to health services, social security and benefits regardless of the degree of affiliation to the job market.

Public measures: These have been regarded as the best means of ensuring a high level of economic security also for the least privileged – and a high level of entitlements. Hence nearly all social welfare services are financed by direct and indirect taxation. Social expenditure (including unemployment benefit, health care, etc.) amounts to 31 per cent of the GDP (the EU average is 27 per cent), or about half of total public expenditure.

Redistribution: Equalisation of incomes via social transfer payments is substantial by international standards. Only 4 per cent of families live below the 'poverty line' (OECD's relative low-income concept). 80 per cent of the transfer payments go to people who would otherwise be below this limit. About 20 per cent of GDP is used for transfer payments.

Expansion of services: There has been a marked growth in services catering for children and the elderly. 5 per cent of GDP is used on social services, exclusive of the health care sector.

Decentralisation and control through framework laws: For the past 20 years or so, a guiding principle of Danish social policy has been to place responsibility for its implementation as close to the people as possible. This means that today, responsibility for important elements of social policy rests with local and county authorities while central government sets up the relevant statutory and economic framework.

'Omnipotent' local authorities. Over half of the local authorities have populations of less than 10,000. The smallest have populations of about 3,000 and the biggest has a population of almost half a million. Nevertheless local authorities all have the same broad responsibility – political, economic and practical – for implementing national social and health policies locally.

Alcohol and drugs

Since 1960, there has been an annual increase in the consumption of alcohol, but for the last 5–6 years it has been stable at around 12 litres of 100 per cent alcohol per capita for those above 14 years of age.

The National Board of Health estimates that 6 per cent of the population over the age of 15, i.e. about 250,000 people, consume alcohol to an extent which damages their health. And around 70,000 people receive treatment for alcohol abuse per year.

The number of people in treatment as well as the number of treatment places in specialist institutions for abusers is decreasing, whereas the number of people receiving outpatient treatment has tended to increase. The number of places in private residential institutions (where the patient often has to pay for the treatment) is increasing.

A characteristic common to drug abusers is that they have experienced disadvantaged conditions while growing up, and very early marginalisation. Drug abuse is therefore made even more complicated because of a poor economic background, poor social conditions and mental problems. As a rough estimate, there are about 10,000 drug abusers in Denmark. The rate of increase has been stable over a number of years.

Mental illness

The most important target group for psychiatric assistance is people suffering from serious mental illness. This group is estimated to comprise 40,000–50,000 people, including more than 1,000 people affected by severe psychiatric and social problems as well as poor motivation.

In the past, these people were generally patients at central institutions. At present, the intention is to help them live a life which is as close as possible to normal, preferably in their own homes. This requires the development of municipal facilities and services for the mentally ill. This deinstitutionalisation process may partly explain the growing proportion of mentally ill people found among the homeless registered by reception centres. The trend is probably only temporary, since the decentralised social system intended for the mentally ill has not yet been fully developed.

Local authority commitment to the mentally ill is not only a question of offering various accommodation facilities but also a question of establishing workshops which are open daily for mentally ill people to provide a variety of activities, advice, guidance and training.

National level responsibility for social policy and health

The State is responsible for overall control and establishing the broad legislative and financial framework of social policy.

Primarily, the Ministry of Social Affairs, the Ministry of Labour and the Ministry of Health take preventive measures and resolve problems in the social sector. Since social issues cover a wide spectrum of fields, such as culture, education, housing and leisure activities, other ministries are also involved from time to time.

The Ministry of Social Affairs

The Ministry of Social Affairs has responsibility for the care of the elderly, children and young people, family policy, retraining and preventive social measures. It is responsible for the physically and mentally disabled, particularly vulnerable groups and for some measures involving the mentally ill and drug and substance abusers.

The Ministry of Labour

The Ministry of Labour has responsibility for social measures in the labour market. These include the work environment, the whole area of sickness benefits, voluntary early retirement pay and transitional allowance to insure unemployed people. It is also concerned with retraining programmes, labour exchanges, educational subsidies and enterprise allowances to the unemployed, wage supplements to employers in the private and public sector who take on the unemployed as part of a retraining programme, leave of absence schemes and other schemes designed to expand employment.

The Ministry of Health

The Ministry of Health is responsible for primary health services and hospitals. Here, too, the system is characterised by extensive delegation to politically elected regional and local boards. Responsibility is divided between three administrative levels: national, regional and local, all working in close cooperation with one another.

Trends and challenges of the 1990s

The main theme of Danish social and public health policy during the rest of the 1990s will be the question of how to mobilise resources for renewed social commitment in all sectors of society.

Poverty in Denmark

Through taxation, the Danish welfare model ensures a reasonable distribution of the nation's wealth among all social groups. Poverty in Denmark affects mainly single parents, the long-term unemployed, pensioners, unskilled workers, recipients of social assistance, large families and students.

Private voluntary agencies increasingly bear the brunt of social commitment. Where the State has been unable or unwilling to provide welfare, voluntary agencies step in, frequently with financial assistance from the State.[11]

Measures for the socially excluded

The most disadvantaged and excluded – homeless (especially children), drug abusers, law breakers, some mentally ill patients, and a number of immigrants and refugees – though constituting only a small group, pose a serious problem.

The Ministry of Social Affairs has increasingly cooperated with and funded voluntary social agencies, whose work in complementing professional approaches, has produced positive results. The Ministry of Social Affairs subsidises innovative practices and activities from earmarked funding. In 1995 activities totalling more than DKK 300 million were financed in this way. Examples are:

- funding for voluntary social work whereby private agencies are granted support for social work

- social policy funding to provide a stronger commitment to the most vulnerable groups

- pilot projects aimed at integrating people with disabilities into the labour market

- support for people with occupational disabilities thereby improving their chances of entering and remaining in the labour market

- pilot projects involving social services for the physically and mentally disabled

- pilot projects involving measures for the senile and their families.[11]

Services for the mentally ill

The expansion of district psychiatry and social measures outside the hospital system, have to a certain extent, failed to keep pace with changes in the health service that have reduced the number of beds and the bed occupancy rate. Thus, local authorities are finding it difficult to shoulder their responsibility for the mentally disabled.

As a result, it has been necessary to set aside additional resources for the purpose of expanding district psychiatry and social services.[3]

Commitment to refugees and immigrants

Refugees and immigrants comprise a group with special problems. Compared with Danes, their unemployment rate, between 25 per cent and 50 per cent, is very high.

Many actions have already been undertaken with the aim of fighting intolerance and fear of foreigners, as well as promoting equality. In the years to come, Denmark will continue to seek new ways of ensuring that refugees and immigrants can participate in Danish society on equal terms.[3]

Better conditions for the elderly

Changes in family structure and working life have made it progressively harder for families to take care of their elderly. On the other hand, their past reliance on the family has been replaced by a more independent life, in which the community takes more responsibility for their welfare. The over-60s make up 20 per cent of the Danish population and the proportion of elderly will grow in the years ahead. The fact that an increasing number of elderly people live in their own homes requires further initiatives and greater resources for home help in the future.

Policy towards the elderly will continue to be based on the principle that older people constitute a very heterogeneous group with widely differing needs and potentials. In terms of services and housing, the most frail will be given the highest priority.[3]

Focus on the patient

There is no indication that demand for health services will decline in the 1990s. On the contrary, growing prosperity means that people will be expecting a higher level of service from the health system. Professional and technological developments will continue to affect conditions for treating a number of diseases.

In recent years, excessively long waiting lists for surgical operations have become a big problem. This is clearly unacceptable. Consequently, central government and the counties that run the hospitals, reached an agreement to the effect that waiting time for surgery should not exceed three months and that the capacity for heart surgery be doubled before the end of 1995. However, neither of these targets have yet been reached.

Reducing waiting lists is part of a government plan, launched under the heading 'focus on the patient'. The emphasis is also on wider measures to advance health care and prevent sickness, both mental and physical, and on improving the quality of health services generally.

Over the past few years, the Danes' average life expectancy has become a matter of increasing concern. While in the 1970s Denmark ranked fifth among OECD-countries in terms of average life expectancy, by 1990 it had plummeted to 20th place.

Studies indicate that the decline in Danish average life span – particularly among women – is due to a number of things, including genetic factors, living conditions, lifestyles and attitudes, all of which have an effect on health, sickness and death. Among the principal findings is that tobacco, alcohol and unemployment play a crucial role. For instance, 46 per cent of all men and 39 per cent of all women above 15, are smokers, while 6 per cent of the population consume such quantities of alcohol as are prejudicial to their health.

A new wave of illness appears to be on its way, involving socially induced diseases. Socially generated problems of cooperation, problems within the family, in school and in the workplace will from now on increasingly affect sickness rates, in the form of psychosomatic disorders and of new complaints caused by the pollution of both natural and work environments. Problems of loneliness, rooted in isolation from the job market, in exclusion and in changing family patterns will lead to more and more people living alone, all of which increase the need for special preventive measures.[4,6,9]

Current and future changes in the health services

Following the government budget of 1996, a Hospital Committee was set up to evaluate the overall organisation of the Danish hospital service and analyse the parameters which would affect the long-term development of the hospital service.

The Committee had also to clarify the present use of technology in the treatment of patients and assess whether a better use of information technology in administrative work would release resources for the actual treatment of patients. On the basis of its findings, the Committee was to describe and evaluate various models for the future planning of the hospital service. The Committee completed its work at the end of 1996.

In 1996, the introduction of a Patient's Rights Act was envisaged. The purpose of this Act is to strengthen the legal rights of patients in relation to the health service and to sustain the relationship of confidence and confidentiality between patients and the health service with its various staff groupings.

The Act will be a comprehensive piece of legislation governing the rights and legal status of individual patients in relation to the health service; particularly regarding examination, treatment and general care.

In January 1996, a new Act concerning preventive health measures for children and young people came into effect. This Act combines three previous Acts concerning preventive health measures for children and young people. The purpose is partly to strengthen and improve the efforts made regarding the most vulnerable children and young people, and partly to improve preventive health measures for them. Progress will be achieved by strengthening the general efforts to improve health and prevent disease by creating better coordination between the various health measures and by emphasising individually tailored schemes.

Conclusions

Health policy and decision-making is shaped by politicians at national, regional and municipal levels. In Parliament each party has a spokesperson responsible for health issues to express the party's view on specific topics. This is true for regional councils as well. Through mass media, patient organisations can encourage politicians to raise questions and discuss issues, so influencing the way health policy decisions are made. Breast cancer screening is an example of this process. There is public pressure in favour of screening but there is political reluctance to introduce it because of the financial consequences and disagreement within the medical profession about the need.

Heart surgery is another area where heated political discussion takes place. Here the main player is the patient based Heart Foundation which has gained the support of the mass media to publicise stories about patient deaths while waiting for surgery. This strategy puts pressure on politicians to allot extra resources.

In spite of such differences, there is a general consensus about how the main priority-setting issues in health policy should be tackled, but this does not exclude debate related to the clear financial limitations that exist.

The medical profession, including general physicians, practising specialists, and hospital physicians, do play an active role in this discussion both in the mass media as well as in the medical press.

Each group tends to fight for the maximum amount of resources to be allotted to the particular group of patients they care for.

The medical weekly press (*Ugeskrift for Læger*) published by the Danish Medical Association (to which all physicians must belong), tries to give a balanced medical view on health priority setting problems as they arise. These official medical points of view definitely have an influence on the decision-makers at different levels in the political system.

The decline in life span in Denmark compared to other countries in the European Union has caused much concern. It is generally agreed that this is linked largely to the fact that the incidence of lifestyle related diseases has not decreased sufficiently.

It has only a limited relationship with the general structure of the health system and the availability of medical examinations, treatment and care.

What is very clear is the fact that it has not been possible to combat effectively tobacco and alcohol related diseases as well as accidents. The reason for this is not at all clear but psychology is likely to play a major part. In spite of the great deal of resources spent on health information aimed at preventing disease, there have been severe problems in getting the message across to people.

Whether the right methods have been used is the subject of much debate. Not everybody reacts to the health messages in the same way; higher social classes have a greater tendency to understand the messages and take proper precautions.

The public health system, which is the dominant form of health care provision in Denmark, is financed by tax payers and there is a very strong public feeling that taxes cannot and should not be increased. Therefore, as resources for health are limited, ensuring proper distribution becomes ever more important. As a consequence, a firm limit has been placed on the number of doctors, both general practitioners as well as specialists, who are allowed to work under the Health Insurance Scheme.

The hospitals are being reorganised to save money by grouping together departments with the speciality from different hospitals. The Copenhagen Hospital Unity, organised in 1996, is an example.

However, it remains to be seen whether this measure will reduce waiting lists and increase efficiency. The financial gain also has to be seen.

The overall impact of these changes in the health system is that there is less room for the care of the chronic ill, the psychiatric patients and the elderly.

References

1. Danish Ministry of Health. The Danish Life Expectancy Committee. *Lifetime in Denmark.* Copenhagen, 1994.

2. OECD. *OECD Health Data 1998* (CD Rom). Paris: OECD, 1998 and Nordic Medico Statistical Committee (Nomesco). *Health Statistics in the Nordic Countries 1994.* 1996;47.

3. Danish Ministry of Health. *Health Care in Denmark.* Copenhagen, 1994.

4. Oplysningsindsats vedr. *HIV og AIDS.* Sundhedsstyrelsen. Copenhagen, 1995.

5. Aarsberetning. *Tobaksskaderaadet 1994.* Copenhagen, 1995.

6. Screening. Hvorfor, hvornaar, hvordan. Sundhedsstyrelsen. Copenhagen, 1990.

7. Danish Ministry of Social Affairs. *World Summit for Social Development.* Copenhagen, 1995.

8. Danish Ministry of Social Affairs. *Social Policy in Denmark.* Copenhagen, 1995.

9. Dansk Institut for Klinisk Epidemiologi. *Sundhed og Sygelighed i Danmark 1994. Udviklingen siden 1987.* Copenhagen.

10. *Retningslinier for tilrettelæggelse af den kommunale tandpleje.* Sundhedsstyrelsen. Copenhagen, 1994.

11. Danish Ministry of Social Affairs. *Social Policy in Denmark. Combating Social Exclusion.* Copenhagen, 1995.

5

Decision-Making and Priority-Setting in Public Health and Health Care in Germany

Reinhard Busse and Friedrich Wilhelm Schwartz

Principles, structures and actors

A key feature of the German political system is the sharing of decision-making powers between the states ('Länder') and the federal government, with further powers governing statutory insurance schemes devolved to non-governmental corporate bodies.[1]

The German constitution (Grundgesetz) requires that living conditions should be of an equal standard in all Länder. However, health promotion or protection is not specifically mentioned as a goal. The Grundgesetz defines areas of exclusively federal legislation (foreign affairs, defence etc.) and concurrent legislation. Health is not an area for exclusive federal legislation and only specific topics relevant to the public's health are included in the concurrent legislation: social benefits, measures against diseases which are dangerous to public safety, protection against ionising radiation, certification of doctors and other health professions, pharmaceuticals and drugs, and the economic situation of the hospitals are among the areas in which federal law – if it exists – takes precedence over Länder legislation. In addition, some environmental policies fall into this category. Implicitly, all other aspects of public health are therefore the responsibility of the Länder.

At the central (i.e. federal) level, the Federal Ministry for Health is the key player. It is divided into the following five divisions, each of which contains two sub-divisions: (1) administration and international relations, (2) pharmaceuticals and social policy (welfare, handicapped etc.), (3) health care and statutory health insurance, (4) protecting health and fighting disease and (5) consumer protection (mainly food-related) and veterinary medicine. Before 1991, the sub-divisions dealing with statutory health insurance were part of the Ministry for Labour and Social Services while most of the other sub-divisions were part of the Ministry for Youth, Family, Women, and Health.

The Federal Ministry for Health is assisted by subordinate authorities in carrying out its tasks in the area of public health.[2] These include: the Federal Institute for Pharmaceuticals and Medical Products, the Federal Institute for Consumers' Health Protection and Veterinary Medicine, the Robert Koch Institute, the Paul Ehrlich Institute (Federal Agency for Sera and Vaccines), the Federal Centre for Health Education, and the German Institute for Medical Documentation and Information. The first three institutions are the successors of the former Federal Health Institute which was dissolved after accusations of mishandling the requirement to test pharmaceuticals for HIV.

In addition, the Ministry is advised by the 'Advisory Council for Concerted Action in Health Care' on medical and economic matters and by the Federal Health Council on matters related to the promotion of health and the prevention of disease.

Other federal ministries relevant to health include the Ministries for Environment and Nuclear Energy and for Research and Technology.

The federal structure is represented mainly by the 16 state governments. In 1997, 13 of the 16 Länder governments had a ministry which mentioned 'health' in its name. However, none has an exclusive health department, and in most Länder it is combined with Labour and Social Services (which is also the case in the Länder which do not mention 'health' in the name of its ministry). In a few cases health is combined with family or youth affairs, and in one 'Land' it is attached to environmental affairs.

Within a Länder ministry of health, 'health' is typically one of four or five divisions. In Lower Saxony for example, the 'health' division is sub-divided into units concerned with: (1) public health services and environmental hygiene; (2) health promotion, prevention and AIDS care; (3) state-owned hospitals; (4) hospital planning; (5) supervision of health professions and their professional institutions; (6) psychiatry and illegal drugs; and (7) pharmaceuticals and supervision of pharmacists and their professional institutions. Most other areas with an impact on health such as traffic, city planning or education are controlled by other ministries.

On the provider side, physicians' associations exist in all Länder. As there are several physicians' associations in three Länder, the total number of associations is 22. (The hospitals are not represented by any legal corporate institution but by private organisations.)

The purchasers' side is made up of autonomous sickness funds which are organised on a regional and/or federal basis. On 1 January 1997, there were 554 sickness funds, 56 of them operating entirely in the east of the country.[3] By law, sickness funds have the right and the obligation to raise contributions from their members, this includes the right to determine what contribution rate is necessary to cover expenditure.

Figure 1
Health-related responsibilities and decision-making in Germany until 1988

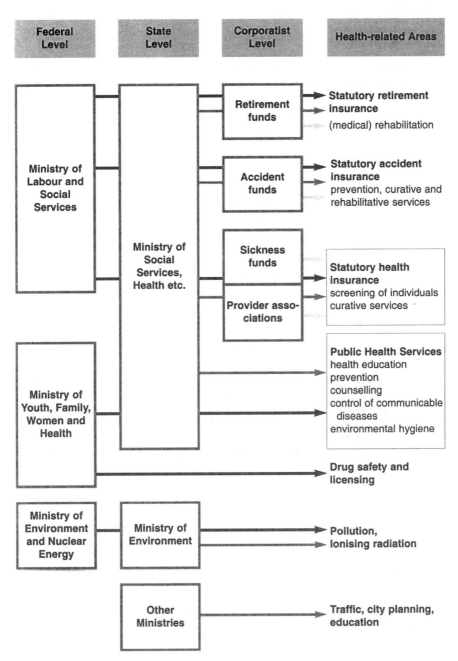

Missions and responsibilities

Federal level

Setting the rules for providing and financing social services and ensuring equity are responsibilities at the federal level. Health-related social services are regulated through several statutory insurance schemes, the most important being statutory health insurance. Others include accident insurance, retirement insurance (which includes responsibility for most rehabilitative measures) and, since 1995, nursing care insurance. All statutory insurance schemes are regulated through the 'Social Code Book' (Socialgesetzbuch, SGB) but fall under the authority of different ministries (Figures 1– 3).

SGB regulates the following areas:[1]

- membership in sickness funds which now covers 89% of the population,

- the content of the sickness funds' benefit package,

- the organisational structure of sickness funds and their associations,

- the goals and scope of negotiations between the sickness funds and providers of health care, notably the physicians' associations, and

- the financing mechanisms.

Currently, the following types of benefit are included by law in the benefits package: disease prevention, screening, diagnostic procedures, treatment (including ambulatory medical care, dental care, medicines, non-physician care, medical devices, in-patient/hospital care, nursing care at home, and certain areas of rehabilitation), and transportation. In addition, sickness funds have to give cash benefits to sick insurees after the first six weeks during which time the employers are responsible for sick pay.

The Ministry's subordinate authorities are responsible for: licensing pharmaceuticals and registering homeopathic products; the evaluation of food-related health risks (e.g. genetically produced food); monitoring diseases; licensing sera and vaccines; providing health education and public information; and collecting and disseminating scientific information.

Other health-related responsibilities at central level include legislation in the areas of pollution and ionising radiation which fall within the remit of the Federal Ministry for Environment and Nuclear Energy.

State ('Länder') level

The Länder governments have a duty to maintain the hospital infrastructure. They draw up 'hospital plans' and finance investment. The investments are paid for irrespective of actual ownership of the hospitals (Figure 4).

Figure 2

Health-related responsibilities and decision-making in Germany 1989 to 1990

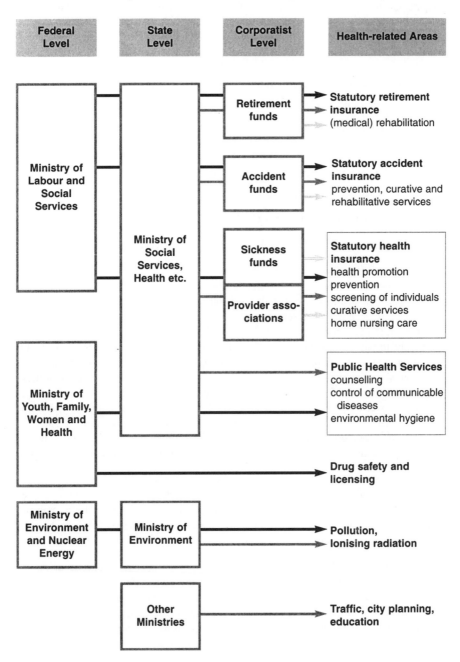

A second major responsibility of the Länder is the organisation of public health services. About 50% of the Länder operate these services themselves while the other half delegate responsibility to local authorities. While the specific tasks of the public health services and the level at which they are carried out differ, they generally include activities such as:

- supervision of employees in health care institutions,

- prevention and monitoring of communicable diseases,

- supervision of commercial activities involving food, pharmaceuticals and drugs,

- certain areas of environmental hygiene,

- counselling in health and social matters,

- providing community-oriented ('social') psychiatric services,

- health education and promotion, and

- physical examinations of school children and certain other groups.

There are approximately 360 public health offices which vary widely in size, structure and tasks.

In the first decades of the Federal Republic's history, the Länder defended their responsibility for public health services against several attempts by the Federal Government to extend its influence to this sector. However, in the 1980's they lessened their resistance and this led to the inclusion of several public health activities in the social code book. Originally, immunisation, mass screening for tuberculosis and other diseases, and health education and counselling were the responsibility of the public health services. However, since the 1970's, the social code book was extended to include many of these services. Similarly, since 1971, screening for cancer has been included in the package for women over 20 years of age and men over 45. At the same time, regular check-ups for children were introduced. Regular health check-ups were introduced in 1989 for sickness fund members over 35 years old. 1989 also saw the introduction of health promotion as a mandatory task for sickness funds (although this was abolished in 1996).

After health promotion and prevention was lost as a responsibility of the public health service, the service became less visible to the public and smaller: the number of physicians working in the service decreased from 4,900 in 1970 to 3,400 in 1995, over the same period the number of dentists in the public health service decreased from 2,500 to 900 and social workers from 4,000 to 2,600.[3]

Health reporting at all levels is still underdeveloped despite the existence of guidelines[4,5] and a common set of indicators.[6] Since the early 1990's, some states have published health reports on selected areas which can serve as models for the future. The reports from North Rhine-Westphalia[7] and Berlin[8] cover the widest spectrum. Currently, federal health reporting is beginning under the auspices of the Federal Statistical Office which comes under the jurisdiction of the Ministry for Internal Affairs.

Figure 3
Health-related responsibilities and decision-making in Germany since 1991

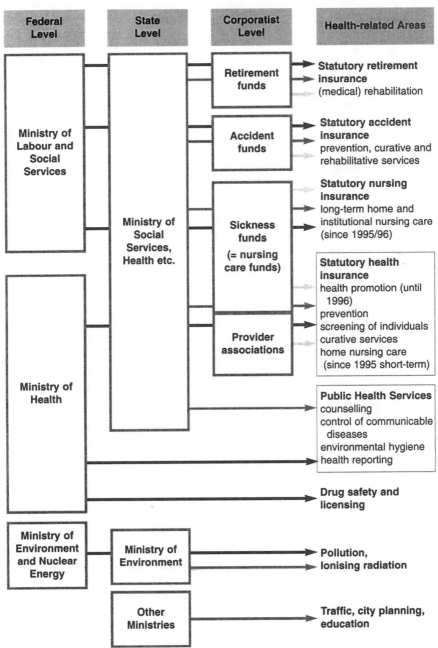

In addition, the Länder are responsible for undergraduate medical, dental and pharmaceutical education and the supervision of the sickness funds operating in the Land, the regional physicians' chamber (with mandatory membership for all physicians) and the regional physicians' association which represent the sickness fund-affiliated physicians (Figure 4).

The Länder coordinate their public health activities through the Working Group of Senior Health Officials (AGLMB) and the Conference of Health Ministers but both are unable to pass binding decisions. In addition, the Länder have established various joint institutions to enable them to perform certain tasks.[2] For example, the Länder of Berlin, Bremen, Hamburg, Hesse, Lower Saxony, North Rhine-Westphalia, and Schleswig-Holstein administer the Academy of Public Health Services in Düsseldorf which trains their public health physicians. Only Mecklenburg-Vorpommern and Saxony-Anhalt organise the training of public health physicians independently.

Corporate level

The corporate institutions on the payers' side, i.e. the sickness funds, have a central position within the statutory health insurance system. The SGB defines the responsibilities of the funds which include negotiating prices, quantities and quality assurance measures with the providers on behalf of all sickness fund members.

The inclusion of health promotion and disease prevention measures in the sickness funds' benefit catalogue, has also led to changes in the responsibilities for service provision. For health promotion, the sickness funds have been the main providers since 1989. However, until 1992, most sickness funds were quite reluctant to offer courses, programmes at work or to give support to self-help groups. With the introduction in the 1993 reform law of mandatory competition between sickness funds for members (as from 1 January 1996; Figure 4), sickness funds identified health promotion as the only area in which they could offer visibly different benefits to other funds. As a result, sickness funds' health promotion activities mushroomed and expenditure grew rapidly (from 600 million DM in 1992 to 1,300 million DM in 1995). The Health Minister used this increase as a pretext to introduce a 'Health Insurance Contribution Reduction Act' in mid-1996 through which health promotion as a sickness fund benefit was abolished from 1997 onwards. The '2nd Statutory Health Insurance Restructuring Act' of 1997 has given sickness funds the right to reintroduce parts of it, but it would have to be financed entirely by members and not through the regular contributions which are shared between employers and employees.

The corporate institutions on the provider side have to provide all direct acute health care services. The most prominent examples are the physicians' and dental physicians' associations which have both the 'Corporate Monopoly and Mission to Secure Ambulatory Care'.[9] This monopoly means that hospitals, communities, sickness funds and others do not have the right to offer ambulatory medical care. The mission includes the obligation to meet the health needs of the population, to guarantee provision of state-wide services in all medical specialities and to obtain a total budget from the sickness

Figure 4

Important missions, responsibilities and decision-making levels within the statutory health insurance system

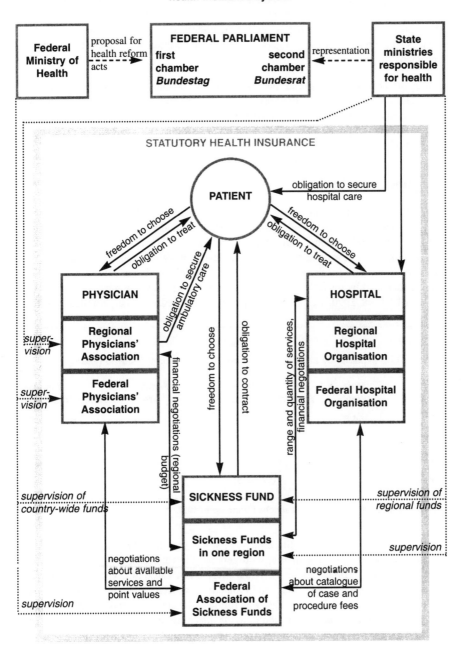

funds which the physicians' associations distribute among their members.[10] The ambulatory care physicians also control a large share of preventive services. For some services, they actually have a legal obligation (screening and check-ups) while for others the physicians are able to negotiate fees with the sickness funds (e.g. immunisations). Thus, preventive services are now delivered under the same regulations as curative services which means they are subject to negotiation between the sickness funds and the physicians' associations.

Due to the absence of corporate institutions in the hospital sector, hospitals contract individually with the sickness fund organisations. A regulation was included in the '2nd Statutory Health Insurance Restructuring Act' giving hospital organisations some legal powers without corporate status (for example, to negotiate the catalogue of prospective care and procedure fees).

The public's health

The public's health in Germany has to be analysed against the background of a 40-year national separation which provides an interesting case-study of changes in health due to political, social and economic influences on an otherwise homogeneous population. The most obvious indicator of differences in the development of public health in the West compared to the East is life expectancy at birth. This initially increased faster in the East but had stagnated by the late 1960s, since when it has continued to improve in the West. Between 1980 and 1990, the gap in life expectancy widened, especially for men (Table 1).

	Male West	Male East (difference)	Female West	Female East (difference)
Table 1 Life expectancy at birth in West and East Germany 1950–95 (years)				
1949/53	64.6	65.1 (+0.5)	68.5	69.1 (+0.6)
1980	69.9	68.7 (-1.2)	76.8	74.6 (-2.2)
1990	72.7	69.2 (-3.5)	79.2	76.3 (-2.9)
1993/95	73.5	70.7 (-2.8)	79.8	78.2 (-1.7)

Sources: McKee *et al.* 1996.[11], Statistisches Bundesamt 1997.[12]

For both sexes, those living in the East fared worse than their Western counterparts at all ages except the first year of life, with generally lower infant mortality rates in the East since the early 1960s (Table 2). When analysed by cause of death, by far the most important contributor to the difference in male life expectancy was circulatory disease, accounting for almost 1.5 years. This was followed by accidents and injuries, accounting for 0.9 years. The leading contributor to the difference in female life expectancy was also circulatory disease, accounting for around two years.[11]

Table 2

Infant mortality in West and East Germany 1950–95 (per 1,000 live births)

	Male West	Male East (difference)	Female West	Female East (difference)
1950	67.7	87.6 (+19.9)	52.0	68.7 (+16.7)
1961	37.6	39.5 (+1.9)	29.2	30.5 (+1.3)
1970	26.5	20.7 (-5.8)	19.8	16.5 (-3.3)
1980	14.5	14.2 (-0.3)	11.5	10.3 (-1.2)
1989/90	8.1	8.5 (+0.4)	6.1	5.9 (-0.2)
1995	5.9	6.0 (+0.1)	4.6	5.0 (+0.4)

Source: **Statistisches Bundesamt 1997.**[12]

Explanations for the widening gap between East and West include differences in diet, better living conditions in the West, differences in access to high technology care, better health care at all levels in the West, and selective migration of pensioners from East to West.[11]

Since unification, the gap in life expectancy and all-age mortality has narrowed (Tables 1 and 3), while infant mortality is now lower in the West than in the East (Table 2).

Table 3

All-age mortality in West and East Germany 1991–95, standardised to the West German population in 1970 (per 1,000)

	Male West	Male East (difference)	Female West	Female East (difference)
1991	8.9	11.4 (+2.5)	7.2	9.5 (+2.3)
1992	8.6	10.9 (+2.3)	7.0	8.8 (+1.8)
1993	8.6	10.7 (+2.1)	7.1	8.5 (+1.4)
1994	8.4	10.3 (+1.9)	6.9	8.2 (+1.3)
1995	8.3	10.0 (+1.7)	6.7	7.8 (+1.1)

Source: **Statistisches Bundesamt 1994, 1995, 1996, 1997.**[12]
Note: no pre-1991 data are available for East Germany.

In 1991, the unified Germany had a life expectancy which was slightly below the EU-12 average both at birth and at age 65. Death rates (standardised to the European population) were above EU average for diseases of the circulatory system (74.1 versus 62.4/100,000 for persons under 65) and for suicide and self-inflicted injury (15.4 versus 11.7/100,000 for all ages) while being at or around the EU average for malignant neoplasms and all external causes of injury and poisoning. Standardised death rates for motor vehicle traffic accidents are below EU average (12.9 versus 14.1/100,000 for all ages) but remain a problem in the East, especially among young males.[13] The incidence of AIDS has been stable since the early 1990s and is among the lowest in the EU (around 2.5 new cases per 100,000/year in 1996). On the other hand, dental diseases remain a problem with Germany having one of the highest DMFT (decayed, missing and filled teeth) index for 12-year-olds of all EU countries.

Decision-making and priority-setting

Due to the complex structure of the German political system and the separation of the health care system into different sectors, decision-making and priority-setting have to be discussed separately for each of the major parts of the system. Here we will deal with the most important sectors: public health services, health promotion and prevention, ambulatory medical and dental care, hospital care, and pharmaceuticals. Figure 4 summarises the important responsibilities and decision-making levels within the statutory health insurance.

Public health

As already mentioned, public health is mainly the responsibility of the Länder and is outside the scope of the social health insurance system. Priority-setting in public health does not figure very highly. Many Länder still operate within the 1935 law which regulates public health services and only one Land, North Rhine-Westphalia, has set targets for public health. Moreover, in no Land are the public health services or the ministries responsible for health truly 'public health agencies' involved in all areas of importance to the public's health, such as nutrition, housing, traffic, city planning or education.

Health promotion and prevention

Until 1988, sickness funds could voluntarily provide supportive measures such as preventive spa treatments for their members. Since 1989, these benefits have been included in the mandatory benefits catalogue which stems from the SGB as part of the standardisation of the benefits' catalogue.

Immunisations covered by the sickness funds are given by physicians in private practice who have the monopoly on delivering ambulatory services. The range of immunisations covered is determined by the sickness funds. However, all immunisations which are 'publicly recommended' by the Länder are usually covered. Immunisations carried out through the public health services are, therefore, only of minor importance for most citizens. Immunisation rates have been decreasing and, in 1996, the 'physicians' parliament' urged all physicians to increase immunisation activities.

The scope of screening examinations is determined at the federal level through negotiations between the sickness funds and physicians' associations. For example, in 1995, the screening for chlamydiae was included in ante-natal care and sonography of the hips was made obligatory within the screening programme for children. Mammography, however, has not been included in the core programme of cancer screening to date.

Encouraging people to participate in screening examinations is largely the task of the sickness funds. After a decrease in attendance in the mid-1980's, participation rates have been increasing. In 1994, in the western part of Germany, 49% of eligible women and 15% of eligible men participated. In the eastern part, the equivalent figures are 43% and 10% respectively. These rates vary widely between the different types of sickness funds which may indicate the importance of both socioeconomic status and the level of screening promotion by the funds. For children, the average participation rates for check-ups were 89% in the western part and 69% in the eastern part in 1995.[3]

Joint efforts in public health, health promotion and prevention – the AIDS example

Due to the complicated structure of public health, health promotion and prevention in Germany, joint efforts to tackle health problems are needed more than in other countries. A good example is the fight against AIDS.[14]

In March 1987 a central AIDS coordination Group was established to coordinate federal activities and also to establish an AIDS Centre to coordinate and support scientific research and public education and information. In addition, the Government provided funding for AIDS specialists to be employed at all public health offices. Lastly, the 1987 agreement called upon the Länder to establish a joint AIDS Commission with federal and local governments and to negotiate a long-term strategy for coordinated measures in their individual areas of responsibility. Shortly afterwards, the Länder Health Ministers held a special meeting at which they requested the Federal Government to cooperate closely with the Länder when implementing its planned measures. The voluntary reporting of AIDS cases was supplemented with a regulation making it mandatory for laboratories to report all cases of HIV-positive blood samples.

In the following years, many governmental and non-governmental institutions were involved including the Federal Ministry for Research and Technology, the Federal Centre for Health Education (providing mass communication programmes), the Paul Ehrlich Institute (developing diagnostic test methods), the German Institute for Medical Documentation and Information, the German Association of AIDS Self-Help Groups and the local AIDS self-help groups. Since 1993, self-help groups have been able to receive funding from the sickness funds according to the regulations for health promotion.

Medical and dental care

Ambulatory medical and dental care are the sectors in which the corporate institutions have the greatest power. The SGB concentrates mainly on regulating the framework, i.e. categories of benefits and scope of the negotiations between the sickness funds and the physicians' and dental physicians' associations. These negotiations determine both the financing mechanisms and the precise details of the ambulatory benefits package. As a general rule, both the scope of reimbursable services and the financing mechanisms are tightly regulated, sometimes legally but usually through negotiations between providers and sickness funds. All patients have free access to all physicians in private practice (Figure 4), i.e. both general practitioners and specialists. However, privately insured patients (around 9% of the population) usually enjoy benefits equal to or better than those of patients covered by statutory health insurance; although this depends on the insurance package chosen.

All services which are paid for by the sickness funds are listed in the 'Unified Value Scale' which also lists the number of points to be reimbursed. Examples are given in the following table (based on the 1996 version of the 'Unified Value Scale'):

Table 4	
The German Unified Value Scale for health services payments	
Service	*Number of points*
Basic fee per patient per 3 months	60–575 depending on specialty of physician and status of patient (working/retired)
Surcharge for regular care (per 3 months) by nephrologists for patients needing dialysis, oncologists for patients with cancer or rheumatologists for patients with rheumatoid arthritis	900
Consultation fee (practice)	50
Diagnosis and/or therapy of psychic disorder through Physician-patient conversation, duration at least 15 min.	450
Consultation fee (home visit)	400 (non urgent)/600 (urgent)
Ante-natal care per 3 months	1850
Cancer screening	260 (men)/310 (women)
Health check-up	780
ECG	250
Osteodensitometry	450

Internally, the physicians' associations modify the actual reimbursement through a 'Remuneration Distribution Scale' which is different for every physicians' association.

The 1989 Health Care Reform Act was an attempt to strengthen the purchasers' side by standardising and centralising all negotiating procedures. It was designed to improve the ability of collective negotiation committees to solve problems, especially the earlier imbalance between sickness funds and provider associations. The law introduced a series of obligations on the sickness funds to foster close and uniform cooperation, and it enhanced the status of the federal associations vis-à-vis the regional associations and the single sickness funds. In doing so, it ignored the fact that the most innovative and decisive developments had been produced cooperatively by executives from the regional associations of sickness funds and by physicians, which were then tested regionally and eventually adopted at national level. The numerous obligations for uniform and joint actions since 1989 proved to be an obstacle to the implementation of further innovations.[9]

Another impediment for innovation was the existence of predetermined budgets which were negotiated or set at the Land level (Figure 4): the physicians' representatives were reluctant to accept new services without an increase in total reimbursement which was legally fixed between 1993 and 1995. On the other hand, the sickness funds argued that the physicians provided too many services which were not mandatory. After a new 'Unified Value Scale' with more lump-sum fees had been introduced in 1996, which could reduce reimbursement for some specialities, the climate both within the physicians' associations and between them and the sickness funds deteriorated. Late in 1996, the Federal Physicians' Association proposed the removal of certain preventive and curative benefits from the benefits catalogue and to offer these services to the patients on a private billing basis (among them were regular check-ups, toxoplasmosis screening during pregnancy, mammography screening, acupuncture and genetic diagnostics).[15]

The most important body, at the national level, for the negotiations between sickness funds and physicians over the scope of benefits is the 'Federal Committee of Physicians and Sickness Funds' (Figure 4).[16] This committee has several sub-committees, one of which was responsible for making decisions on the effectiveness of new diagnostic and therapeutic methods until 1997. The 2nd Statutory Health Insurance Restructuring Act widened its mandate to the evaluation of technologies already included in the benefits catalogue. The sub-committee was then renamed the 'Medical Treatment Sub-committee' and passed new guidelines for its evaluation process. It remains to be seen whether this will lead to more rational decision-making. In the past, the inclusion of new services has often been determined more by informal decision-making, rather than by formal, often time-consuming mechanisms.[17] Another joint committee of physicians and sickness fund representatives makes decisions on the relative weight of all services in the ambulatory part of the benefits catalogue (the 'Unified Value Scale').

One weakness of the 'Unified Value Scale' is that it only lists services and not the indications which justify these services. This mechanism has preserved the comparatively high level of clinical freedom of German physicians which has been limited only by control mechanisms within the physicians' associations. Through these control mechanisms, physicians who claim more services of a certain kind than their colleagues have to justify these services to escape financial penalties.[18]

An area which has been directly regulated by law since 1993 is the number of ambulatory physicians who may treat sickness fund members (while every physician may treat private patients). An upper limit has been set for every major specialty for comparable cities and counties which is based on 110% of the average number in 1990.

Hospital care

The range of services provided in the hospital sector is determined by two factors: the hospital list of the State Government, and the negotiations between the sickness funds and each individual hospital. While the decision of the State Government determines the flow of capital for investment, the negotiations determine whether the costs for running the services are reimbursed by the sickness funds (Figure 4). These mechanisms have ensured the provision of hospital services without waiting lists except for transplantations and other highly specialised treatments.

After fighting against standards and guidelines for a long time, the scientific medical associations have recently begun to publish guidelines (such as Deutsche Gesellschaft für Innere Medizin 1996[19]). However, these guidelines are rather unsystematic and, perhaps more importantly, are influenced by technologies available in secondary and tertiary care setting, such as lung functioning tests for diagnosis of chronic bronchitis.

Pharmaceuticals

Regulations concerning the pharmaceutical market present a dichotomy. On the one hand, the distribution of drugs through wholesalers and pharmacies and their respective surcharges on ex-factory prices are regulated in great detail. On the other hand, the pharmaceutical industry is remarkably unregulated concerning pricing and the need to prove efficacy. The growing realisation that a significant proportion of drugs were of questionable value led to the introduction of the mandate for drug licensing in the 1976 Pharmaceutical Act. Prior to this, products only had to be registered with the Federal Health Office as drugs. Registration regulations only required minor examinations concerning possible toxic effects. However, the 1994 Pharmaceutical Act Amendment Law extended the deadline for licensing pharmaceuticals already on the market to the year 2005. Therefore, out of the estimated 56,000 pharmaceuticals available in Germany, only some 22,000 are currently approved as effective and without serious side effects.[20]

Federal legislation has mainly concentrated on cost-containment issues. The first step in attempts at reducing the impact of pharmaceutical expenditure on health care costs was the development of guidelines for reference prices for pharmaceuticals and the introduction of a limited 'negative list' in 1989. A second step was the introduction of significant cost-containment measures in 1993, i.e. a price cut for pharmaceuticals, higher co-payments by the patients and a spending cap on sickness funds' pharmaceutical expenditure.[21]

Some physicians' associations have recently initiated their own 'positive lists' and the Federal Physicians' Association passed recommendations to initiate far-reaching changes to the prescribing of pharmaceuticals. However, these could not be published as planned due to legal action taken by the pharmaceutical companies.[22] The 2nd

Statutory Health Insurance Restructuring Act has replaced the spending caps for pharmaceuticals by 'target amounts' per practice from 1998 onwards. In addition, the Federal Committee of Physicians and Sickness Funds is revising its pharmaceutical guidelines which will probably lead to more prescription exclusions.

The Advisory Council for Concerted Action in Health Care

As well as the major players, there are also advisory bodies in the field of health. The most prominent is the 'Advisory Council for Concerted Action in Health Care' which was formed in 1986. This committee consists of seven experts in the areas of medicine and economics appointed by the Federal Minister of Health following proposals by the states.

The tasks of the Advisory Council are: to analyse the development of the health care system and its medical and economic effects; to establish priorities for the reduction of health care deficits and existing excess health benefits, taking into account the current financial situation and available economic reserves; to propose data collection on medical and economic trends; and to suggest possibilities for further development of the health care system.[23]

In January 1993, the Health Minister requested the Advisory Council to prepare a report on the development of social health care provision for the next century and to give advice about possible future directions. The main questions to be addressed in this report were:[24]

1. What effects on the use and provision of health care are generated by demographic developments, changes in morbidity and medical and medical-technical advances?

2. Is it necessary to set ethically justifiable medical priorities and to limit benefits?

3. Which benefits should remain an essential part of the social health insurance after the year 2000? Are some benefits no longer justified for reasons of health and social policy based on the principle of solidarity and subsidiarity? Should new benefits be provided?

4. How can more incentives for prevention and promotion of a healthy lifestyle be incorporated into social health insurance?

5. Which are the medical and health-policy requirements which existing diagnostic and therapeutic procedures should meet?

In its 1994 interim report, the Advisory Council identified areas for health targets as a precondition for an outcome-oriented health care policy and grouped them into three categories: medical targets, strategies and areas of support. In 1995, it looked at two examples in more detail, ante-natal screening and care.

However, the Advisory Council mainly considered the financial situation of the health care system, contribution rate stability, and the four proposals for determining a new package of benefits.[25] All were based on a core package to be defined mainly by law and which would either explicitly exclude existing benefits or include only a certain range of defined benefits.

Around the core the sickness funds would develop a differentiated menu of tariffs with more choice for the consumer. In any case, the consumer would either have to pay for more co-insurance, for more co-payments or for more services not covered by the social health insurance. From a health system perspective, the measures would change the balance of health care power since the corporate bodies of both physicians and sickness funds would no longer be needed for negotiating the range of benefits. A weakness of these proposals was the inability of the Council to provide details about which benefits should be considered unnecessary, especially since the current Social Code Book specifically includes only 'necessary and economical measures'.

After identifying possible areas for health promotion and prevention in 1994, the Advisory Council recommended in 1995 that 'primary prevention in terms of both health promotion measures and general measures affecting the entire population should be financed from other sources',[26] for example, using the public health system for the prevention of communicable diseases but also using biology teachers to teach healthy nutrition or personal hygiene. However, individualised primary, secondary and tertiary prevention aimed at protecting people against infections, enabling early diagnosis and preventing the worsening of disease in individual patients were considered to be medical tasks and therefore an appropriate part of the social health insurance benefits.

In October 1995, the Health Minister asked the Advisory Council to produce a further special report examining the effects on employment and economic growth of expenditure and contribution-rate changes in the health care system and the statutory health insurance system. The first part of that report was delivered in October 1996 and analysed demographic and morbidity effects and trends, capacity for efficiency and the impact of the health care sector on employment.[27]

Regarding the influence of the Advisory Council, the support of the Minister and the political parties which have to take up its proposals has weakened. This reflects the current political priorities on health which are often more concerned with financial issues than improving the public's health.

Research

As the role of federal authorities in health care decision-making about individual health care technologies and health care delivery is very limited, the funding of research to produce evidence about diseases, technologies and health care structures is one of the few possibilities for the Federal Government to influence the decision-making process of the corporate institutions.

Health research primarily occurs within the 36 university medical faculties in collaboration with related departments. University-based health research is supplemented by non-university health research at National Research Centres and federal and state institutes.

The two most important ministries which fund health research are the Federal Ministry for Research and Technology (BMFT) and the Federal Ministry for Health (BMG). In 1993, they spent around 780 million DM for basic funding of the non-university research institutions and around 280 million DM for project funding in the area of health research.

The funding priorities of the BMG are promoting health, controlling disease, health care, and health insurance.[28]

BMFT's health research funding aims 'to foster health and to control disease'[29] and focuses on prevention and preventive care, disease control and health services. Initially, it was purely oriented towards funding individual projects. Since the late 1980s, it has also aimed at correcting the structural weaknesses of health research which have been identified by institutions like the German Research Association and the German Science Council.

The BMFT has funded five public health research associations since 1992. The associations are based in Berlin, Hannover (North German Research Association), jointly in Bielefeld and Düsseldorf (Northrhine-Westphalian Research Association), Munich (Bavarian Research Association), and Dresden (Research Association Saxony). They are built around the postgraduate programmes in public health in these cities. While it is still too early to judge the impact of the individual projects on decision-making and priority-setting processes, public health as a whole is increasingly being recognised both inside and outside the science community.[30]

Conclusions and prospects

While there is evidence of joint efforts to solve problems or to tackle specific areas of public health interest, there is generally inadequate coordination of services so that specific improvements in the public's health or the achievement of health objectives in the area of health care can be achieved. Ambulatory and hospital services are, for example, not coordinated – except for the attempt to coordinate planning for high technology which was abolished in 1997. In addition, the scientific basis of existing health care services and often for newly introduced ones is, as in other countries, often weak or non-existent. However, the Federal Ministry for Health has realised this situation and, in response, commissioned a report which gathers information on effectiveness and outcomes research and health technology assessment in four EU and two North American countries and which makes recommendations for strengthening these activities in Germany.[31]

Health objectives and targets gained (renewed) attention early in 1997 by the sickness funds which are looking for new tools to be used for competition. Schönbach – a senior manager of the Federal Association of Company-based Sickness Funds – proposed that sickness funds set their own individual health care targets which they should try to pursue through managed care and disease management tools.[32] Health system analysts supported the use of health care targets by the sickness funds but argued for common targets on which sickness funds' performance may be judged.[33]

Meanwhile, the Advisory Council elaborated on its earlier proposals in its 1997 report.[34] It incorporated the idea of an outcome-orientation in reimbursement schemes to promote the pursuit of outcome-oriented health care,[33,35] i.e. to modify existing input- and process-oriented remunerations (e.g. budgets and fee-for-service) by the degree to which a provider (or providers in a given region) reach defined targets. This will, hopefully, integrate the improvement of public health into health care on a regular institutionalised basis.

Acknowledgement: The authors wish to thank Gunta Nickel for the excellent technical preparation of the figures.

References

1.   Busse R, Howorth C, Schwartz F W. The future development of a rights based approach to health care in Germany: more rights or fewer? In: Lenaghan J (ed.) *Hard Choices in Health Care – Rationing and Rights in Europe.* London: BMJ Publishing Group, 1997: 21–47.

2.   Federal Ministry for Health. *Health care in Germany – the health care system in the Federal Republic of Germany.* Bonn, 1994.

3.   Bundesminister für Gesundheit. *Daten des Gesundheitswesens.* Baden-Baden: Nomos, 1997.

4.   AGLMB (Arbeitsgemeinschaft der Leitenden Ministerialbeamten der Länder). *Gesundheitsberichterstattung der Länder – Konzept, Themen, Pilotbericht.* Hamburg, 1989.

5.   Forschungsgruppe Gesundheitberichtserstattung. *Aufbau einer Gesundheitsberichterstattung – Bestandaufnahme und Konzeptvorschlag.* Sankt Augustin: Asgard (in 3 volumes), 1990.

6.   AGLMB (Arbeitsgemeinschaft der Leitenden Ministerialbeamten der Länder). *Indikatorensatz für den Gesundheitsrahmenbericht der Länder.* 1991.

7.   MAGS (Ministerium für Arbeit, Gesundheit und Soziales des Landes Nordrhein-Westfalen). *Gesundheitsreport Nordrhein-Westfalen 1994.* Bielefeld: Institut für Dokumentation und Information, Sozialmedizin und öffentliches Gesundheitswesen, 1994.

8.   Senatsverwaltung für Gesundheit. *Jahresgesundheitsbericht 1994.* Berlin, 1995.

9.   Schwartz FW, Busse R. Germany. In: Ham C (ed.) *Health Care Reform: Learning from International Experience.* Buckingham-Philadelphia: Open University Press, 1997:104-18.

10. Schwartz FW, Busse R. Fixed Budgets in the German Ambulatory Care Sector. In:

Schwartz FW, Glennerster H, Saltman RB (eds.) *Fixing Health Budgets – Experience from Europe and North America*. Chichester: Wiley & Sons, 1996:87-108.

11. McKee M, Chenet L, Fulop N, Hort A, Brand H, Caspat W, Bojan F. Explaining the health divide in Germany: contribution of major causes of death to the difference in life expectancy at birth between East and West. *Zeitschrift für Gesundheitswissenschaften* 1996;4: 214–24.

12. Statistisches Bundesamt. *Statistisches Jahrbuch 1997.* Stuttgart: Metzler Poeschel, 1997. [published annually].

13. European Commission. *The State of Health in the European Community*. Luxembourg: Office for Official Publications of the European Communities, 1996.

14. Federal Ministry of Health. *The Fight Against AIDS in the Federal Republic of Germany*. Bonn, 1993.

15. Irrimmel L. *Kostenerstattung und Individuelle Gesundheitsleistungen*. Köln: Deutscher Ärzte-Verlag, 1998.

16. Busse R, Schwartz FW. Herausforderungen an den Bundesausschuß der Ärzte und Krankenkassen. *Arbeit & Sozialpolitik* 1997;51(11/12):51-57 (English abstract: p.7).

17. Schwartz FW. Die Rolle formeller und informeller Beratungsgremien bei der Implementation neuer Technologien im deutschen Gesundheitswesen. In: Schölmerich P (ed.) *Fortschritte in der Medizin und Erwartungen der Gesellschaft*. Stuttgart-Jena-New York: Gustav Fischer Verlag, 1995:255–67.

18. Henke K-D, Murray MA, Ade C. Global budgeting in Germany: lessons for the United States. *Health Affairs* 1994;13(4):7–21.

19. Deutsche Gesellschaft für Innere Medizin. *Rationelle Diagnostik und Therapie in der Inneren Medizin*. München: Urban & Schwarzenberg, 1996f.

20. Schwabe U, Paffrath D (eds.) *Arzneiverordnungs–Report '96*. Stuttgart-Jena: G. Fischer, 1996:15.

21. Busse R, Howorth C. Germany's Spending Cap for Pharmaceuticals – Effects on Cost and Quality. In: Schwartz FW, Glennerster H, Saltman RB (eds.). *Fixing Health Budgets – Experience from Europe and North America*. Chichester: Wiley & Sons, 1996:109–27.

22. KBV (Kassenärztliche Bundesvereinigung). Die KBV informiert. *Deutsches Ärzteblatt* 1996;93:B2210.

23. Advisory Council (for the Concerted Action in Health Care). *Health Care and Health Insurance 2000. Individual-responsibility, Subsidiarity and Solidarity in a Changing Environment*. Expert Opinion Report 1994 (abbreviated English version). Bonn, 1994. Complete version in German: Sachverständigenrat für die Konzertierte Aktion im Gesundheitswesen. *Gesundheitsversorgung und Krankenversicherung 2000. Eigenverantwortung, Subsidiarität und Solidarität bei sich ändernden Rahmenbedingungen*. Baden-Baden: Nomos, 1994:52.

24. Advisory Council (for the Concerted Action in Health Care), *Op. cit*, 1994:5.

25. Advisory Council (for the Concerted Action in Health Care), *Op. cit,* 1994:36ff.

26. Advisory Council (for the Concerted Action in Health Care). *Health Care and Health Insurance 2000. A Closer Orientation towards Results, Higher Quality Services and Greater Economic Efficiency.* Summary and Recommendations of the Special Expert Report 1995. Bonn, 1995. Complete version in German: Sachverständigenrat für die Konzertierte Aktion im Gesundheitswesen. *Gesundheitsversorgung und Krankenversicherung 2000. Mehr Ergebnisorientierung, mehr Qualität und mehr Wirtschaftlichkeit.* Baden-Baden: Nomos, 1995:21.

27. Advisory Council (for the Concerted Action in Health Care). *The Health Care System in Germany: Cost Factor and Branch of the Future. Vol. I: Demographics, Morbidity, Efficiency Reserves and Employment. Special Report 1996* – Summary. Bonn, 1996. Complete version in German: *Sachverständigenrat für die Konzertierte Aktion im Gesundheitswesen (1996). Gesundheitswesen in Deutschland: Kostenfaktor und Zukunftsbranche. Band 1.* Baden-Baden: Nomos. 1996.

28. BMFT (German Federal Ministry for Research and Technology). *Health Research 2000.* Bonn, 1994:132f.

29. BMFT (German Federal Ministry for Research and Technology). *Health Research 2000.* Bonn, 1994:15.

30. Schwartz FW, Badura B, Leidl R, Raspe H, Siegrist J (eds.). *Das Public Health Buch: Gesundheit und Gesundheitswesen.* München-Wien-Baltimore: Urban & Schwarzenberg, 1998.

31. Bitzer E, Busse R, Dörning H, Duda L, Köbberling J, Kohlmann T, Lühmann D, Pasche S, Perleth M, Raspe H, Reese E, Richter K, Röseler S, Schwartz FW: *Bestandaufrahme, Bewertung und Vorbereitung der Implementation einer Datensammlung 'Evaluation medizinischer Verfahren und Technologien' in der Bundesrepublik.* Health Technology Assessment Volume 1. Baden-Baden: Nomos, 1998.

32. Schönbach K-H. Marktorientierung der Krankenkassen. *Die Betriebskrankenkasse* 1997;85(1):9–17.

33. Busse R, Wismar M. Funktionen prioritärer Gesundheitsziele für Gesundheitssysteme. *Arbeit & Sozialpolitik* 1997;51(3/4):27–36 (English abstract: p. 6).

34. Advisory Council (for the Concerted Action in Health Care). *The Health Care System in Germany: Cost Factor and Branch of the Future. Vol. II: Progress and Growth Markets, Finance and Remuneration. Special Report 1997* – Summary. Bonn, 1997. Complete version in German: Sachverständigenrat für die Konzertierte Aktion im Gesundheitswesen. *Gesundheitswesen in Deutschland: Fortschritt und Wachstumsmärkte, Finanzierung und Vergütung. Band 2.* Baden-Baden: Nomos, 1997.

35. Schwartz FW, Haase I, Busse R. Erfolgsorientierung – Eine neue Dimension in der Vergütungsdiskussion. *Arbeit & Sozialpolitik* 1995;49(5/6):29–34.

6

Public Health Policies and Priorities in Greece

E Petridou, E Mossialos, G Papoutsakis, Y Skalkidis,
Y Tountas, A Velonaki and E Velonakis

Introduction

Greece's health system is characterised by a surplus of specialists and a deficit of primary health care services. The latter are mainly provided by the outpatient departments of hospitals and a network of state-employed, but mostly transiently serving and inexperienced, physicians in the rural areas. Likewise, public health services in this country have never reached the level of development that citizens of other European Member States have long enjoyed.

The Greek health care system is confusing and confused, corroded by special interests, exploited by powerful groups and yet quite generous. It is surprisingly more human than the health care systems in other developed countries and, apparently, quite effective with respect to ultimate outcome criteria. Despite deficiencies in the health care delivery, health indicators in Greece are among the best in the world.

Information included in this chapter has been derived from a number of reports and papers. Moreover, interviews were conducted with leading experts in health policy from the government and the opposition, senior public servants and academics.

This chapter is divided into four parts. The first part describes the decision-making process in developing priorities in health policy. Part two focuses on and analyses specific policies and priorities including official priorities, inequalities in health and health services and the provision of health care, community care and preventive services. Part three examines the regulation of technology and technology assessment. Finally, part four discusses the need for developing a coherent public health policy in Greece and suggests a number of policy objectives.

Developing priorities in health policy

The Ministry of Health and Welfare is responsible for over 90 per cent of activities relating to health. Figure 1 illustrates the decision-making process concerning health policy developments. Several other Ministries and Agencies are involved in various direct or indirect ways: the Ministry of Defence is responsible for medical care of the Armed Forces, the Ministry of Education for school health education, the Ministry of Environment for air pollution monitoring and control, the Ministry of Labour for health in the workplace and occupational safety, the Ministry of Energy, Technology and Research for a large segment of biomedical research, the Ministry of Commerce for consumer protection, the Ministry of Agriculture for pesticide control, the Ministry of Transportation for driving licensing and the Greek Standardisation Organisation (ELOT) for setting and approving standards etc.

Greece has numerous health committees; most of them are established on an ad hoc basis, but there are also Standing Committees concerned with some major health issues like AIDS and other communicable diseases, drugs or health promotion (Committee of Health Education Planning), which have an inter-ministerial component.

Parliamentary committees are frequently established in order to gather information and develop technological expertise to be used in framing legislation.

There is a Directorate for Foreign Relations at the Ministry of Health, responsible for international contacts. According to a former President of the Central Scientific Health Council (KESY), the Directorate is understaffed and is unable to meet the standards imposed by the international nature of many of the missions of the Ministry and required within the EU and is understaffed.

Relationship between policy development at the national, regional and local levels

In the early 1980s KESY was established with a mission to develop national health and health services plans. KESY was supposed to be largely independent from the Ministry of Health; however, it has lost many of its privileges and responsibilities over the last ten years. Currently, it is an administrative rather than scientific body and usually considers routine issues that are forwarded at the discretion of the Ministry. Decisions made by KESY are not binding.

Many legislative initiatives have been named 'national health plans' by the respective ministries, or even governments, but the only scientifically based and reasonably complete plan was prepared almost 20 years ago.[1] Many subsequent efforts have never been completed. However, the problem with the national health plans, complete or incomplete, is that they rarely influence the decisions of political leaders. The regionalisation of health services was planned in 1979 but never implemented. More recently, the country has been divided into major administrative divisions that have a substantial

Figure 1
The decision-making process in health policy development

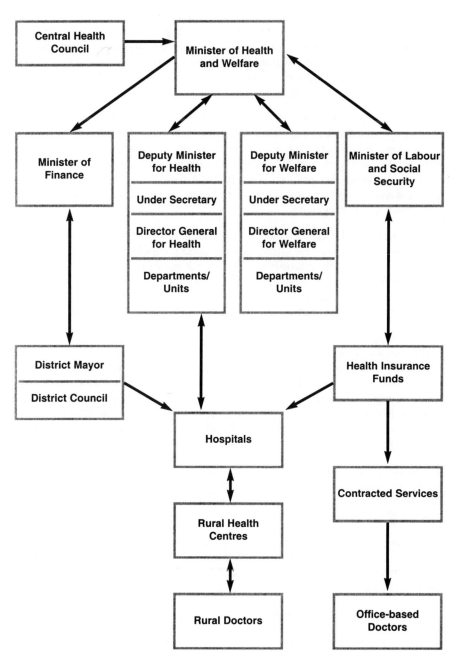

degree of independence even in matters related to health. Whether this new effort will be more successful than the earlier one remains to be seen.

The process of policy development and priority setting is mostly determined by negotiation, frequently non-transparent, between groups that possess considerable political or monopolistic power. This is not to say that decisions are irrational, contradictory or incompatible with objectively-defined health priorities. However, there is no tradition in Greece of using objectively-defined health criteria in order to develop priorities, and cost effectiveness is not usually considered.

A typical example is that the widely-heralded law establishing a national health system, that was presented as being modelled on the British National Health System, does not focus on prevention and is mainly concerned with career trajectories and compensation to hospital medical personnel. When preventive services are instituted, this is usually in response to public pressure. Nevertheless, basic preventive services are eventually provided and the system is reasonably accessible and in some areas, such as childhood immunisations, quite effective.

Regionalisation and decentralisation are recognised as important issues in Greece and several political leaders have attempted to promote them.[2] However, there are major obstacles, including poor data on needs and demands and concentration of health professionals, particularly medical doctors, in large cities and tertiary health centres. Several communities have instituted screening programmes although many of them did not meet the WHO criteria for continuity and integration with other components of the health system.

AIDS educational programmes and other health promoting activities have been initiated by local governments, but again few of these programmes have remained active over a long period. WHO-initiated programmes, for example 'Healthy Cities', have been received enthusiastically, but never evaluated. It seems unlikely for the moment, that any city in Greece is becoming much healthier than previously, and certainly not on account of these programmes. It will also be difficult in the future to attribute any positive changes to the project since there is practically no concurrent evaluation.

In the context of health-related research and action programmes, regions and local governments can liaise at a national level. However, such liaison activities are unusual and exceptional. Ultimately, however, it may be that the influence of the European Union will eventually modify that attitude.

The University of Crete has undertaken certain research activities. Health services research is also carried out by the Department of Hygiene and Epidemiology of the University of Athens, the National School of Public Health and other scientific associations and institutions.

The role of research-based evidence

Most research projects in Greece are supposed to indicate how the results of the project will influence development and policy issues in their respective fields. However, there is no evidence that this has ever been formally done in the health field. Nevertheless, Greece is somewhat unusual in that the right decisions are often taken through unusual processes or for the wrong reason. Thus, publicity, even disproportional publicity, about the health effects of air pollution has led to government-initiated corrective measures. The early introduction of widespread vaccination against hepatitis B was in response to the realisation that chronic active hepatitis and liver cancer are very common in the country. Perhaps more importantly, a very successful programme for the control of thalassaemia through prenatal diagnosis and identification of heterozygotes has been initiated in response to extensive research work on thalassaemia by Greek and other investigators.

Consumer and other interest group involvement

Public debate on health issues in Greece is mainly between political parties, the health professional associations and the trade unions. Spontaneous mobilisation of large segments of the population is rare in Greece and most people take either the party line or follow the narrow priorities associated with their own profession.

Trade unions are frequently involved in negotiations concerning health benefits and their insurance coverage. Members of central governing boards sit on the KESY Executive Board and other health committees together with representatives of the Greek Orthodox Church. Patients' associations are gradually acquiring increased power. Among these associations, the most influential are those of 'Kidney Failure Sufferers', 'Haemophiliacs', 'Thalassaemics', 'Spastic Societies' and 'Families of Children with Cancer'.

Budget setting and implementing priorities

The budget of the Ministry of Health is formulated principally in negotiations with the Minister of Financial Affairs. Within a given budget, it is theoretically possible for the Minister of Health to transfer resources from secondary to primary care, but in practice this is very difficult. There is increasing demand for secondary health services caused in part by the ageing of the Greek population, and hospital budgets are not flexible. During recent years the overall health budget has been increased moderately in an effort to strengthen primary health.

Some major changes may require legislative measures but the Minister of Health and Welfare has wide scope to make administrative decisions. In any case, the development of primary health services almost always requires satisfactory levels of management and marketing as well as assurance of consumer participation.

The main incentive for shifting emphasis to primary care, a common objective for all governments since 1975, has been the overproduction of medical doctors and a restriction of available positions for medical training in hospital-associated specialties. Many rural primary care centres have also been established and minimal financial incentives for doctors to staff them have been provided. The main obstacle has been the tradition for Greek patients to approach directly a specialist without referral from a primary care physician. Perceptions about the superior competence of specialists versus that of generalists have been an additional hindrance to shifting emphasis from secondary to primary health care.

The total health budget is divided into running expenses and capital investment. It cannot exceed a specific percentage of the total budget of the country. However, the actual ceiling can be negotiated and depends on the balance of political power among ministers. Specific items in the health budget are derived from the amount specified in the budget of the previous year with revisions, which must be justified, submitted by the directors of the various departments of the ministry, the governing boards of hospitals and other institutions reporting to the Ministry of Health.

Following the recent creation of major administrative regions in the country with an increased level of financial independence, the regions can now directly submit their own budgets. These cover their own running expenses, excluding those of hospitals, but including running expenses of personnel employed in the peripheral headquarters, as well as earmarked allocations for health emergencies and specific health programmes in response to local demand. In spite of this partial decentralisation, most demand for primary and secondary care is covered by the central budget and under the control of the ministry.

Despite efforts to introduce more objective processes, it is essentially the Minister of Health who decides the allocation of the health budget between primary and secondary care and specific institutions. Authorities in peripheral regions can submit their budgets directly to the Ministry of Financial Affairs but shortfalls, which are the rule rather than the exception, are covered by the Ministry of Health. The Ministry of Commerce takes the lead when purchase of major technological equipment for the hospitals is required, according to requests submitted by the governing boards of the public hospitals.

Regional financing is made on the basis of the projected expenses for salaries and other inflexible expenses of the Regional Health Authorities. Supplementary financing may be awarded by the Ministry of Health if requests fall within programmes covered by the budget or with executive action of the minister for retrospective coverage of expenses with transfer of funds among the budget items. There are no health indicator-based prospective formulae for resource allocation and, as indicated, allocation is guided by previous patterns that can be revised under exceptional circumstances or on the basis of political dynamics and spontaneously by public pressure.

At the national level, decisions are made by the leadership of the Ministry of Health following requests submitted by peripheral regions and recommendations by the responsible ministry personnel. At present, however, there is a tendency to foster the independence of the peripheral regions which are encouraged to submit adequately justified region-specific budgets to the Ministry of Financial Affairs. Parliamentary representatives influence changes in the regional allocation of resources, on the basis of political rather than health indices-derived criteria.

Capital developments are funded from the national budget, taking into account regional priorities with respect to primary or secondary health care. Considerations for capital development funds are: region-specific developmental priorities, in theory special health-related needs and, in practice, political influence. The European Union is an important source of capital development funds.

Major acquisitions of new equipment and technologies – mostly through imports – requires approval from the Ministry of Commerce in what is usually a time-consuming process. Investment in the private sector is not restricted, provided it respects legislation for public health employment and protection of the environment. However, legislation is very prohibitive for the operation of new privately owned hospitals. According to OECD, public spending for health was 5.9 per cent of GNP in 1996. However, data from the national accounts indicate that health care expenses for 1992 were 8.29 per cent of GNP, 60 per cent of which were provided by the state and 40 per cent from private sources. A large section of private health spending is believed to be channelled outside the formal taxation system.

Non-governmental organisations, insurance companies, the pharmaceutical industry and other interest groups can influence components of the health budget but most of the influence is exercised outside formal channels. The degree of influence is a function of political connections, access to the media and public sensitivity to the issues invoked by the particular group, person or company.

Policies and priorities in practice

Official health priorities

There have been no comprehensive official health targets set by the government, and one of the health experts interviewed by us has interpreted this as a manifestation of a rather unrealistic attitude: 'let's just do as well as we can'. In defence of the Greek attitude, it should be pointed out that over the last 20 years infant mortality has been declining fast and is now less than 10/1000 live births, and death rates from major disease categories, including cancer and cardiovascular diseases are among the lowest in Europe. Therefore, citizens and politicians alike have been preoccupied with processes like elimination of waiting lists and coverage of marginal services such as skin grafting.

Only recently, has there been such an emphasis on some of the key health status issues, in particular the major problem of the high level of injury morbidity and mortality. The Centre for Research and Prevention of Injuries among the Young has been established in the Department of Hygiene and Epidemiology, Athens University Medical School. Administrative structures have also been established for the control of drugs and communicable diseases. Previous implicit objectives such as adequate vaccination rates of children, elimination of zoonoses and reduction of thalassaemic births through primary or secondary prevention have largely been accomplished.

There have been no official discussion documents on priorities, the Greek attitude being to address problems once they arise or as they are recognised with notable disregard of cost effectiveness considerations. 'Health for All' and 'Europe against Cancer' have been widely discussed but mostly in academic circles. Nevertheless, under the pressure of the international community, successive Greek governments have taken steps to control the tobacco epidemic which is particularly acute in Greece. However, the per capita tobacco consumption in Greece still remains higher than in any other European country. Healthy eating has also been considered during the last few years.

Health professional associations have been supportive of prioritising health problems so long as these priorities do not impinge upon their narrowly defined interests or political objectives. Single issue pressure groups (for instance, the Association of Patients with Kidney Failure) have been generally successful because health demands are rarely considered in competition with other real or perceived health needs.

Formal evaluations of health initiatives have not been undertaken on a large scale. Academic groups regularly point out successes in particular areas, whereas concerned professionals warn continuously about two major health-related 'epidemics', those of tobacco smoking and of injuries. As a general rule, government and opposition provide different evaluations of the processes related to delivery of services.

Inequalities in health and health services

The focus of concern is on inequalities in health care rather than on health.[3-5] Inequality in health status is not a major issue, perhaps because rural populations have, with a few exceptions, better health indicators than those of urban residents despite the fewer services made available to them.[6-10] There are very large variations in the quantity and quality of provision in different parts of the country, only partly due to the way in which the population makes use of the services. Inequalities of health services, however, are frequently considered, particularly in respect to the contrast between the major urban centres and the peripheral regions or between groups with different health coverage.

In 1994, expenditure from the public health budget varied from 18,310 drachmas per head in Central Greece to 43,124 drachmas in Attica.[3] While there was one doctor working in a health centre per 1,510 persons in Attica, there was one doctor per 3,284 persons in the Peloponnese. The provision of hospital beds varied from 2.9 per 10,000 in Western Greece to 6.9 in Attica. Social differentials in morbidity and mortality are not major issues, perhaps because relevant health statistics are not available. Two important issues that dominate the public debate are health coverage of migrants, particularly illegal migrants, and the widely considered need to 'oil' the system in order to get prompt service or bypass waiting lists.

The Greek health system has in general been responsive to the need to reduce inequalities, although the focus has been on inequalities in health care rather than on health and its social determinants. Part of the problem is that documentation of health needs has been more difficult than documentation of availability of health care services because of the lack of tradition and respect in the country for high quality health statistics. This situation now appears to be changing.[11]

The power of resource allocation as a tool to address health and socioeconomic inequalities is recognised but it is exercised in response to more readily documented socioeconomic inequalities than to health variations. What is lacking in Greece in this context is an organised voluntary sector. Corrective measures are expected solely from the government and even large organisations like the Red Cross depend on government subsidies.

Basic facts – implied priorities and coverage of health care services

More than half of the Greek population are covered by the General Security System (IKA) and another 30 per cent are covered by two other major health funds (OGA for insurance of the rural population and TEBE for small businessmen). There are also many more health funds for the remaining population and a small percentage including indigents have only in-patient care. Health coverage varies, being more extensive for public servants and banking system employees as well as for employees of the telecommunications (OTE) and of the electrical power system. However, the IKA is also remarkably comprehensive, covering long-term care, mentally ill, optical tests, pharmaceuticals, dental care (excluding sophisticated prosthetics) as well as most specific interventions including kidney dialysis, in vitro fertilisation and organ transplantation. There is no coverage for homeopathy and some forms of cosmetic surgery. A nominal contribution on the part of the insured person is usually required but it can be as high as 25 per cent for less essential services. There are lists of recommended drugs but no drug is specifically excluded. With the exception of indigents, coverage is least extensive among those who are insured in TEBE or OGA. Lastly, TEBE pensioners are switched to IKA when they retire.

There are variations in the extent of coverage. Over the last 25 years, successive governments have failed in their intention to integrate the health sectors of the social security funds. Differences in social care reflect the extent of coverage with respect to health care. In most cases insured persons can transfer their rights between different health funds.

When a patient receives treatment in another country he is compensated if there has been prior authorisation by senior Greek medical professionals, or if proof is otherwise provided that there was a need for such an intervention. Concern has been frequently expressed that the flow of patients for treatment to other countries is largely unjustified.

Provision of health care services

Health care in Greece is provided by the National Health System, the public and private insurance organisations and the private sector.[12] The National Health System was established in 1983 and consists of primary, secondary and tertiary care. Primary care is provided by a network of 170 rural health centres which work in conjunction with 1,311 rural health stations. Primary care in the urban areas is provided by the outpatient departments of the public hospitals. Secondary care is provided by the general hospitals located in almost every one of the 52 Prefectures of Greece. These hospitals all have basic medical specialties. Tertiary care is provided by the university hospitals of the seven medical schools of the country, as well as by the regional hospitals. Most of the tertiary care is concentrated in the Greater Athens area or Thessaloniki.

From the rural stations and the health centres, cases in need of hospitalisation are referred to the secondary or tertiary care hospitals according to need, following a formal referral procedure. There is relatively free choice of doctors and hospitals, so patients are able to seek care in hospitals other than those of their Prefecture or Region.

There are 370 social insurance funds in Greece.[13] About forty of these provide medical coverage in addition to a wide range of social services. There are wide variations in quality and distribution of care between these funds. As indicated, 93 per cent of the population is covered by the six most important insurance organisations. The largest insurance organisation of the public sector is IKA, with 5.3 million persons insured out of the 10,260,000 total population of Greece. IKA has its own network of health services. It has 105 polyclinics at district and regional level and 137 local surgeries. IKA employs 6,900 medical personnel and 2,500 nursing personnel.

Primary care. Primary care within the Greek National Health System is provided by the rural health stations, the rural health centres and the outpatient departments of the hospitals. Primary care is also provided by the polyclinics of insurance organisations. Furthermore, there are private doctors who are private contractors of insurance organisations and accept insured patients in their private surgeries.

Non-specialist care. Within primary care settings there are specialist doctors such as internal medicine specialists, paediatricians, cardiologists, etc. As the specialty of general medicine was only recently established by law, there are few general medicine practitioners in Greece.

Dental care. Dental care within the Greek National Health System covers fully only those aged 0 to 18 years. The remaining population groups are offered merely emergency dental care. IKA offers a wide range of dental care free at the point of delivery to all age groups; however, in general, the services are not considered to be of high quality. Other insurance organisations cover dental care irrespective of age, but the level of out-of-pocket contributions differs according to the insurance organisation.

Distribution of pharmaceuticals. Pharmaceuticals are distributed through the pharmacies which are all private enterprises. The public obtain the pharmaceuticals after paying an out-of-pocket contribution which differs according to the insurance organisation; the pharmacies are reimbursed by the insurance organisations. A large proportion of pharmaceuticals do not require a doctor's prescription, and can be bought over the counter. In such cases the patients have to cover the whole cost.

Optician services. As with pharmacists, opticians are private professionals outside the

National Health System. The insurance organisations cover a variable proportion of the cost of optician services.

In-patient care. In-patient care services are provided by a total of 414 hospitals with an overall capacity of 53,388 beds. Within the National Health System there are 128 hospitals (119 general, 9 psychiatric). In 1996, the mean duration of hospitalisation for the general hospitals is 5.9 days, while for the psychiatric hospitals it is 119 days. The annual bed occupancy rate was 69 per cent and 97 per cent respectively.

There are 37 public hospitals outside the National Health System, with a mean hospitalisation duration of 10.5 days, and bed coverage of 63 per cent. In the private sector there are 249 hospitals (209 general, 40 psychiatric). Currently, the mean duration of hospitalisation for the general private hospitals is 9.1 days and the bed coverage is 47 per cent. The mean duration of hospitalisation in the private psychiatric hospitals is 97 days.

On average, there are 5.2 hospital beds per 1,000 population and 12.6 hospital admissions per year. Hospitalisation per person is 1.1 days, and the overall mean duration of hospitalisation is 9.8 days. It has to be noted that there are great geographical variations in the availability of hospital services, as well as variation between the public and the private sector. More than 60 per cent of the hospital beds and manpower are located in the Greater Athens area. Also, the mean number of days of hospitalisation for the private general hospitals is 9.1 days, while the corresponding figure for the National Health System general hospitals is 5.9 days. In the public sector the ratio of doctors to beds is 1:2, and the ratio of nurses to beds is 1:1. In the private sector the corresponding figures are 1:5 and 1:3.

Community care services

Long stay in-patient services – mentally ill and mentally handicapped, physically handicapped, elderly. These categories of services are provided mainly by the private sector. Within the public sector there is a National Rehabilitation Centre for the physically handicapped, and a few residential institutions for the aged. More institutes for the aged are offered by the voluntary sector or the church. For the mentally ill there are nine hospitals of the National Health System, two outside the National Health System, and 40 private hospitals.

Day care centres: There is a limited number of day care centres for children of employees of Hospitals within the National Health System, but the vast majority of day care centres are under the auspices of the Patriotic Institution of Social Welfare and Insurance (PIKPA), the National Welfare Organisation EOP, the municipalities, the Ministry of Education or they are licensed on a private basis.

Social services: For the elderly, there are Open Care Centres (KAPI) in every municipality, which are popular and successful.

Services for children: Apart from maternal and child health services provided by the system, services for children are delivered free of charge by PIKPA and the polyclinics of some municipalities as well as by the 48 Units of Maternal and Child Health and the ten Family Planning Centres for those insured in IKA. Moreover, immunisations are provided by the 54 regional health departments of the respective prefectures.

Within the last decade, the number of hospital beds has decreased as many small private clinics have closed down. The number of in-patient care beds per 1,000 population dropped from 6.2 in 1981 to 5.0 in 1994. The number of diagnostic centres and doctors has risen significantly. This has resulted in increases in the use of primary care services and diagnostic tests carried out. The mean number of medical visits per person annually is more than six.

The consumption of pharmaceuticals has increased. From 1987 to 1992 the pharmaceutical market increased 320 per cent. The expenditure on pharmaceuticals represents almost 15 per cent of the expenditure of hospitalisation. There has also been an increase in the number of the patients who travel abroad for hospital care. The latter is a result of the recently adopted policy of most of the insurance organisations to cover this kind of cost.

In relation to overall public expenditure, there has been an increase in the public expenditure for hospital care. In 1992, total health expenditure amounted to 8.29 per cent of the GNP, 3.42 per cent being private expenditure, and 4.87 per cent public expenditure. The expenditure for treatment abroad increased by 318 per cent during the period 1985 to 1991.

Preventive services

Child immunisation services are offered free of charge for diphtheria, tetanus, pertussis, poliomyelitis, measles, mumps, rubella and tuberculosis vaccines. Hepatitis B vaccine is offered free of charge for special population groups but it has to be purchased. Haemophilus influenza b vaccination rates are increasing, but this vaccine is not offered free of charge either. Vaccination for travellers in high risk countries are offered free of charge.

A recent ad hoc study[14] indicates that rates of fully vaccinated children are close to 90 per cent for diphtheria, tetanus, polio and measles, somewhat lower for rubella and mumps, close to 60 per cent for pertussis, just over 40 per cent for tuberculosis and 20 per cent for hepatitis for children of two years of age, apart from BCG vaccine which is mostly offered at the age of six years. Data from other studies provide similar overall rates.[15-19] Vaccination coverage is known to be deficient in children of migrants and small population pockets exist around the country.[18,19] The situation is not unsatisfactory but there is room for improvement to meet WHO objectives for year 2000.

Most vaccines, with the exception of vaccines for hepatitis B and haemophilus influenza b, are provided free of charge and they are available at health centres, polyclinics of municipalities, IKA, PIKPA, the regional health departments of the prefectures and pharmacies. There is no charge for immunisations performed in primary health care

settings and most family paediatricians, even when they are performed in private practice, do not overcharge for this service which is carried out in the context of a well baby
visit. An obstacle is that most services are only available during morning hours, especially in the urban areas.

Family planning services are provided in primary health centres, well baby clinics and
outpatient services of most gynaecology and obstetrics departments in the hospitals, but
many women receive advice from their own obstetrician, because the private sector is
very strong in this specialty. Contraceptive pills and IUDS are free. An important issue
in Greece is the high frequency of induced abortions. Although these abortions are legal
in Greece, the high frequency implies ineffective utilisation of contraceptive methods.
A possible explanation is that many services, although available, do not have effective
outreach components and they are not appropriately tailored to the needs of young
people.

Antenatal services are provided by primary care centres, well baby clinics, outpatient
clinics of obstetrics and gynaecology hospitals and by the many obstetricians in private
practice.[20] In public settings these services are provided free of charge, whereas obstetricians in private practice sometimes incorporate these visits in their follow-up after the
delivery. When indicated, prenatal diagnosis is provided free of charge in the designated
centres; however, women have to join a waiting list, or they are frequently referred to
the thriving private sector. Formal quality control systems for the private sector do not
exist.

Screening programmes

Screening for inborn errors of metabolism is provided free of charge for all new-
borns delivered in public or private maternity hospitals.[21] Tests are done in the Institute
for Child Health in Athens and cover phenylketonuria (performed since 1973), G6PD
Deficiency (1977), congenital hypothyroidism (1980), and galactosaemia (1994). This
programme is considered as a major accomplishment of the Greek health services.
Prenatal screening for thalassaemia is also freely available and quite effective, although
a handful of children suffering from thalassaemia are born, either because screening has
not been undertaken, or more frequently because the tests are not sensitive enough in
some unusual situations, such as intermediate forms of disease.[22] Moreover, selective
screening is available for cystic fibrosis, Downs syndrome and familial hyper-
cholesterolaemia.

Screening for adults, mostly Pap tests for cancer of the cervix and mammography for
breast cancer, are available in most primary settings but the system is poorly organised
on a national basis, has limited outreach components and has never been thoroughly
evaluated.[23]

Many women prefer to be guided by their obstetricians into the private sector where
tests are performed for a fee and usually there is no assurance of follow-up or continuity. There are no country-wide data on the proportion of women who have ever been

screened and no estimates for the proportion of those regularly screened.

Health promotion

Health promotion has not yet been fully developed in Greece and national institutions for health promotion or health education do not exist.[24] Instead, initiatives are taken by certain scientific, non-governmental, not-for-profit organisations such as the Institute of Child Health, the Greek Heart Foundation, the Research Foundation on Child Health, the Greek Cancer Society, the Society for Health Promotion and Health Education, the Hellenic Society of Social Paediatrics and Health Promotion, the Anti-Smoking Society, the Institute of Social and Preventive Medicine etc.

Thus, despite the fact that several health promotion and health education activities are undertaken, the efforts are fragmented, and not adequately coordinated. Recently, in the context of the decentralisation, regional health education committees have been established at a regional level or in the context of non-governmental institutions supported by the municipalities. In the Ministry of Health, there is a Department of Health Education which mostly undertakes rather traditional prevention activities such as the protection of child and maternal health. Since 1992, this department has been supported by the Committee for Health Education Planning. The National School of Public Health, which is supervised by the Ministry of Health, offers postgraduate training in public health and undertakes other training activities in the field of health education, such as nutrition seminars targeting day care and primary school teachers.

The university departments in the seven medical schools of the country are active in health promotion. Specific activities are carried out by the Department of Hygiene & Epidemiology of the University of Athens which leads national work on injury prevention, the University Community Mental Health initiative etc.

Specific governmental organisations active in the field of AIDS education/health promotion are the Centre for the Control of Special Communicable Diseases (KEEL) and the Drug Control Organisation (OKANA). The establishment of a National Centre for Health Promotion and Health Education has been suggested by an expert committee and proposals for the aims, responsibilities and organisational logistics of the centre have been submitted to the Ministry of Health, but a final decision is still pending.

Most of the above mentioned bodies produce ad hoc health promotion materials to support their health education activities. The Ministry of Health, department of Health Education is also responsible for the production and distribution of health education materials, which mostly consist of brochures and posters of moderate quality.

Health education in schools is undertaken by the specific organisations/institutions which embark on such activities, and they are usually supported by the Ministry of Health department of Health Education, the Ministry of Education and the local authorities. A School Health Education department has been established within the Ministry of Education, which has recently appointed a Health Education officer in every educational district. Preliminary evaluation of this effort has yielded very encouraging results.

There is adequate legislation prohibiting smoking in hospitals, schools, banks and public service settings. However, it cannot be claimed that legislation is enforced, even in hospitals, both on the part of health professionals, the patients and the visitors.

Taxation is used more as a means of collecting funds than as a means of controlling consumption. However, tobacco and alcohol taxation has recently increased substantially. In the context of environmental protection policies, leaded petrol is sold cheaper than unleaded petrol. Other specific issues include:

AIDS: KEEL is the main organisation responsible for formulation of strategies on AIDS education and prevention. National campaigns are organised on a regular basis with extensive use of mass media as well as campaigns targeting young age groups or specific occupational groups (e.g. marine workers). Campaigns are also organised at local level.

Cigarette consumption: There are no on-going campaigns, but tobacco advertising through television is banned. There is no age limit for the purchase of cigarettes but the price of cigarettes is rising. The successful campaign led by S. Doxiadis, former Minister of Health during 1979–80, should be pointed out, however.[25]

Alcohol consumption: The price of alcohol is rising because of taxation, but campaigns are limited and mainly target the harmful effects of drinking and driving. Last year a video on alcohol and road traffic accidents was produced (supported by the European Commission – DGV) which has been distributed to every high school in the country. Entry to bars is prohibited by law to those aged under 17 years, but the law has never been enforced. More alcohol tests are performed by the police to detect drunk drivers. Some legislative efforts at the national level for stricter regulation of drinking and driving have not been fruitful so far.

Accident prevention: Road traffic accidents are a major public health problem in Greece; which is why this type of injury receives priority over accidents in the workplace, or home and leisure accidents. The wearing of seat belts is obligatory by law, as well as helmet use by motorcyclists. However, these measures are not enforced by the traffic police and Greece ranks last among other European countries with regard to seat belt use; less than one in four adult passengers and about one in ten children are safely restrained in the car. An effort is currently being undertaken by the Centre for Research and Prevention of Injuries among the Young and other interested parties to pass a law on child restraints as part of a campaign for 'Safe Child Transportation'. From July 1996, motor insurance has been linked to driving behaviour; this measure is expected to yield positive results. The issue of accident prevention gets mass media attention from time to time but a comprehensive campaign has not been undertaken.

Diet: Nutrition education campaigns have not been given great prominence, because Greece is considered to enjoy the benefits of the Mediterranean diet. Healthy diet is promoted among young people as there is legislation determining the kind of foods sold at the school canteens. A special Bureau for Nutrition is functioning in the Ministry of

Health, which aims mostly at supervising preventive activities and establishment of healthy nutrition policies. The Department of Nutrition and Biochemistry of the National School of Public Health plays an instrumental role.

Health needs of ethnic minorities: Greece has not traditionally been a multi-ethnic society. Only in recent years have migrants from the former Eastern European countries and countries from the far-East settled in the country. Therefore, services aimed at the special health care needs of these population groups are organised only on a local basis. National initiatives concern mainly the children and the elderly.

Drug abuse: In Greece all drugs (narcotics) are illegal. A pilot programme for the use of methadone was started recently, and there is also a programme for needle exchange. Health education campaigns are organised on a regular basis generally targeting young people. Drug-related activities are mostly coordinated by the newly founded national para-governmental organisation against drugs abuse (OKANA).

Technology regulation and assessment

According to members of the faculty of the Radiology Department of Athens University, Greece has approximately 120 CT scanners throughout the country. (It should be noted that this figure does not coincide with other sources of information e.g. from the Department of Technology of the Ministry of Health, which refer only to the publicly-owned ones or from other sources of information, e.g. IKA.) Eighty per cent of CT scanners are concentrated in the Greater Athens area which has a population of about 4 million people but also serves the needs of a significant number of patients who are referred from other areas of the country. This means that around 25 CT scanners per million population are available. For the rest of the country, this figure is estimated to be approximately five CT scanners per million population. In terms of ownership, less than 50 per cent of CT scanners belong to the public sector. Thus, the public sector, when it needs to, buys these services from the private sector. A typical example of the utilisation of CT scans in Greece is that during 1995 IKA, which covers 60 per cent of the Greek population, spent 5 million ECUs on CT scans.

There are no positron emission tomography scanners in the country. But there are approximately 20 magnetic resonance scanners. Finally, there are nine lithotripters in Athens, (three publicly-owned) two in Thessaloniki (one publicly-owned) and there is also a publicly-owned one in Heraklion, Crete.

Some regulations exist on medical technology and provision of relevant equipment, but a comprehensive national plan based on specific needs assessment is lacking. Controlling mechanisms are set mainly according to financial constraints, especially in the public sector. For private hospitals there are quantitative restrictive regulations for purchasing high technology equipment. However, the private diagnostic centres are not restricted in this way, which is why the supply of high technology equipment has grown so fast. An example of the absence of planning and regulation on national or regional level is the case of lithotripters, the number of which grew very rapidly until the major national insurance organisation (IKA) bought its own. Thereafter, the work load of the privately-owned lithotripters fell dramatically.

With regard to mechanisms for protection from potentially hazardous emissions from medical equipment, there are some quite strict regulations which concern equipment with a potential radioactive impact. Control is implemented by the 'Demokritos' Institute for Nuclear Technology and Radio-Protection, a para-governmental scientific and research organisation, which renews licences for laboratories with such equipment. Newly acquired medical equipment is also approved by a committee of radio-protection experts. A representative of the Environment Division of the Ministry of Health also sits on this committee. No advisory bodies exist concerning technology in the biomedical domain, but the National Drug Organisation (EOF) provides advice on pharmaceuticals, and the General Chemical Laboratory is responsible for food control and market control.

Developing a framework for public health policy in Greece

Despite a number of significant developments over the last 20 years, the Greek public health system still presents a series of problems. However, while recognising these deficiencies, it should be noted that Greek health indicators continue to be among the best in the world. The health care system is quite flexible and responsive to the needs of citizens and is interwoven with traditional value systems with extended family and friends assuming much of the responsibility when a medical need arises. This paradox poses a series of questions about the most appropriate method to develop a framework of public health policy in Greece.

Proposals to upgrade the system should take seriously into account existing structures and current norms for provision of public health services. The system could and should utilise the rich experience of other countries but the simple transfer of foreign models has never been particularly successful in Greece; moreover, it often elicits resistance from those who are expected to implement the new model. In addition, the public sector is already overextended and relatively ineffective in Greece. An effort to upgrade public health activities could therefore degenerate into new bureaucracies that produce reports rather than accelerate action.

Although individual prefectures each employ doctors to work in public health departments, most of them are newly trained doing their one year of compulsory service. The distribution of those doctors doing public health work is not always related to the needs of the population. The role of public health services in Greece is largely old-fashioned and bureaucratic, e.g. licensing restaurants, hairdressing establishments, swimming pools etc.

The public health services are not really related to, nor do the public health doctors feel responsibility for, the health of defined populations. The relation between the public health doctors and the rest of the health service is administrative rather than managerial or professional. Thus, public health doctors have no authority to review, comment on or evaluate the services provided by the other health sectors.

A number of problems associated with structure, definition of tasks and responsibilities, provision of population registers, inadequate laboratory facilities, and under-developed inter-sectoral links and programmes continue to hinder progress in the public health system. Two serious ones are that:

- The public health system lacks an effective system of medical records or a health information system designed to show how health resources are used, or how they affect the outcome of care. There is also virtually no system to assess services for quality or appropriateness, let alone cost-effectiveness, anywhere in the health services.

- The status, pay and conditions of service of public health doctors are low in comparison to that of clinical doctors, even at the Ministry of Health. Thus the quality of individuals in public health is perceived as second rate and many are thought of as 'drop outs' from clinical practice.

In Greece there is a crucial need to develop a cadre of public health doctors who can contribute to the improvement of health and the formulation of health and health service policy. They could make a significant contribution to the following tasks.[3] To:

- Define and describe the health needs of the population;

- Identify environmental and social hazards to health;

- Elucidate localised predisposing conditions and consequences of disease;

- Undertake surveillance of communicable and non-communicable disease control activities;

- Provide advice to those concerned with setting priorities and planning services;

- Participate in the development of policy on disease prevention, health promotion and health education;

- Evaluate the implementation and outcome (efficiency and effectiveness) of health policies and services provided in populations.

Public health specialists are required at all levels of a health system, both in a strategic role as well as in an operational capacity to implement policies.

In view of the crucial contribution that public health professionals make to health policy and the improvement of the population's health, it is essential to recruit well qualified and committed professionals to the discipline. This can only be achieved by ensuring that they have adequate status within the system, are not burdened with unnecessary bureaucratic tasks, are rewarded at least as well as other specialists, are adequately supported and have an appropriate career structure.

At the central level, major functions that will need to be fulfilled are:

- Monitoring the nation's health and the outcome of health care;

- Seeking a greater understanding of what influences and determines health, ill health and the quality of life;

- Implementing the changes required to achieve improvement.

Public health medicine should be introduced into a variety of settings to be effective, including:

- The central ministry or health department;

- The local health departments;

- Hospitals and other health services' administrations.

A way to focus activity at each level could be the preparation of a report on the health of the population which would spell out areas of unmet need, inefficient provision and opportunities for more effective resource use.

Although the health of the population of Greece is satisfactory, there is still a need to develop a strategic approach to public health planning which requires the identification of specific goals for improvements in the population's health. A priority should be the development of policy objectives, not only for health but also for the important determinants of health and the processes that lead to changes in those factors. The development of objectives and targets can be used to highlight areas of a public health strategy and help in the process towards converting policy into programmes. This would also enable Greece to develop a more coherent health policy and enable options and choices to be considered within an agreed framework. There are clear problems and real needs in Greece in the field of public health. The challenging task is to integrate the lessons we learn from other countries and systems into our own traditions and social functions. Transplantation is never a risk-free operation.

References

1.   Trichopoulos D, Liaropoulos, L, Ritsataki A, Gana A (Rapporteurs). *Health and Health Services in Greece*. A five-year plan. Report of a Committee (Chairman M Violaki-Paraskeva). Athens 1976, pp. 1–292 (in Greek).

2.   Gana A, Ritsataki A, Trichopoulos D, (Rapporteurs). *Regionalisation of Health Services in Greece*. Report of a Working Group of the Center of Planning and Economic Research (Chairman G Mericas) KEPE, Athens 1979, pp. 1–231 (in Greek).

3.   Abel-Smith B, Calltorp J, Dixon M, Dunning A, Evans R, Holland W, Jarman B, Mossialos E. *Report of a Special Experts' Committee on the Greek Health Services*. Ministry of Health, Welfare and Social Security. Pharmetrica, Athens, 1994.

4.   Mossialos E. *The Consumption of Health Services in Greece*. Doctoral Thesis, University of Athens, 1989 (in Greek).

5.   Report of a Working Group for the Greek Ministry of Health, Welfare and Social

Insurance. *The Health of the Greek Population.* Athens 1992.

6. Malamitsi-Puchner A, Minaretzis D, Tzala E, Economidou O, Papathoma E. Pregnancy Outcomes of Migrant Women in Greece. Proceedings of the 7th National Congress of the Hellenic Society for Social Paediatrics and Health Promotion, *Children in New Home Countries.* Alexandroupoli 1997. Forthcoming (in Greek).

7. Petridou E, Valadian I, Trichopoulos D, Tzonou A, Kyriopoulos Y, Matsaniotis N. Medical services and socioeconomic factors: determinants of infant mortality in Greece. *International Journal of Health Education* 1989;VIII:20–23.

8. Petridou E, Kosmidis H, Haidas S, Tong D, Revinthi K, Flytzani V, Papaioannou D, Trichopoulos D. Survival from childhood leukaemia depending on socioeconomic status in Athens. *Oncology* 1994;51:391–95.

9. Petridou E, Davazoglou A. Proceedings of the 7th National Congress of the Hellenic Society for Social Paediatrics and Health Promotion. *Children in New Home Countries. Alexandroupoli* 1997. Forthcoming (in Greek).

10. Petridou E, Kotsifakis G, Revinthi K, Polychronopoulou A, Trichopoulos D. Determinants of stillbirth mortality in Greece. *Soz Praventivmed* 1996;41:70–78.

11. Ministry of Health and Welfare. Central Scientific Health Council. 1993 *Yearbook. Concentrated and Analytical Operational Data on Public Hospitals.* Athens, 1993.

12. Tountas Y, Stefannson, Frissiras S. Health reform in Greece: planning and implementation of a national health system. *International Journal Health Planning Management 1995;*10:283–304.

13. Ministry of Health and Welfare. Department of Social Relations. *The Greek Health System.* Athens, 1995 (in Greek).

14. Valassi-Adam H, Anterioti P, Apalaki H, Zaimaki H, Laurentzou A, Markopoulou B, Boukouvala H, Papahirakli H, Solou O, Tsatsouli H, Fotinou M. Assessment of the vaccination status of the hospitalised population. *Ann Clin Paediat University Atheniensis* 1995;42:82–86.

15. Ministry of Health, Welfare and National Security. *The Greek National Immunisation Programme. Health Education.* Athens, 1991 (in Greek).

16. Department of Public Health. Ministry of Health, Welfare and Social Security and the National School of Public Health. *National Immunization Programme in Greece.* Athens, 1994 (in Greek).

17. Kanariou M, Petridou E, Liatsis M, Revinthi K, Mandalenaki-Lambrou K, Trichopoulos D. Age patterns of immunoglobulins G, A, & M in healthy children and the influence of breast feeding and vaccination status. *Pediatr Allergy Immunol* 1995;6:24–29.

18. Skalikidou A, Petridou H, Velonaki A, Papoutsakis G. Secular trends in hospital morbidity of infectious diseases in children and young people in Greece. *Pediatriki* 1996;59:174–84, 1996 (in Greek).

19. Tsoukana P, Birbili H, Flytzani V, Stoikidou M, Petridou E. Immunization coverage and vaccine preventable infectious diseases among children of Greek migrants.

Proceedings of the 7th National Congress of the Hellenic Society for Social Paediatrics and Health Promotion. *Children in New Home Countries*. Alexandroupoli 1997. Forthcoming (in Greek).

20. Valassi-Adam H, Nakou S and Trakas N. *Perinatal Care in Greece*. Proceedings of a National Working Group, Institute for Child Health, Athens, 1986 (in Greek).

21. European Parliament. Scientific and Technological Options. *Prevention and Treatment of Genetic Diseases*. Brussells, May 1995.

22. Petridou E and Loukopoulos D. Thalassaemia. In: Silman AJ, Allwright SPA (Eds) *Elimination or Reduction of Diseases? Opportunities for Health Services Action in Europe*. Oxford University Press, 1988, pp. 211–26.

23. Garas I, Pateras H, Triandafilou D, Georgountzos V, Mihas A, Abatsoglou M, Trichopoulos D. Breast cancer screening in southern Greece. *European Journal of Cancer Prevention* 1994;3:35–39.

24. Tountas Y. Greece (Country Report). *Promotion and Education* 1995;.II(2-3).

25. Doxiadis S, Trichopoulos D, Dimou-Phylactou H. The Impact of a nationwide anti-smoking campaign. *Lancet* 1985;2:712–13.

7

Public Health in Spain

Andreu Segura Benedicto

Introduction

Spain is the third largest country in western Europe. The population is 39 million, with a surface area of nearly half a million square kilometres and an average density of 78 inhabitants per square kilometre, one of the lowest densities in Europe. The unequal distribution of the population throughout the country has created an imbalance between regions. There is a growing tendency for the population to concentrate in the coastal regions, with the exception of Madrid and a few other cities. There are 20 cities with populations of over 200,000, where a third of the total population is concentrated.

Since 1975 the live birth rate has diminished more than 50 per cent. The figure for 1995 is 9.18 per thousand inhabitants. The fertility index estimated in 1996 was 1.15 children per woman. 15.45 per cent of the population was aged over 64 years in 1991. The aging trend has thus become the main demographic characteristic of the Spanish population.

The total budget for social protection was 22.7 per cent of Gross Domestic Product (GDP) in 1995, whereas the EU average was 28.4 per cent.[1] Total expenditure for health was estimated at 7.6 per cent of GDP in 1995. Public spending on health represents 6.22 per cent of GDP.[2]

Political organisation in Spain since 1978 has changed dramatically with the introduction of parliamentary democracy and political decentralisation to regional governments – Autonomous Communities. In addition to the central government and parliament, there are 17 regional governments accountable to their regionally elected parliaments. This political organisation has led to a very diverse situation regarding legislation, which in turn affects the health system.

This chapter describes the main health problems of the Spanish population, the basic characteristics of the health system and the role of public health services. After an

149

overview of policy and priority setting, it considers some specific issues about prevention and health promotion activities.

Health problems

In recent years, the health situation has changed for the better. Spanish epidemiological patterns are now similar to those of other EU populations. However, some particular features must be mentioned.

Spain's global health indicators are among the best in the European Union. For example, in 1996 life expectancy at birth was 73.4 years for males and 81.3 years for females. Life expectancy at 65 was 15 years for men (6.8 years corresponding to disability-free life) and 18.4 years for women (6.5 years disability free). The figure for the perinatal mortality rate was 6.0 deaths (under one year old) per thousand live births.

In recent years the crude mortality rate has stabilised, but the standardised rate has shown a continuous decrease. As in most developed countries, mortality rates due to cardiovascular disease are also diminishing. Furthermore, the baseline rates of ischaemic heart disease were lower in Spain and the current rates are still better than in many EU countries. The overall cancer mortality rate is increasing. Now cancer is the main cause of death if cardiovascular disease and stroke are considered separately. Again, cancer mortality is lower than the European average. Lung cancer in men and breast cancer in women are the most important causes of cancer mortality. For cancer of the cervix, Spain has one of lowest mortality rates in Europe. However, for chronic respiratory diseases, AIDS, suicide and occupational injuries mortality is increasing. The occupational injuries rate is the highest in the EU.[3]

Spain's morbidity pattern corresponds to that observed in developed countries, with an increase in chronic, degenerative and mental health problems, and disability. AIDS and HIV infection are also very important health problems, as are traffic accidents and injuries.

The pattern of health problems reflects differences among the autonomous territories, most of them as a consequence of social and gender inequalities.[4] For example, in 1995 the infant mortality rate in Asturias (7.0/1,000 live births) was 75 per cent higher than that of Cantabria (4.0/1,000). There were similar differences in perinatal mortality, with the highest registered in La Rioja (8.7/1,000 live births) and the lowest recorded in the Canary Islands (3.4/1,000).[5]

The Spanish standardised mortality rate for ischaemic heart disease was 58.664/100,000 inhabitants in 1994. The highest rate was found in the Canary Islands (88.61) and the lowest in La Rioja (40.37).

The average rate for all cancers at national level was 154.69/100,000 inhabitants in 1994. The Basque country had a standardised rate of 165.19 and Murcia 143.28. Lung cancer mortality rate was between 24.14 in Castilla-León and 35.96 in Extremadura. The average figure for all of Spain was 30.26. The breast cancer mortality rate was

20.99 per 100,000 women in Spain as a whole, but at the regional level the highest value was found in the Balearic Islands (28.12) and the lowest in Castilla-León (17.37).

Standardised cancer incidence rates from nine population registries in Spain in 1991–92 showed that the highest values (excluding skin cancer and other melanoma) were among men in the Basque country (294.7/100,000 men) and Mallorca (Balearic Islands) with 286.1/100,000. The lowest were for Albacete (Castilla-La Mancha) with 199.0 and Granada (Andalucia) where the figure was 228.0. The corresponding highest rates for women were 182.4/100,000 for Navarra and 178.4 for Mallorca, and the lowest for Granada (138.8) and Albacete (142.4). Regional differences for male lung cancer were greatest between Asturias (63.5/100,000 men) and Albacete (34.1). Breast cancer incidence rates for women were highest in Navarra (61.7/100,000 women) and lowest for Granada (37.4).[6]

Approximately 30 per cent of the population over 15 years of age reports fair, bad or very bad health (32 per cent in 1987, 31 per cent in 1993 and 32.5 per cent in 1995). Differences on the way health was self-perceived are relatively small among Autonomous Communities. The Canary Islands used to have the highest value, close to 37 per cent and Navarra the lowest with 25 per cent.[7] There are, however, important differences in self-perceived health according to socio-economic status and level of education. The 1995 data shows a large difference between the figures for people belonging to the highest socio-economic class, with 14.6 per cent of this strata of the population falling into the three categories mentioned above (fair, bad and very bad) and the lowest socio-economic groups, where 41.4 per cent of people reported that they perceived their health to be fair, bad or very bad. The same ratios can be observed for education levels. Thus, people with university degrees who perceived their health to be fair, bad or very bad was 14.1 per cent while the figure for members of the population without any formal school qualification was 41.4 per cent.[8]

Higher levels of drug abuse are present in urban communities where there are higher rates of unemployment and social marginalisation. Conversely, the highest incidence rates of AIDS, mostly among drug users, are in Madrid (298.5 new cases/million inhabitants in 1995), Balearic Islands (265.9), the Basque Country (232.5) and Catalonia (230.6). Extremadura and Castilla-La Mancha have the lower rates at 43.6 and 73.9 respectively.[9]

Although all Autonomous Communities formally have had full responsibility for health protection and promotion activities for more than 15 years, the response to public health has been generally poor. There are some differences between Autonomous Communities in the organisation of public health services, but they have little relevance with regard to health promotion interventions.

Main characteristics of the health system

The current health system in Spain evolved from the historical development of the Social Security system since 1944, and the reforms introduced by the Health Act (Ley

General de Sanidad-LGS) in 1986. The 1986 Health Act was a response to the 1978 Constitution which established the right of all Spaniards to enjoy health protection. The Act established the National Health System (Sistema Nacional de Salud-SNS), which has responsibility for protecting health and guaranteeing equity of access to health care.

The SNS acts as the universal public insurer, and is responsible for financing and providing most health care services, mainly via the National Health Institute of Social Security (Instituto Nacional de Sanidad y Seguridad Social-INSALUD). Furthermore, there are other public health insurers, such as Work Accident and Occupational Diseases Insurance Companies (Mutualidades de Accidentes de Trabajo y Enfermedades Profesionales) or Army and Civil Servants Public Insurance Companies (Mutualidades de Funcionarios de las Administraciones Publicas), which are financed by social security and provide health care through either their own resources or not-for-profit service organisations. The SNS services cover nearly 99 per cent of the population. In addition, 6 per cent of the population use non-public services. Five per cent of the population has double coverage,[10] although in some autonomous regions like Catalonia this proportion approaches 21 per cent. Private facilities are mainly devoted to dentistry and obstetric care services.

Total health expenditure has increased continuously since 1960, from 1.5 per cent of GDP to 7.60 per cent in 1995. Currently, public health spending represents 81.8 per cent of total health expenditure. This accounts for 6.22 per cent of GDP. During the 1980s, public spending increased at a rate of 4.9 per cent per year. Until 1989, public financing of the health budget was provided through social security contributions. However, general tax revenues currently account for 95 per cent of total health funding and taxation will become the only economic source for public health expenditure from the year 2000.[11]

There are important differences in per capita public health expenditure among Autonomous Communities according to a recent report by the Ministry of Health. For example, Navarra spends 100,000 pesetas per capita, whereas Galicia spends 70,000.[12]

Hospital care uses nearly 60 per cent of the health budget and pharmaceuticals more than 20 per cent. Primary health care expenditure represents less than 19 per cent. Only 1.2 per cent is devoted to formal public health services which are responsible for health protection and promotion at the community level.

In 1996, Spain had approximately 800 hospitals with a total of 170,000 beds (4.4/1,000 inhabitants). The SNS owns a quarter of the centres and 50 per cent of beds. Seventy-one per cent of in-patient admissions were to public hospitals.[13] Currently there are 410 medical doctors, 425 nurses, 100 pharmacists, 40 veterinarians and 30 dentists per hundred thousand people. The number of health professionals has increased greatly since 1975. The number of nurses has increased by five times and dentists by three. Half the doctors and just over half the nurses work in hospitals.[14] Nearly 28,000 physicians and a similar number of nurses are involved in primary care.

The SNS includes all public health care providers. Part of them come from INSALUD and part from other state (public) institutions. In addition, the SNS contracts with other providers. Health care services are organised into primary and secondary levels. At secondary level, there are in-patient and out-patient hospital services and also specialist ambulatory centres, provided mainly through INSALUD. Psychiatric hospitals, mental health centres and nursing homes mainly belong to provincial and local authorities.

As a consequence of the reform process which began in 1984 (before the enactment of the Health Act 1986)[15] primary health care is provided mainly by INSALUD. There are two different patterns of primary care provision.[16] The first is the pattern that was developed by the reform measures and involves the organisation of primary health care into teams, working in Primary Health Centres (PHC) with full-time staff. These teams include physicians, General Family and Community Medicine specialists, nurses and, in some cases, other medical specialists and health workers. Their care activities include disease prevention (immunisation and case-finding for some diseases) and health promotion activities such as health counselling. In 1994 the average population coverage for this pattern of primary health care provision was 61 per cent, although there were wide regional differences. For example, in Galicia the reform process had only reached 21 per cent of the population, whereas Navarra had achieved 83 per cent.

Secondly there is the pre-reform primary health care scheme which remains in operation for about 40 per cent of the population. General practitioners and paediatricians work at INSALUD ambulatory care centres for only two and a half hours a day. Emergency home care is carried out by special services.

Since February 1995, plastic surgery (excluding previous injuries, disease or congenital malformations) transsexual surgery, psychoanalysis, hypnosis and cures have been formally excluded from public health care interventions through an explicit list of health care practices offered through the public health system that is issued by the Health Ministry.[17] The main criteria used to justify these exclusions are the lack of scientific evidence on the safety and efficacy of the health interventions. Moreover, dental care has historically been excluded from social security health care. It is regularly offered only in the Basque Country.[18]

The National Health System is divided into 128 Health Areas within the Autonomous Communities, but only in a few cases have Health Areas been developed. In seven of the Autonomous Communities (Catalonia, Andalusia, the Basque Country, Valencia, Navarre, Galicia and the Canary Islands) covering 60 per cent of the Spanish population, health care services are now fully devolved and provided through an Autonomous Health Service (AHS), the regional equivalent to the National Health System in each Autonomous Community. In these cases, the AHS finances and provides public health care services. The remaining 10 Autonomous Communities, covering the remaining 40 per cent of the population, still have their health care systems under the direct control of the national administration.

The National Health Service also includes other kinds of services, including public health services, mainly devoted to community health protection from environmental hazards, epidemiological surveillance, immunisation and collective health promotion. The public health services system has formed part of the Autonomous Communities' responsibilities since the start of the political reform process.

These services, devolved from the former centralised Spanish public health organisation, were restructured into provincial divisions. Each province has a public health headquarters and in some cases, several public health centres within its territory. In addition, government employed physicians, nurses, pharmacists and veterinarians work part-time at the local level.

The development of these services differs among the Autonomous Communities.[19] In general, under the former structure of public health services, personnel work part-time, but local public health workers, such as physicians and nurses are slowly being integrated into primary health care teams. In the Autonomous Community of Valencia pharmacists and veterinarians work at newly created community health centres. The governments of Autonomous Communitiess have the responsibility to authorise and monitor all kinds of activity related to health care services.

Health policy and priority setting

Health policy responsibilities are divided between the National Health Service and Autonomous Communities' authorities. Municipal authorities play a secondary role, falling under the Autonomous Communities' authority with the exception of Barcelona, Madrid and some other large cities. Figure 1 provides an outline of the division of health-related responsibilities.

Equity is a central tenet in current health policy in Spain. Universal access to health care is assumed by the Health Act and fostered by the establishment of the National Health System during 1986–90. However, until now the focus has been on accessibility rather than on the reduction of health inequalities. There are several groups[20] concerned with this topic and the Spanish Epidemiological Association has set up a working group.[21] During the last period of socialist government, the Health Ministry supported the preparation of a report on health inequalities under the direction of professor Vicente Navarro and Joan Benach.[22] However, no formal global health policy on inequalities exists except for programmes related to Women's Health which are carried out by several autonomous health services and in some places by INSALUD. Only social services departments and the NGOs work on social inequalities.

The Ministry of Health is responsible for the public health budget which is presented to the central parliament as part of the general budget. Social Security is under the Ministry of Labour and besides health spending it determines retirement pensions and unemployment benefits.

The size of the overall health budget is determined historically on an incremental basis. Increases in recent years are due to promoting universal health care and the increase in

Figure 1
Health-related responsibilities in the Spanish health and social security system (1998)

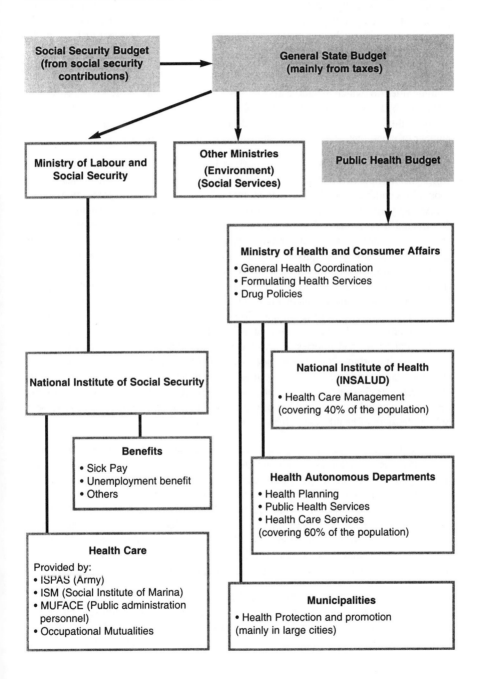

health services actually used by the population. There is no criterion to establish the required size of the health budget except for demand for health services. With respect to health prevention and promotion there is no specific budget because many these activities are integrated into the Primary Health Care Reformed Network. However, specific public health services have a budget which represents only 1 per cent of total public health expenditures.[23]

The health budget is allocated by the Treasury (Exchequer) to the Autonomous Communities to which health care has been devolved and to the National Health Institute which administers health care in the other Autonomous Communities where responsibility has not yet been devolved. The budget allocations are based on the number of inhabitants, without any adjustment for age or health needs.

According to the Health Act, health priorities have to be established in a health plan which includes the health goals, activities and time schedules. The Spanish Health Plan should be a combination of all the Autonomous Communities' health plans compiled by the Ministry of Health. However, to date, only 13 Autonomous Communities have constructed a preliminary health plan, among them the seven with devolved health care.[24] In practice, only in Catalonia has the plan been applied to manage the Catalan Health Service which is equivalent to a National Health System at the autonomous (regional) level. On the basis of these plans, in 1995 the Ministry of Health published a strategy document aimed at the process of completing the new National Integrated Health Plan. The Spanish Health Plan considered 14 intervention areas: ageing; HIV infection and AIDS; cancer; respiratory diseases; digestive diseases; locomotive disturbances; communicable diseases; tuberculosis; diabetes; mother and child health; mental health; oral health and injuries. Each of these areas includes general goals to reduce mortality and morbidity but they do not have quantitative targets. For each intervention area, the plan considered specific measures related to health promotion and prevention; health care; professional training and coordination among health services and other services like social services and so on. Until now, the practical consequences have been only in the field of health research and development.

The national research and development strategy is defined by the Science National Plan which includes a section on health and quality of life related to health. Moreover, the health system itself has a specific agency, named FIS (Fondo de Investigacion de la Seguridad Social: Social Security Research Foundation) to fund the research activities in accordance with defined priorities based on Ministry of Health Policies. Related to the FIS there is REUNI, a network of research units located in the National Health System. The network has a hundred research units devoted to clinical epidemiology or experimental research.[25] The papers published by these research units influence health policy. Clinical researchers can therefore have a direct influence on health practice.

Public and institutional participation in policy issues were included in the Health Act. Such participation occurs at the Health Area, Autonomous Communities and central levels. The slow development of the Health Areas organisation has limited effective participation at this level. However, Autonomous Community health services, as well as

INSALUD, have representative bodies which include public and corporate institutions. Lastly, the SNS has, at its central level, an Inter-territorial Council where central and Autonomous Community health administration representatives meet to analyse public health policy issues.

In addition, health professionals have influence through unions and colleges, as well as in academia. In the case of medical specialties, there is a national board for each medical specialty which determines the training requirements for professional practice. Their influence is specially orientated towards pay questions and labour relations, but also towards clinical practice as they are more orientated to treatment than prevention.

On the other hand, public health services have little influence on health policy because planning and management is not within their competence. However, the recent development of the health information system (health surveys, mortality and morbidity statistics, cancer registry etc.) could increase their influence, since obviously health information is necessary for planning. In this context, the Ministry of Health has published health indicator reports in relation to the Health For All strategy,[26] and we expect a new report from the Public Health Directorate of the Health Ministry. This report deals with the population health problems and their determinants, as well as public health priorities.[27] Moreover, the Spanish Society of Public Health and Health Administration (SESPAS) has also published three biannual reports 'La salud y el sistema sanitario en España'.[28,29,30] These provide an overall assessment of the main issues in public health in Spain. The last report was devoted to public health and the future of the welfare state. These reports are prepared as a contribution for the biannual SESPAS meetings and they represent an external evaluation of the health situation and health politics.

Health professional undergraduate training in public health subjects such as planning, management, evaluation and epidemiology is still inadequate. However, postgraduate specialisation training in family and community medicine and in preventive medicine and public health is increasing in demand in areas related to health policy. Since 1985, four new public health schools have been created which together with the National Public Health School (founded in 1924) provide numerous postgraduate education programmes in these areas.

The pharmaceutical and technological industries act as lobbies influencing pharmaceutical prescription and medical interventions. The mass media disseminate news of the advances in medical technologies, thus increasing both professional and general expectations. So far citizens have had little influence on decision making, though patient and customer associations are growing. Patients with particular diseases and their relatives are concerned with the effective coverage of care and consumer associations are interested in malpractice.

Formal influence on health policies on the part of interested groups is rare. There is an agreement between the Health Ministry and the pharmaceutical industry about the total amount of pharmacy expenditure, and with the medical unions about salaries. In fact, the role of these lobbies is indirectly influencing clinical decisions. The 'Informe Abril' (the report of the Parliamentary Commission on the reform of the Spanish Health Care System) which was published in 1991,[31] shows that such an influence persists.

In accordance with the Health Act, a declaration defining patients' rights was issued by the INSALUD in 1986. It contains 16 items and refers to health care characteristics needed to preserve confidentiality, avoid discrimination and so on.[32] In some autonomous communities there are similar documents. There are ethical committees at the hospital level, which, in a few cases, include population representatives.

During recent years, interventions to introduce a kind of 'internal market' among public and private providers of SNS have been taken in Catalonia and the Basque Country. Their autonomous health services have established a formal contract with the providers, prioritising health objectives and activities, with part of the payment being related to the achievement of these objectives. However, up to now insufficient information on this exists and it is too early to evaluate its impact on health policy and health expenditure.

In summary, the decision-making process to establish priorities at the central level has been, until now, an informal one. There is no explicit framework for priority setting and consultation.

The most important influences on health care policies are the medical establishment and the pharmaceutical and medical industries. Another important influence comes from the Autonomous Communities with their devolved health care services, particularly among those which give their political support to the central government.

Budgets are fixed at the beginning of each year with an annual increment. However, the final annual budget has frequently been higher than the initial budget decision as a consequence of pharmaceutical expenditure and other non-controlled health costs. These deviations from the original budget have led to substantial adjustments as happened in 1983, 1989, 1992 and 1994. The parliamentary agreement on health financing reached in the 1994–97 period avoided these deviations. Since 1998 there has been another Parliamentary agreement, which will be in effect until the year 2000. The criteria for resource allocation among the Autonomous Communities with healthcare responsibilities is based upon population distribution (capitative) with some amendments, including the proportion of people moving from other Autonomous Communities to obtain health care, adjustments made for regional (ie. Autonomous Community) GPD and the number of university hospitals.[33]

Most of those involved in policy agree that cost containment measures are needed. Unfortunately, the lack of experience in setting priorities and the current absence of any explicit framework results in poor rationalisation.

It is difficult to predict the consequences of cost containment policies but the main result would probably be a fall in public expenditure on health. If it were possible to restrict health interventions which lack evidence of effectiveness and safety, the consequences could be positive in terms of the population's health and the financing of the health care system.

Equity policies like positive discrimination are non-existent. In fact, the allocation of resources to the autonomous communities depends on the number of inhabitants and is not based on need. Only some social services departments, which are independent of the health care system, have developed interventions such as cash benefits for those under the poverty line. At central level there is a form of social subsidy for people without social security protection.

However, the recent universalisation of health care services has actually resulted in social redistribution. In Catalonia, for example, people from deprived social classes are the main users of public health care services, after adjusting for gender, age and health perception.[34]

Preventing disease and promoting health-specific activities

Preventive activities in primary health care have been undertaken in several Autonomous Communities, although these have been insufficiently coordinated with the public health services. The Spanish Society for Community and Family Medicine has been carrying out a programme of Preventive Activities and Health Promotion in Primary Health Care (PAPPS) since 1988. Expert panels make specific recommendations that are updated yearly. More than 400 primary health care centres (from a total of 1,700 in Spain) follow these guidelines, covering a population of 6 million. These activities are regularly evaluated in around 200 centres.[35] Moreover, Public Health Services promote activities addressed at smoking, drug use and other lifestyle risks.

Immunisation

Childhood immunisation against infectious diseases is recommended and provided free of charge in primary care centres. Since October 1995, a common immunisation schedule has been adopted for the whole country. The Basque Country unilaterally added the Haemophilus influenza vaccination in March 1996. According to official data,[36] the proportion of immunised children in 1996 was: poliomyelitis 91 per cent; pertussis, tetanus and diphtheria 90.2 per cent, and measles, rubella and mumps 89.7 per cent (in 1995). The Balearic and Canary Islands showed the poorest immunisation rates (under 60 per cent and 70 per cent respectively). Since 1996, 16 of the 17 Autonomous Communities have introduced hepatitis B immunisation. In five of them the target population is new-borns, and in the rest, 12–13 year old children. 85 per cent of the teenage population was covered.

Influenza vaccine is also recommended to people over 65 and patients with cardiovascular and chronic respiratory diseases.

Antenatal care

Out-patient services in hospitals and obstetricians at ambulatory centres play an important role in the follow-up of pregnancies. General physicians in some primary health centres also provide ante-natal care as part of their preventive activities. Furthermore, the majority of women use private services for their deliveries, probably because of the comfort they provide. Routine ultrasound is widely used in ante-natal care.

Family planning

Family planning centres were developed in the 1970s by local councils as part of social services and have since been integrated into the health services system. In 1992, there were 208 public family planning centres to support primary care, maternal health counselling and contraceptive prescriptions. According to the last fertility survey (1985),[37] which contains the latest data available, 60 per cent of women knew of the existence of family planning centres but only 32 per cent of women used them. Abortion is permitted under three conditions (rape, foetal health risk, mother's health risk) and is provided mainly in private clinics. In 1996, the abortion rate was 5.69/1,000 women between 15 and 44 years old, with wide regional differences, Asturias had the highest rate (9.65) and Navarra the lowest (2.08).[38]

Breast and cervical cancer screening

Although no national breast cancer screening programme exists, several Autonomous Communities have developed their own programmes. In Navarra, the programme has operated since 1990 with a participation rate of 85 per cent of the target population, and in Galicia and Rioja since 1992 and 1993 with participation rates of 70 per cent and 82 per cent respectively. Eight Autonomous Communities have recently initiated screening activities.[39] Some physicians prescribe preventive mammography to women younger than provided for by the programme. Although cervical cancer incidence and mortality rates are low in Spain, six Autonomous Communities have developed screening activities, Extremadura and Castilla-Leon having a population-based programme.[40] Case finding is common in gynaecology services particularly in women with a high educational level.

Smoking

More than 30 per cent of the adult Spanish population are smokers and 13 per cent of non-smoking people are ex-smokers. Overall smoking prevalence has slowly declined since 1985, but prevalence in women is increasing. The declining trend in men is associated with better education.[41]

Prevention policies are based on increasing tobacco taxes, limiting publicity, restricting purchases by young people and restricting the places where smoking is permitted. However, compliance with these regulations is, in most cases, limited.[42] In addition, cigarette packets include health warnings, central and regional health authorities undertake sporadic educational campaigns in the media, and health educational programmes at primary schools include anti-smoking advice.

The PAPPS programme includes smoking counselling among its preventive and health promotion activities. General practitioners are encouraged to ask whether their patients smoke, and in some cases they are asked to give smoking advice.

Alcohol and drug abuse

Currently, 61 per cent of the adult Spanish population drink alcohol regularly, consumption being more frequent in men (67 per cent) than women (44 per cent). Since 1987 the trend has been falling, with the population of moderate drinkers increasing from 30 per cent in 1987 to 39 per cent in 1993, while the number of excessive drinkers falling from 9.7 per cent to 4 per cent. Alcohol preventive policies are based on fiscal measures, advertising controls and purchase restrictions. But alcohol consumption has no geographic limits. In 1994, EU Directive 89/552 on publicity rules was incorporated into the Spanish regulations. Taxes on alcoholic beverages were raised in July 1996. Since then the most significant change has been the reduction of the maximum level of alcohol in the blood stream permitted for drivers, from 0.8 mg/L to 0.5 mg/L.

At the national level, the SNS has promoted intersectoral cooperation with the Agriculture, Commerce, Justice and Economy Departments to make recommendations for reducing alcohol availability as well as improving research and statistical information.[43]

In relation to traffic accident risks associated with alcohol consumption, maximum alcohol levels in blood have been reduced for truck drivers. Since 1992 the maximum level permitted for these drivers has been 0.3 g/l.

Some Autonomous Communities have specific regional policies. Catalonia forbids the sale of alcoholic beverages to those under 18 years old from midnight to 6am, although compliance appears to be rare.

The PAPPS guidelines include identifying excessive drinkers and offering counselling. These initiatives have just been initiated and an evaluation is not yet available.

With regard to control and prevention measures for illicit drugs, the situation is quite different. Since 1985, the National Drug Plan (NDP) has coordinated policy strategies and activities with the Autonomous Communities. A specific information system (SEIT) was created in 1987 which produces information on treatment, emergency services and mortality due to heroine and cocaine abuse.

There are 325 centres providing care to drug users who notify SEIT of their activities. Over half of them prescribe methadone. Forty seven specific care units are located at the hospital level.[44] In addition, therapeutic communities mainly organised by Non Governmental Organisations (NGOs) are operating.

Initially, the NDP policy centred on abstinence, but the increase in the incidence of AIDS has led to a new strategy based on reduction. The NDP and other institutions frequently support mass media campaigns against drug use.

AIDS

AIDS is a big health problem in Spain. The incidence rate was 159 cases per million in

1996 and 108.1 per million in 1997, the highest rate in the EU and an important cause of premature death. Since the beginning of the epidemic drug users have been the most significant risk group. The trend in heterosexual incidence is increasing. The AIDS National Programme supports a specific information system and makes recommendations on prevention and treatment policies. According to a recent survey, in 1996 the estimated prevalence of infected people between 15 and 39 years of age was 4.3 cases per thousand inhabitants. The total number of people infected with HIV, excluding AIDS cases, came to between 100,000 and 120,000.[45] Despite a number of preventive interventions, such as needle exchange, free condom distribution and mass media information campaigns, the trend has been less satisfactory than in other European countries. As Alvarez-Dardet and Hernandez have pointed out, this situation may be the consequence of insufficient public health intervention since the efforts made have been too timid, too few and tardy.[46]

Motor vehicle accidents

According to 1995 figures, nearly 650,000 people have motor vehicle accidents annually, with 420,000 needing emergency medical care. 92,000 accidents give rise to hospital admissions. Traffic accidents cause 6,500 deaths per year.[47] These figures should be considered as underestimations because they only include the accidents that involved police.[48] The rapid increase in the number of vehicles, particularly motorbikes, and the slow road building programme are key determinants of this situation. At this moment, it is impossible to know the role played by alcohol consumption because no data is available.[49]

Traffic authorities have responsibility for prevention policies. Safety activities based on speed limits, compulsory helmet and seat belt use and blood alcohol level control are their responsibility. Although health authorities are concerned with the problem, no specific activities of primary prevention are carried out, other than some mass media campaigns and most of these are organised together with traffic authorities. Medical emergency facilities (ambulance and helicopter) have been expanded over recent years but they have been developed without sufficient planning and evaluation.

Health needs of immigrants and ethnic minorities

The gypsy population is Spain's most important ethnic minority numbering some seven hundred thousand people. Although there are no legal restrictions on their access to health services, cultural differences and social marginalisation make access difficult. The health consequences of drug abuse is one of the main health problems for the gypsy population.

In addition, in recent years immigration from North Africa and Latin America has increased. Although the immigration rate is lower than the European average, according to the official estimates more than 20,000 immigrants per year are expected until 2005. Migrants who have work permits can use the National Health System without restrictions. Health care for refugees is organised by the Red Cross which makes agreements with the National Health System. For other migrant populations, no formal health care policy exists, but health services deal with emergencies. Access to ambulatory care is at the professionals' discretion. However, there is a 'Forum on the social integration of migrant people' at the central level and equivalent institutions in Autonomous Communities like the 'Migrant Advisory Council' in Catalonia which address the health care problems of the migrant populations.

Healthy Cities Project (HCP)

Barcelona and Seville were among the 35 European cities which began the HCP in 1987. Now the Spanish network includes 30 cities, located in 14 Autonomous Communities, covering 27 per cent of the total population. There are five networks involving 226 cities working at the AC level.[50] Periodic meetings to debate health services and health problems of urban populations are their main activities. Their influence on public health policies and activities depends basically on the economic resources available to the local administrations and on the scope of local services. The involvement of other sectors of the local administration as well as community participation are low.[51] In 1995, during the International healthy and ecological cities congress held in Madrid, Manzanera, Moncada and Artazcoz considered the change of strategy towards a more comprehensive perspective of sustainable cities, which includes health aspects.[52]

Summary

The Spanish health system is still undergoing a process of change. The financing of the health system is not definitively fixed. The current parliamentary agreement is only in effect until the year 2000. The primary health care reform and the decentralisation process should already have been completed but as yet there is no definite date for this completion. Another important question will be social security reform and the decentralisation of the National Institute of Social Security with changes for special social security agencies like MUFACE, MUGEJU, ISFAS and the Instituto Social de la Marina. Public health services need to be integrated effectively into the National Health System though there is little interest in them from political organisations.

The priorities of the health plans are being implemented only by Autonomous Communities with full health care responsibility, such as Catalonia and the Basque Country. The main concern of health policy are cost containment and professional involvement in management. The debate on equity will be one of the more important issues in the political arena in Spain together with the possibility of establishing some restrictions on the health care services currently provided. Private providers could begin to play a more important role than they have up until now either within the public system or as a complementary sector without public finance. Public participation is at an early stage of development.

Acknowledgement

I am indebted to Fernando G Benavides, Carlos Alvarez-Dardet, Albert Oriol and Esteve Fernandez for their comments and assistance.

References

1. Proyecto de Presupuestos de la Seguridad Social. *Anexo al Informe economico-financiero 1999*. Ministerio de Trabajo y Seguridad Social.

2. Ortún V. Sistema sanitario y estado del bienestar. In: Catalá Villanuev F, de Manuel Keenoy E. (eds.) *La Salud Pública y el Futuro del Estado del Bienestar*. Informe SESPAS 1998. Granada: Escuela Andaluza de Salud Pública, 1998.

3. Alonso I, Regidor E, Rodriguez C, Gutierrez-Fisac JL. Principales causas de muerte en España 1992. *Medicina Clinica* (Barc) 1966;107:441–5.

4. Regidor E, Gutierrez-Fisac JL, Rodriguez C. *Diferencias y Desigualdades de Salud en España*. Madrid: Diaz de Santos, 1994.

5. Regidor E, Rodriguez C, Gutierrez-Fisac JL. *Indicadores de Salud. Tercera Evaluaciòn en España del Programa Regional Europeo Salud para Todos*. Madrid: Ministerio de Sanidad y Consumo, 1995:23.

6. Parkin DM, Wehlan SL, Ferlay J, Raymond L, Young J. (eds.) *Cancer Incidence in Five Continents*. Lyon: IARC Scientific Publications, 1997.

7. Subdireccion General de Informacion y Estadisticas Sanitarias (Direccion General de Aseguramiento y Planificacion Sanitaria). Encuesta Nacional de Salud 1993. *Rev Sanid Hig Publica* (Madr) 1994;68(1):121–78.

8. Navarro V, Benach J. Desigualdades sociales en salud en España. *Rev Esp Salud Publica* 1996;70:505–636. See also Ministerio de Sanidad y Consumo. *Encuesta Nacional de Salud de España. 1995*. Madrid, 1996.

9. Sida en España. *Tasas por millón de habitantes*. Fecha de actualización: 31 de diciembre de 1996. Madrid: Centro Nacional de Epidemiologia, 1997.

10. Direccion General de Aseguramiento y Planificacion. *Plan de Salud 1995*. Madrid: Ministerio de Sanidad y Consumo, 1995.

11. Ortún V. Sistema sanitario y estado del bienestar. In: Catalá Villanuev F, de Manuel Keenoy E. (eds.) *La Salud Pública y el Futuro del Estado del Bienestar. Informe SESPAS 1998*. Granada: Escuela Andaluza de Salud Pública, 1998.

12. Marrón A, Jimenez J, Aliaga F, Garcia D. El *Sistema Nacional de Salud en la década del 2000*. Barcelona: SG Editores, 1994:34.

13. Prieto A (Dir). Sistema Nacional de Salud. *Servicios de Salud*. Datos y cifras. Madrid: Ministerio de Sanidad y Consumo, 1996.

14. Regidor E, Rodriguez C, Gutierrez-Fisac JL. *Indicadores de Salud. Tercera Evaluación del Programa Europeo Salud para Todos*. Madrid: Ministerio de Sanidad y Consumo, 1995.

15. The 1984 Royal Decree established the basic health structures and began the reform of primary health care.

16. Aranda JM (ed.). *Nuevas Perspectivas en Atención Primaria de Salud. Una revisión de la aplicación de los principios de Alma-Ata.* Madrid: Diaz de Santos, 1994.

17. Real Decreto 63/1995, de 20 de enero, sobre ordenacion de prestaciones sanitarias del Sistema Nacional de Salud. BOE No. 35 de 10 de febrero de 1995:4538–43.

18. Conde J. Las prestaciones del Sistema Nacional de Salud: criterios de racionalizacion. *Gac Sanit* 1995;9:5–10.

19. Mata E, de la Puente ML, Ramis-Juan O, Segura A, Tresserres R, Villalbi JR. *Los Servicios de Salud Publica en las Comunidades Autonomas: Semejanzas y Diferencias en 1995.* Barcelona: ISP, 1996.

20. Rodriguez JA, Lemkow L. Health and social inequities in Spain. *So Sci Med* 1990;31:351–8.

21. Grupo de trabajo de la Sociedad Espanola de Epidemiologia. *La Medición de la Clase Social en Ciencias de la Salud.* Barcelona: SG editores, 1995.

22. *Informe de Comisión Científica de estudios de las desigualdades sociales en Salud en España.* Madrid: Ministerio de Sanidad y Consumo, 1996.

23. Girón B, Santamaria P, Biglino L, Jimenez P, Prieto A, Sevilla F. Gasto sanitario publico en España 1991:1993: Cuentas satélite. *XVI Jornadas de Economia de la Salud.* Valladolid 5–7 junio de 1996.

24. Dirección General de Alta Inspección y Relaciones Institucionales. *Estudio Descriptivo de los Planes de Salud en España.* Madrid: Ministerio de Sanidad y Consumo, 1994.

25. Centro coordinador de REUNI. *Anuario REUNI 1994: Catálogo de la Red de Unidades de Investigación.* Madrid: Instituto de Salud Carlos III, 1995.

26. Mata de la Torre M (Dir). *Indicadores de Salud.* Madrid: Ministerio de Sanidad y Consumo, 1990.

27. Dirección General de Salud Pública. *Estado de Salud de los Españoles.* Madrid: Ministerio de Sanidad y Consumo, 1998.

28. Segura A, Benavides FG, Alvarez-Dardet C, Spagnolo E. (eds.) *Informe SESPAS 1993: La Salud y el Sistema Sanitario en España.* Barcelona: SG editores, 1993.

29. Navarro C, Cabases JM, Tormo MJ. (eds.) *La Salud y el Sistema Sanitario en España: Informe SESPAS 1995.* Barcelona: SG editores, 1995.

30. Catalá Villanuev F, de Manuel Keenoy E. (eds.) *La Salud Pública y el Futuro del Estado del Bienestar. Informe SESPAS 1998.* Granada: Escuela Andaluza de Salud Pública, 1998.

31. Comision de Análisis y Evaluación del Sistema Nacional de Salud. *Informe y Recomendaciones.* Madrid: Ministerio de Sanidad y Consumo, 1991.

32. Romeo C. Configuración sistemática de los derechos de los pacientes en el ámbito del derecho espanol. In: Instituto Nacional de la Salud. *Jornadas Sobre los Derechos de los Pacientes 1990.* Madrid: Ministerio de Sanidad y Consumo 1992:171–98.

33. Argenté M. El nou acord de finançament autonomic del la sanitat. *Fulls Econòmics* 1998;21:7–10.

34. Segura A, Vicente R. (dirs) *Enquesta de Salut de Catalunya 1994.* Barcelona: Servei Catalá de la Salut, 1996.

35. Brotons C, Iglesias M, Martin-Zurro A, Martin-Rabadan M, Gené J. Evaluation of preventive and health promotion activities in 166 primary care practices in Spain. *Fam Practice* 1996;13:144–51.

36. Dirección General de Salud Pública. *Evolución de la Cobertura Vacunal en España 1992–1995.* Madrid: Ministerio de Sanidad y Consumo, 1996.

37. Instituto Nacional de Estadistica. *Encuesta de Fecundidad.* 1985. Madrid: INE, 1990.

38. Dirección General de Salud Pública. *Interrupción Voluntaria del Embarazo. Datos Definitivos Correspondientes a 1996.* Madrid: Ministerio de Sanidad y Consumo, 1997.

39. Direccion General de Salud Pública. *Informe Sobre Actividades de Control y Prevenciòn del Cáncer en España y sus Comunidades Autonomas.* Madrid: Ministerio de Sanidad y Consumo, 1995.

40. Ascunce N, del Moral A. Detección precoz del cáncer de mama y del cáncer de cuello de útero. In: Navarro C, Cabases JM, Tormo MJ. (eds.) *La Salud y el Sistema Sanitario en España: Informe SESPAS 1995.* Barcelona: SG editores, 1995 pp. 46–55.

41. Dirección General de Salud Pública. *Encuesta Nacional de Salud 1993.* Madrid: Ministerio de Sanidad y Consumo, 1995.

42. Mendoza R. El tabaquismo. In: Segura A, Benavides FG, Alvarez-Dardet C, Spagnolo E. (eds) *Informe SESPAS 1993: La Salud y el Sistema Sanitario en España.* Barcelona: SG editores, 1993 pp. 133–45.

43. Robledo T, Rubio J, Gil E. Alcohol y salud. In: Navarro C, Cabases JM, Tormo MJ. (eds.) *La Salud y el Sistema Sanitario en España: Informe SESPAS 1995.* Barcelona: SG editores, 1995 pp. 101–11.

44. De la Fuente L, Barrio G. Prevencion de los problemas asociados con el uso de drogas ilegales. In: Navarro C, Cabases JM, Tormo MJ. (eds.) *La Salud y el Sistema Sanitario en España: Informe SESPAS 1995.* Barcelona: SG editores, 1995 pp. 90–100.

45. Anónimo. *Estudio de la Seroprevalencia de VIH en una Muestra Representativa de la Población Española, 1996.* Madrid: Dirección General de Salud Pública, 1998.

46. Alvarez-Dardet C, Hernandez Aguado I. AIDS in Spain: lessons learned from a public health disaster. *J Epidemiol Community Health* 1994;48:331–2.

47. Plasencia A, Ferrando J. Accidentes de trafico. In: Navarro C, Cabases JM, Tormo MJ. (eds.) *La Salud y el Sistema Sanitario en España: Informe SESPAS 1995.* Barcelona: SG editores, 1995 pp. 72.

48. Plasencia A, Ferrando J. Epidemiologia de los accidnetes de tráfico. In: Alvarez González FJ. (ed.) *Seguridad Vial y Medicina de Tráfico.* Barcelona: Masson, SA., 1997 pp. 1–21.

49. Plasencia A. La medida del alcohol en los accidentes de tráfico: hasta cuando la estrategia del avestruz? *Gac Sanit* 1996;10:51–4.

50. Dirección General de Alta Inspección y Relaciones Institucionales. *Ciudades Saludables: Informe 1995.* Madrid: Ministerio de Sanidad y Consumo, 1995.

51. Artazcoz L, Moncada S, Manzanera R. El proyecto ciudades saludables casi una década despues. In: Navarro C, Cabases JM, Tormo MJ. (eds.) *La Salud y el Sistema Sanitario en España: Informe SESPAS 1995.* Barcelona: SG editores, 1995 pp. 1475–6.

52. Manzanera R, Moncada S, Artazcoz L. *L'experiència de la xarxa espanyola de ciutats saludables (XESCS).* International Healthy and Ecological Cities Congress. Madrid: 1995 pp. 215–24.

8

Decision-Making in Public Health Policy in France

Claude Rumeau-Rouquette and Gerard Breart

Introduction

Decisions about health policy are greatly influenced by the political, social and cultural context, and, in particular, by the health care system. This chapter begins with a brief description of the French health care system, followed by an examination of the information that fuels the decision-making process, finally it looks at the interplay between political forces and interest groups that leads to the decision.

The scientific bases that underlie public health decision-making have been described,[1,2] and we know that the following are required:

- an assessment of needs and resources,

- a forecast of positive and negative effects,

- cost evaluation.

Furthermore, decision and evaluation are intertwined, for all health measures ought to be evaluated, and this evaluation may, in turn, lead to new decisions. All of these operations are based on information and its processing by various techniques, statistical, economic, epidemiological and others.

In reality, the decision-making process is much more complex: it is sometimes consensual and rests most often on an interplay between various groups and their relative power. These include elected officials, government bodies, the medical profession, trade unions, the media and consumers, as well as industry and other market forces. The relationship between power and interest groups depends on the type of decision and its political and economic context.

The French health care system[3]

Before describing the health care system, it is necessary to outline the general setting in which it operates. In 1990, France had 56.4 million inhabitants and a population density of 103.1 persons per square kilometer, lower than that of Germany, the United Kingdom, or Belgium. In 1988, 18.6 per cent of the population was under the age of 20. In 1986, there was one hospital bed for every 80 inhabitants, and, in 1990, 2.6 doctors per thousand inhabitants. These figures are similar to those for Germany and Belgium and distinctly higher than those for the United Kingdom, where there was, during the same period, one hospital bed and 1.4 doctors per thousand inhabitants. By 1991, French women had attained a long life expectancy (80 years), while that for men was in the middle range for the European Community.

General characteristics

The French health care system is characterised by *freedom of choice*: patients choose the doctor they wish to consult, they can consult several for the same disorder, and can change doctors as often as they wish. There are no limits on access to specialists and hospitals. In the same spirit, doctors may choose where they practise and what they prescribe. Nonetheless, fees for doctors who are 'conventionne' (that is, eligible for insurance practice) are negotiated between representatives of the medical profession, the government, and the 'Sécurité Sociale', described below. Only a few doctors, who practise outside the insurance system, can set their fees freely. Many consider that this 'liberal' system increases costs, and that it will become more restrictive in the near future.

The French social security system is based upon the *principle of solidarity* and comprises three branches: health insurance (sickness fund), family allocations, and old-age pensions. The health branch reimburses the insured for health expenses paid to the doctor, hospital, or pharmacy. However, the practice of third-party payment is becoming more widespread. In this case, the patient pays only the co-payment, that is, the portion that would not in any case be reimbursed (0 to 30 per cent, even 60 per cent, according to the rate of reimbursement), and the doctor or hospital is directly reimbursed for the balance by the 'Sécurité Sociale'. This statutory insurance covers 75 per cent of health expenses, and additional reimbursement is available from private insurance companies (often trade-union based non-profit 'mutuelles').

The second branch of the 'Sécurité Sociale' distributes certain benefits for families with children. The third is a retirement or pension system.

The 'Sécurité Sociale' is a private entity funded by those insured with it, their employers, and the government. Participation is mandatory and 98 per cent of the population are covered. Nonetheless, because of unemployment, and despite measures to aid the unemployed (unemployment insurance benefits, and a minimum income, the RMI), a growing proportion of the population may no longer have social protection, especially young people who cannot find a first job and the homeless. Charitable associations are setting up new systems, and some have suggested that 'two-track medical care' may be appearing.

The growing deficit of the 'Sécurité sociale' has increased the role of the State. As the government is making up the shortfall with new taxes, it wants a greater role in the Sickness Fund's administration. The introduction of the current plan to redress the finances of the 'Sécurité Sociale' was marked by social unrest. This was the case in April 1997 in protest against measures to contain health costs in which an overall budget is to be approved each year and sanctions applied if this is exceeded.

Public health

The health care system has long *favoured treatment over prevention*. Medical facilities focus mainly on diagnostics and care for the sick. This tendency is especially obvious in hospitals, where consultations for prevention are not generally available, except in maternity wards. It is less true among private practitioners, who have an increasingly important role in providing health and hygiene advice and in screening for various diseases.

Medical education devotes more attention to curative than preventive medicine. However, there have been recent efforts to adjust this imbalance, including the creation of a public health internship analogous to that in standard medical programmes, and the promotion of graduate programmes in the field by advanced degrees (DEA) and dissertations in public health.

Research in public health has evolved unevenly in France. Although epidemiological research has advanced steadily over the past 30 years, other disciplines, in particular the economics and the sociology of health, still do not receive enough attention.

Two categories of health providers include prevention among their goals. First, those who deal with population groups with particular risks. These include occupational or industrial physicians as well as those in school settings. Industrial medicine is more highly developed and involves, in particular, systematic examinations at the time of hiring staff and for monitoring purposes. Nonetheless, it has only a very limited role in monitoring occupational risks related to particular work situations. At the initiative of the 'Sécurité Sociale', some facilities for carrying out systematic examinations among the general public have been established.

The second type of organisation deals with prevention and includes those bodies that survey and monitor environmental air and water pollution, air quality, and work-related risk factors. These agencies, although outside the health system, can contribute to it. Recently, the health system has set up bodies to monitor the negative effects of health care and health care facilities, including, for example, drug side effects and iatrogenic infections in hospitals.[4]

The role of the state and centralisation

Figure 1 provides an outline of the organisation of public health in France. The national government plays an important role: within the Ministry for Health, the 'Direction Générale de la Santé' is responsible for monitoring, supervision and evaluation in the area of public health; other ministries are also involved in health issues; the most important of these being Environment, Labour and Agriculture.

Also, within the Ministry for Health, the High Committee for Public Health contributes to defining goals and proposing policy, for example, by issuing reports. Other bodies involved with health policy include: the Pharmaceuticals Agency (Agence du Medicament), the French Blood Agency, the General Delegation against Drug Addiction, and the French Committee for Health Education. The Pharmaceuticals Agency gives the authorisation for marketing, and is in charge of post-marketing surveillance. The other bodies propose preventive action and are in charge of surveillance. A proposal to create two agencies along the lines of a French Food and Pharmaceuticals Administration has been put forward and approved by Parliament.

The State has an active policy that promotes public health on several different fronts. Public health research takes place at INSERM (National Institute for Health and Medical Research), in universities, and also in a new organisation, the National Network for Public Health. This research is financed mainly by the State and local authorities, with some contributions from the various Sickness Funds ('Caisses d'Assurance Maladie') and several private foundations, especially in the domains of cancer and AIDS.

The State organises prevention programmes such as those set up for perinatology and for AIDS. Other measures target more directly populations with specific problems. The State also promotes health monitoring by setting up the information systems described below, as well as evaluation systems, in association with the National Agency for Development of Medical Evaluation.

The French health care system remains quite centralised. Decisions made by the State are supposed to apply equally to all, and even those provisions that refer to populations considered to be at high risk are, in theory, uniformly applicable throughout the nation.

Some State responsibilities such as maternal and child health and prevention of alcohol abuse have been devolved to the local level, where they are managed by the regional and departmental divisions for Health and Social Services. Alongside these agencies, the regional Health Observatories, which are officially private entities (non-profit associations), are intended to provide a sort of one-stop shopping centre for health information.

Decentralisation has endowed local elected authorities (mayors, general and regional councils) with power and responsibilities in the administration of health care and preventive services. A balance between local and central power is still difficult to achieve sometimes, as illustrated recently by the dispute between the Ministry for Health and local officials about hospital closures.

Figure 1
Organisation of public health at national level in France

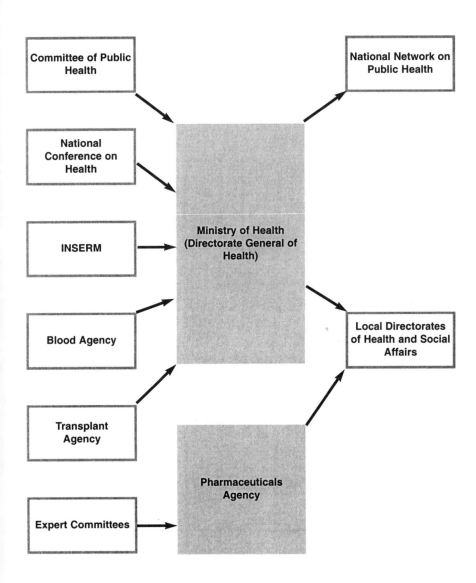

Defining priorities

Defining priorities is an essential stage in health policy-making, as it is a necessary step in planning decisions. The Ministry of Health has relied for many years on groups of experts. Over the past 20 years, it has set up procedures based on health information, research and studies designed specifically to lay the groundwork for decisions.

Permanent sources of information

These information sources allow an assessment of the significance of health problems, by tracking their frequency and seriousness. They can also uncover trends and shifts and identify inequalities. Although information about the population's health status has long been underdeveloped in France in comparison with the Nordic- and English-speaking countries, it has expanded considerably over the past 20 years.[5]

The National Institute for Statistics and Economic Studies (INSEE) keeps good demographic statistics, and its demographic panel allows a sample of the French population to be tracked, along similar lines to the English 'longitudinal survey'. Although these demographic data include no medical information, they are useful for health policy planning, as they supply the bases for rate calculations and also provide information about such health determinants as population density and socio-economic characteristics. These data do, however, present the problem of how to keep them up-to-date between censuses, since France does not have local population registers. Data are updated annually for each 'département' or county, taking into consideration births and deaths, but migration inflow and outflow are not taken into account. It is hard to know the population of small geographic areas, for example, those around a pollution source or industrial zone. However, very specific decisions may be necessary to protect the health of these populations.

Cause-of-death statistics are kept by INSERM, in liaison with INSEE.[6] These data are confidential, and obtaining the names of the deceased requires special authorisation. The quality of these statistics and their accessibility have improved substantially, and they are an important element in decision-making. In particular, they allow the stability or changes in certain rates to be observed and geographic disparities to be measured. Since deaths are reported in the place of residence (town and 'département'), they can be analysed for fairly small areas, but the mortality rates cannot be calculated routinely if population changes are not updated regularly. Another disadvantage of these statistics is that they exist in a relative vacuum: because there is no linkage between the demographic data and the causes of death, the study of differential mortality is limited. This disadvantage is a general characteristic of the French health statistics system, which places great stress on preserving confidentiality.

The quality of the registration of infectious diseases is, in France as in many other countries, very uneven and often mediocre. For this reason, alternative systems have been set up, for instance for AIDS. Registration of AIDS cases is mandatory and is handled by a special centre which is also a WHO Reference Centre for Europe.[7] Particular care is taken with the validation and analysis of these data, which are consistent and coherent. However, decision-making also requires information on the incidence of HIV diagnoses, so that the progress of the epidemic can be forecast. The results of various forecasting attempts have varied according to the quality of the data, the models used, and the hypotheses. Decision-making also requires more specific knowledge about the epidemic in small geographic areas and among high-risk groups.

For contagious diseases, especially influenza, information is drawn from networks of volunteer doctors. This method does not guarantee representative data, but it does allow an epidemic to be detected and the necessary emergency measures to be taken in the affected zones.

Although there is no national morbidity register in France, such registers have become more frequent at the 'département' level.[8] They cover cancer (about ten different registers), congenital malformations, children's disabilities, and cardiovascular diseases, and are used for monitoring and for research. The registries of congenital malformations, which were initially created to uncover increases in prevalence, have also facilitated the evaluation and improvement of intra-uterine diagnoses and research on teratogenic factors. Cancer and cardiovascular disease registers have usually been intended to allow the long-term trends of prevalence and geographic distribution to be studied.

Other permanent sources of information are the standard indicators of capacity and functioning of organisations and facilities that provide treatment and prevention. The quality of these data is uneven.

Much information about the environment, and pollution in particular, is available, but is generally kept by relatively independent bodies, as is also the case with the economic data gathered by INSEE. Surveys of household consumption do include a section on health, and INSEE is considering a major survey of handicaps.

Besides the permanent sources of information that have been described, various ad hoc investigations take place at national and regional levels but cannot be detailed here.[9,10]

Health research

The study of health determinants, through both basic and epidemiological research, is well developed in France and has an excellent reputation. France also participates extensively in European and international cooperative projects. There are nonetheless some gaps, notably in the study of such disorders as rheumatism and some important general health determinants. It is regrettable that there has not been more interest in research on socio-economic factors as health determinants over the past 20 years. Centres of research on health economics are rare. French epidemiologists concentrate primarily on the study of risk factors that are either biological or related to lifestyle (smoking, drinking, but also working conditions). There has also been too little research into risk factors related to pollution.[11]

Despite these problems, priority setting increasingly takes research-based evidence into account. A recent survey, described in the following section, showed that a relationship between health determinants and health problems is a primary criterion in the selection of priorities.

Evaluating health interventions is fundamental in deciding whether to introduce new interventions and new measures.[12] Evaluation methods, which first assessed drugs in randomised trials, have undergone considerable development.[13] These techniques have since been adapted for evaluating prevention methods promoted among the general population. Comparisons of various rates before and after an intervention are widely used; evaluations based on geographic comparisons are less common in France, because of the relatively centralised nature of decisions.

The creation of the 'Agence Nationale pour le Dévelopement de l'Evaluation Medicale' is a sign of the particular concern that the administration of the French health care system has for this area. Nonetheless, health programmes are not always evaluated, nor does quality control of their routine operations always take place. Evaluation of simple interventions such as some screening methods and the introduction of new procedures is probably becoming more widespread.[14] This is not true, however, for other measures, such as information campaigns.

Setting priorities: a specific approach

Elected and appointed officials and physicians have long played a predominant role in defining priorities. A scientific approach to this process began with cost-benefit analyses of health choices.[15] In 1969, the Ministry of Health launched a major survey to lay the groundwork for budgetary choices in several areas which had been selected in advance by a group of experts, mainly professors of medicine. These fields included health problems linked to childbirth, ageing, and accidents, specific diseases (mental disorders, alcoholism, rheumatism) and the functioning of the health care systems. After this initial choice of priorities, measures to be taken in the perinatality domain were chosen by a more scientific approach that included the following stages: evaluation of the problem, inventory of possible choices, and assessment of resources, costs, and expected effects. Decisions to institute measures in perinatal health, the necessary funding and evaluation of the effects of the programme all followed. Despite this success, the procedure has not often been used as exhaustively since then. It has also been criticised for its quantifying of benefits, costs and the value of human life. Despite these limitations, such analyses have had a positive effect by making clear the necessity of assessing needs and resources accurately, forecasting costs, and evaluating the steps taken.

During the 1980s, the general priority areas have continued to be set through cooperation and consultation between government officials and experts. The development of organised expert appraisals, especially, for example, consensus conferences, has furthered the scientific approach.[16] Furthermore, evaluation techniques have grown in number and provide the basis for new decisions.[17]

In 1994, the Ministry for Health used the Delphi technique in a survey to define national priorities in public health.[18] This method allows the insights of a large group of people to be solicited, in a process that enables them to exchange opinions. The use of written questionnaires prevents group phenomena from influencing opinions. The first steps involve narrowing down the subject, identifying and contacting the respondents, and choosing the sample size. This survey included three questionnaires and was supervised by a committee of six senior civil servants from the ministries of health and research. The questionnaires were filled out by 125 experts, ranging from health care administrators, to members of the High Committee on Public Health, research and teaching institutions (INSERM, universities, The National School of Health etc.), and specialists from information systems within the Health Ministry, the regional Health Observatories, and finally health insurance funds (the primary statutory insurer and supplemental 'mutuelles').

The first questionnaire asked for a list of eight health problems considered particularly important in France, another list of four major determinants of health problems (besides sex and age), and, finally, the criteria used in compiling both lists. The second questionnaire called for a selection and ranking of the health problems and determinants suggested by the first; it also included a question about problems in the organisation of the health care system. The third questionnaire asked for a final ranking of the highest priority health problems and concrete suggestions for improving the four most important problems of organisation. There was also a question on measures that might improve the quality of life.

In summary, the highest priority problems were judged to be: accidents, the major types of cancer, AIDS and other sexually transmitted diseases, mental illness, senility and dependence, perinatal issues, iatrogenic and nosocomial disorders and infections, child abuse and neglect, pain and backaches. The priority determinants were lifestyle habits (alcohol, smoking and careless risk-taking), socio-economic conditions (exclusion, extreme poverty, problems of access to health services, curative, preventive, and informative). The problems of organisation were also extensively considered: lack of a structured public health policy, lack of coordination between decision centres, inappropriate professional training and organisation of care, insufficient facilities and systems for prevention, information and evaluation. Other problems raised included the need for better integration of health projects into social policies, for promoting initiatives, commentary and public debate, and for improvements in the quality of life for the handicapped.

This procedure was notably different from those used since 1970. For the first time, a large group of experts was consulted about setting priorities, a task previously limited to official commissions or small selected ad hoc groups. This group contained a variety of viewpoints although health care consumers were not included as such. The use of questionnaires prevented the kind of domination that so often occurs in meetings. It is, nonetheless, striking that the main health problems were so similar to the 1970 list, with, of course, the addition of AIDS, as well as other sexually transmitted diseases and drug addiction, and also iatrogenic disorders, pain, and child abuse. The most novel and interesting aspect is the examination from all angles, beginning with the second questionnaire, of the problems of the organisation of health care. The responses sum up well the current shortcomings and aspirations.

The report's conclusions have been used to design specific programmes on ageing and perinatal programmes which were implemented in 1997. The public debate is focusing more on specific programmes than on setting priorities.

Decision-making

Setting priorities would be an academic exercise were it not accompanied by decisions to allocate the necessary resources.

The form of decisions

In France, it is the State that decides health policy. In the most important cases, decisions take the form of a law debated and voted by the Parliament and, in rare cases, of an ordinance, if Parliament so authorises the government. It should be remembered that the social security system was enacted by ordinance in 1945. Most often, however, health programmes are initiated under the authority of pre-existing laws and can lead to either regulatory measures (decrees, 'arrêtés', circulars) or to incentives (recommendations, financial measures, etc.).

Health policies effective throughout France are enacted by the Ministry of Health, and other Ministries, if appropriate. Some local measures are taken by local authorities, that is, local representatives of the national government, or local elected bodies.

The decision-makers

In such a system, the primary role belongs to those with political power. Those with such power include civil servants and administrators as well as elected officials. This power is supposed to represent the will of the people but is also sensitive to pressure from the medical profession, trade unions and the media.

The senior management of the Ministry of Health and the committees and agencies that surround it also have important roles. Their enthusiasm determines how much support a given project receives. This group is fairly stable in comparison to the more ephemeral political personnel, and its stability is one of its strengths.

The Ministry of Finance acts as arbiter, keeps an eye on cost estimates and tries to reduce them as much as possible. It has a key role and undoubtedly contributes to the rigour of the decision-making process. Although it is often considered to be the cause of stagnation, it is sometimes only the excuse.

The medical profession's role is also very important. As the only advisors to health ministers for many years, physicians influenced most decisions to such an extent that one could talk about 'medical power'. But the profession is far from homogeneous.

The medical professors who used to make up most of the Consultative Committees of the Ministry of Health were generally more oriented towards curative services than public health. In the past, several exceptions to this rule have led movements such as that for family planning. Often dissidents within the profession, these public health leaders, with the help of the media, have been able to contribute towards setting priorities and have even influenced decisions. Currently, support for public health is fairly strong within medical academia. Practising physicians, numerous in France, appear open to the kinds of preventative medicine that they can practise in their own offices, but few participate actively in the setting of priorities or evaluation of choices. Furthermore, the consequent diminution of their income and social role is inducing many to adopt fairly conservative attitudes in response to what they perceive as threats to their pockets and prestige. The physicians most involved in public health (school and industrial physicians) have not yet fully comprehended the scope of their role.

Alongside the traditional participants in health policy-making, the many components of the so-called 'market economy' are playing an increasingly important role. Health issues affect major economic and financial interests and involve enterprises (the pharmaceutical industry, medical engineering, public works etc.) in a system in which the reimbursement of expenses prevents market laws from applying. Preventive measures that involve industrial production and mass consumption are welcomed more warmly than others. Thus, in the 1970s, methods of non-invasive intrauterine diagnosis were more successful than those involving good health practices. It is sometimes difficult for politician/decision-makers to resist these pressures, especially in periods of high unemployment.

Trade union influence is manifested in two ways: directly, when unions feel their members are threatened, by certain organisational reforms for example; and indirectly, to the extent that unions are involved in the administration of the 'Sécurité Sociale'.

Finally, both the media and public interest groups and associations play an increasingly important role. The media has a major effect on public opinion and information in the area of health care. It is regrettable that they so often give in to a hunger for sensationalism and high ratings. They can influence policy directly or indirectly.

General consumer groups are less important and influential in France than in other countries. Their activity mostly involves bringing to public attention flaws and faults in the sale or manufacture of products. Specialised groups, which defend the interests of those who suffer from medical malpractice and discrimination, are acquiring more influence, as are groups representing patients and their families.

In conclusion, there has been a recent change in France regarding decision-making in health policy. Recommendations and proposals are more often based on a scientific approach rather than on expert opinion only. The development of surveillance systems and evaluation studies have allowed epidemiology to play an increasing role in decision-making.

References

1. Holland WW. *Evaluation of health care*. Oxford: Oxford University Press, 1983.

2. Battista RN, Lawrence RS. Implementing preventive services. *American Journal of Preventive Medicine* 1988;4 (supplement).

3. Duriez M, Sandier S. *Le système de santé en France, Organisation et fonctionnement*. Paris: Service de l'information et de la communication. Ministère des affaires sociales, de la santé et de la ville, 1994.

4. Brüker G, and Fassin D. *Santé Publique*. Paris: Ellipses, 1989.

5. Haut Comité de la Santé Publique. *La santé en France, rapport général*. Paris: La Documentation française, 1994.

6. Bouvier-Colle MH, Vallin J, Hatton F. *Mortalité et cause de décès en France*. Paris: INSERM-Doin, 1990.

7. European Centre for the epidemiological monitoring of AIDS. *HIV/AIDS surveillance in Europe, quarterly report, 48*. Paris, 1995.

8. Paccaud F, Raymond L. Les registres de morbidité. *Revue d'Epidémiologie et de Santé Publique* 1988;36:267–382.

9. Blondel B, du Mazaubrun C, Bréart G. *Enquête nationale périnatale 1995. Rapport de fin d'étude*. Paris: INSERM U-149, 1996.

10. Rumeau-Rouquette C, du Mazaubrun C, Rabarison Y. *Naître en France, 10 ans d'évolution*. Paris: INSERM-Doin, 1984.

11. Cordier S, Dab W. Epidémiologie des risques liés à l'environnement. *Revue d'Epidémiologie et de Santé Publique* 1995;43:393–4.

12. World Health Organization Europe. *Prevention in primary care*. Copenhagen: WHO, 1994.

13. Schwartz D, Flamant R, Lellouch J. *Clinical trials*. London: Academic Press, 1980.

14. *Fonds d'intervention en Santé publique. Résumé des projets*. Saint-Maurice: Réseau National de Santé Publique, 1994.

15. Rumeau-Rouquette C, Blondel B. Influence des politiques sociales et de santé sur l'évolution future de la mortalité. Le plan périnatal français. In: J Vallin, A Lopez (eds.) *La lutte contre la mort Paris:* P.U.F., 1985:293–304.

16. Tournaire M, Bréart G, Delecour M, Papiernik E. *Apport de l'échographie en obstétrique*. Paris: Vigot, 1987.

17. Philippe HJ. *L'évaluation en gynécologie*. Paris: Masson, 1995.

18. Direction Générale de la Santé. *Les priorités nationales en santé publique, Etude Delphi*. Paris: Dossier documentaire, 1995.

9

Public Health Policy and Priorities in Ireland

Bernadette Herity and Patricia Fitzpatrick

Introduction

The Republic of Ireland has a population of 3.5 million and covers an area of approximately 69,000 sq. kilometres. About half the population lives within 60 kilometres of Dublin, the capital. Only three other cities, Cork, Limerick and Galway, have populations greater than 50,000, while the rest of the country has in the main a scattered rural population.

Life expectancy in Ireland has increased substantially over the past 50 years. For males life expectancy at birth is 72 and for females 77.5 years; however life expectancy still remains below the EU average (Figure 1). Infant mortality has fallen from 46/1,000 live births in 1950 to 8.2/1,000 in 1991, just above the EU average of 7.5/1,000. Mortality

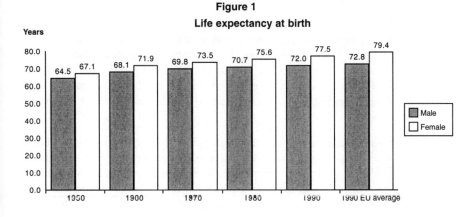

Figure 1
Life expectancy at birth

rates for heart attack and stroke have fallen; for stroke the rate is below the EU average, while for heart attack the rate remains above the average.[1] The death rate from accidents in the years 1988–92 was 35/100,000 population, below the EU average of 55/100,000 (1991). The death rate from cancer is rising and at 273/100,000 for 1988–92 is above the EU average of 245 (1991).

The prevalence of smoking has fallen from 43 per cent of adults in the 1970s to 28 per cent, but there has been an increase in the number of females smoking and smoking-related disease still accounts for 6,000 deaths in Ireland per year.[1] While recorded consumption of pure alcohol per capita in Ireland is low compared to many other European countries, alcohol-related problems are still prevalent in Ireland.[2]

Structure of health services

In order to comprehend the context in which public health policy and priorities are decided in the Republic of Ireland it is necessary to give a brief account of the structure and organisation of the health services.

The current organisation of health services results from the Health Act 1970 which transferred responsibility for the administration of health services from local authorities to eight regional health boards with populations varying from 200,000–1,000,000 people. The boards are responsible to the Minister for Health, are funded directly by the Department of Health through central taxation, and moneys must be spent in accordance with Department of Health policy. Each board has a Chief Executive Officer (CEO) and most powers and functions of the board are vested in him/her. Membership of the board (of about 30–35) includes local political representatives (50 per cent), representatives of health professions and nominees of the Minister for Health.

Each board runs 'programmes' with the titles of Acute Hospital, Special Hospital and Community Care Programmes and each programme has a programme manager. Smaller boards have only one hospital programme. The majority of public health functions are carried out under the Community Care Programme. The 1970 Act also introduced the choice of doctor scheme to replace the dispensary service which required patients entitled to free general practitioner (GP) care to attend a designated doctor in the area in which they lived.

Health care is provided by a mix of publicly and privately funded services; eligibility for free services is based on income. Approximately 40 per cent of the population is entitled to totally free services (category I), and all women are entitled to obstetric care without charge. The remainder (category II) are entitled at no cost to hospital services in a public ward, infectious disease services, some child health services and to rebates on drug and long-term illness costs. Those in employment pay social insurance at 1 per cent of earnings for these services. Many category II persons are also privately insured with Voluntary Health Insurance (VHI), a semi-state company which runs five schemes with benefits directly related to annual subscriptions.

GP services are provided free to category I persons by the health boards. This arrangement is based on agreement with participant GPs and is called the General Medical Service (GMS). Payment is on a capitation basis with fees for some special items of service. Within geographical constraints there is a choice of doctor but GPs do not have automatic right of entry to the GMS since there is a fixed number of GMS practices. The remaining 60 per cent of the population pay their GP from their own resources on a fee per service basis. There are approximately 2,000 GPs in the country, i.e. 1/1,750 population.

The public hospital service consists of health board hospitals and voluntary hospitals. The former are funded and run directly by the health boards and the latter by boards of management. The voluntary hospitals were largely founded by charitable organisations, such as religious orders, in the 19th century and predate the establishment of state-run hospitals. They are privately owned and at present receive funding directly from the Department of Health. The largest of these hospitals are in Dublin and are teaching hospitals and tertiary referral centres. However, in a proposed reorganisation of the hospital services, it is proposed that these hospitals will also be funded through the health boards. There are also a number of privately run hospitals which are not state supported.

Public health structure

Recent years have seen changes in the hierarchy and staffing of public health in Ireland, following the publication of a review of public health.[3] This report advocated a restructuring of the staffing structure of public health in Ireland; the designated changes are now being implemented.

In 1995, Regional Departments of Public Health were established in each health board. Each department has a director and a number of specialists in public health medicine, the number in each health board proportional to the size of the population. The Director of Public Health is a member of the management team of the health board.

Each department is concerned with the following: epidemiology of disease; environmental health, including monitoring of potential hazards and cluster analysis; communicable disease, including surveillance, dissemination of information and policy for disease control; needs assessment; chronic disease surveillance and health promotion. National health promotion policies are established and implemented by the Health Promotion Unit of the Department of Health, while the role of the Departments of Public Health is to cooperate with the Health Promotion Unit in advising on priorities and evaluating outcomes.

Each health board is divided into a number of community care areas. Until 1996, the medical team within each area consisted of a Director of Community Care/Medical Officer of Health, a Senior Area Medical Officer and a number of Area Medical Officers. Under the revision of the staffing structure the post of the Director of

Community Care/Medical Officer of Health is being abolished. Each community care area medical team will be led by a Senior Area Medical Officer, while the management of the area will transfer to an Area Manager, a new post.

The role of the Senior Area Medical Officer is to plan and implement the provision of community medical services for the community care area; these include childhood developmental examination, school medical examinations, medical examinations of children entering into the care of the health board, cervical screening clinics, investigation of infectious disease outbreaks and control of tuberculosis through contact tracing and treatment. In addition the medical services include coordination of services for the elderly and people with disabilities. The Area Medical Officers work with the Senior Area Medical Officer in the provision of these services. The Senior Area Medical Officer will have a close collaborative working relationship with the Regional Department of Public Health to facilitate policy implementation and information exchange.

Public health research

There are five departments of public health medicine or related areas in Irish universities, each of which undertakes research in public health. Public health research is also carried out by the eight health boards, and by the Economic and Social Research Institute. Frequently collaborative research is undertaken by those bodies. It is expected that the newly established All Ireland Institute of Public Health will initiate and coordinate north-south collaboration in public health research. Government funding for all health research is awarded through the Health Research Board, a statutory agency established in 1987. It advertises annually for applications for grants, scholarships and fellowships in medical and allied disciplines and disburses approximately £IR 2,500,000 annually. Funding for public health research also comes from medical charities, EU research programmes and international agencies.

Public health policy

Since the 1960s a number of policy documents have been published on various health issues, which have directed the development of specific services. These documents include: report of the Commission on Itinerancy,[4] report of the Commission of Inquiry on Mental Handicap,[5] 'Outline of the future hospital system',[6] report of Commission of Inquiry on Mental Illness,[7] Child health services,[8] 'Care of the aged',[9] 'Training and employing the handicapped',[10] report of the working party on prescribing and dispensing in the General Medical Service,[11] 'Task force on child care services',[12] report of the working party on the General Medical Service,[13] 'Psychiatric Services – planning for the future',[14] 'Irish medical care resources: an economic analysis',[15] 'Health – the wider dimensions',[16] 'Promoting health through public policy',[17] 'The years ahead – a policy for the elderly',[18] report of the Commission on Health Funding,[19] 'Needs and abilities, a policy for the intellectually disabled',[20] 'Community medicine and public health. The future',[3] and the third report of Dublin Hospital Initiative Group.[21]

However, an overall plan encompassing all aspects of health care was not published until recently. The Department of Health in 1994 produced the first national strategy for health 'Shaping a Healthier Future – a strategy for effective healthcare in the 1990s'.[1] Figure 2, overleaf, portrays diagrammatically the main pathways and interactions between key shareholders in policy formation.

Advances in technology and therapeutic options, although welcomed, have increased the cost of health care in Ireland as elsewhere. In Ireland there has been a large increase in the number of people over the age of 65 years, with an increase of 4.8 per cent between 1986 and 1991, from 384,000 to 403,000; this doubling of the projected increase meant that the number of elderly people had reached by 1991 a level not expected until the next century.[22] The principal cause was a greater than expected fall in mortality rates. In addition there has been an increase in patient expectations of medical care.

These factors have contributed to the spiralling cost of health care. Funding of health care has to compete at governmental level with funding of all other public services; while as a proportion of Gross Domestic Product Ireland spends a comparable amount on health care (8 per cent) as other countries, the actual amount per capita is considerably lower than in the more affluent countries.[1] In order to address the problems of funding of health services, a central element in the national strategy is the emphasis which has been placed on achieving the greatest possible benefit from whatever resources are available.[1]

In 1998 the Department of Health & Children published their Strategy Statement 1998–2001 entitled 'Working for health and well-being'.[23] This strategy statement builds upon the process of health strategy commenced with the publication of the national strategy in 1994.

Disease surveillance and screening

In Ireland certain infectious diseases are notifiable by the diagnosing doctor under statutory regulations (Appendix 1). The Director of Public Health in each area has responsibility for implementing the statutory requirements for the monitoring and control of infectious diseases. A National Infectious Disease Surveillance centre will soon be established and will facilitate disease surveillance on a national basis. Surveillance of tuberculosis takes place at national, regional (health board) and local (community care area) level through the Department of Health and the health boards. Non-statutory sources of information (e.g. laboratories, prescriptions of anti-tuberculous medications) are local in nature and are important supplementary surveillance procedures to ensure complete case reporting.[24] Currently, surveillance of HIV infection and AIDS is via linked testing of presenting patients and unlinked anonymous surveillance on antenatal bloods from some maternity hospitals.

Two regions in Ireland contribute to Eurocat, a programme supported by the European

Figure 2
Main pathways and interactions between key stakeholders in policy formation

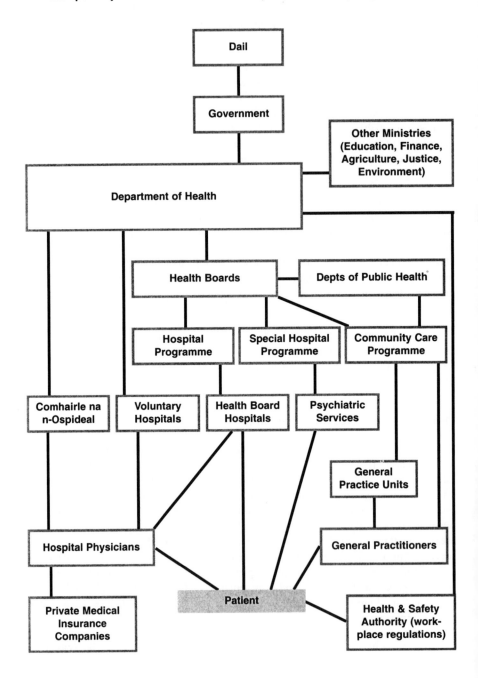

Community for the epidemiological surveillance of congenital anomalies in Europe.[25] Dublin began transmission of data to the Eurocat central registry in 1979 and Galway in 1981. The Dublin registry covers all births to mothers resident in the Eastern Health Board area, while the Galway registry covers births to mothers resident in Galway county.

All new-born children in Ireland are screened for the following diseases (prevalence in parentheses): phenylketonuria (1/4,500); congenital hypothyroidism (1/3,300); galactosaemia (1/18,700); homocystinuria (1/64,500); and maple syrup urine disease (1/123,500).[26] All children are invited to a developmental screening at nine months of age; this is carried out by Area Medical Officers. All children in public primary schools are screened for vision and hearing.

Following the publication of the national strategy for cancer[27] the Minister for Health has funded the development of national screening programmes for breast and cervical cancer on a phased basis. The screening programme for breast cancer has commenced in the North-Eastern Health Board and will be extended to the rest of the country. Cervical screening has been available on an opportunistic basis through GPs, special clinics and maternity hospitals. A pilot programme of population screening has commenced in one of the health boards. Funding for the pilot and for additional cytology support has been made available. Steering committees have been established for both screening programmes and legislation to enable the creation of a population register for screening purposes was passed in 1997.

The national strategy 1994

The main theme of the national strategy for health is the reorientation of the health care system towards improving the effectiveness of the health and personal social services by reshaping the way that services are planned and delivered. The strategy was accompanied by a Four Year Action Plan, mapping out the detail of the implementation of the strategy over the years 1994–1997. 'Shaping a Healthier Future' signified a watershed in Irish health care; no previous document had ever set out the plans and policies in such a specific way and with such emphasis on quality, equity and accountability.

The strategy was formulated by the Minister for Health and the Department of Health. It was drafted by the planning unit of the department and developed in consultation with the other subdivisions of the department. A number of key reports already published were used in the development of the strategy (see under Public Health Policy). These included the 'Report of the Commission for Health Funding',[19] 'Health – the Wider Dimensions'[16] and many other sectoral reports covering areas such as public health, the elderly, child care, acute hospital services, mental health and mental handicap.

In producing each of these forerunner documents, submissions had been invited from the general public and from all interested parties and an exhaustive consultative process ensued. In the formulation of the strategy, the Department of Health drew on these prior consultations and in the interest of expediency did not seek fresh consultation with the general public. However, key individuals in various sectors of the health services were consulted informally. After publication of the document, consultation was invited from all appropriate parties on how best to implement the details of the policies outlined.

In addition, the Department of Health drew on routine sources of information to prioritise services and plan the national policy, including data from the Central Statistics Office and the Hospital In-patient Enquiry system (HIPE), which provides valuable information on service provision, documenting diagnosis, procedures and discharge status of all in-patients and day patients in acute hospitals.

The Report of the Commission on Health Funding[19] was the work of a commission established by the Minister for Health to examine the financing of the health services and to make recommendations on the extent and sources of the future funding required to provide an equitable comprehensive and cost effective public health service and on any changes in administration which seem desirable for that purpose. The members of this commission included senior members of the Departments of Health and the Taoiseach (Prime Minister), senior economists, accountants, a senior medical representative of the Irish Medical Organisation, a senior trade union official, and senior members of health boards. The commission concluded that the solution to problems facing the Irish health service did not lie in the system of funding but rather in the way that services are planned, organised and delivered. It highlighted inadequate accountability, insufficient integration of related services and a lack of information systems to facilitate decision-making about choices.

'Health, the Wider Dimensions' was a document produced by the Department of Health.[16] It was drafted by the Planning Unit of the department and developed in consultation with the other subdivisions of the department. It emphasised reorientation of the health services in keeping with the Ottawa Charter and highlighted the multisectoral dimension to health. In preparing the strategy, the Department of Health took account also of the themes and targets of the World Health Organisation's (WHO) 'Health for All 2000' (1985) and of the potential for strengthening EU cooperation in line with Article 129 of the Maastricht Treaty.

The three principles underpinning the strategy are equity, quality of service and accountability. The concepts of health gain and social gain are used to focus the health care services more clearly on improvements in health status or the quality of life. The emphasis in priority-setting in service development and provision is on application of resources to yield maximum benefit. The main causes of premature mortality in Ireland, cancer, cardiovascular disease and accidents, are prioritised as areas in which major health gain is achievable.

The strategy emphasises the need for a change in the basis upon which choices are made, with emphasis on evaluation of the health care needs of the population and of the relative effectiveness of the available responses to different forms of need. A need for a critical evaluation of the outcome of health services and medical intervention is also identified; this includes measurement of patient satisfaction with and public preference for services. Such an approach necessitates comprehensive and good quality information on needs, quality, activity and outcomes. There are deficiencies in the current information systems in operation in Ireland; development of good quality information systems is a focus of the strategy and a priority for the newly established Regional Departments of Public Health. The Hospital In-patient Enquiry System (HIPE) provides information on patients discharged from acute hospitals; however, this is an episode-based rather than a person-based system. Resources have been committed to the computerisation of general practices on a pilot basis, with the objective of accessing good quality, timely, person-based epidemiological data.

The strategy was launched in 1994; since then there has been a change of government with a new Minister for Health. However, the strategy remained the national policy without any change in direction, reflecting consensus between the political parties. In response to the strategy, the health boards developed corporate strategies which incorporate the central themes and give priority to quality and the measurement of outcomes.

Strategy statement 1998–2001

In 1998 'Working for health and well-being', a strategy statement for the years 1998–2001, was launched by the Department of Health & Children.[23] The change of title of the Department occurred in 1997, and is intended to reflect the commitment of Government to improvement of services for children and coordination of policy for children. The strategy statement has been developed in response to certain key challenges facing our health care services: there is growing consumer awareness and demand for high quality service; the disease risks associated with food and with blood products; ethical issues in reproductive medicine; an ageing population; public concern regarding care of children. Reflecting these challenges the key priorities set out by the Department are as follows:

(1) services for children;

(2) food safety, in the light of the bovine spongiform encephalopathy crisis and other food safety problems;

(3) enhancement of standards of safety in relation to blood and blood products; recent discovery of past contamination of Anti-D with hepatitis C has brought this issue to the fore in Ireland;

(4) continuing action to reduce mortality and morbidity from cardiovascular disease, cancer and accidents;

(5) development of a coherent policy position on the issue of abortion;

(6) development and improvement of services for older people and for persons with a mental handicap;

(7) structural and administrative reform with the health services.

The Four Year Action Plan

The strategy is accompanied by a Four Year Action Plan for the period 1994–1997, which sets out specific developments across a range of services and actions to improve linkages between community-based and acute hospital services in particular. National targets for reductions in risk factors associated with premature mortality and for improvements in other indicators of health status are stated, as are national objectives for service development on the basis of the directions and principles of the strategy.

Health promotion

The priority targets for health promotion are outlined in the Four Year Action Plan and further developed in the subsequent publication of 'A health promotion strategy, making the healthier choice the easier choice'.[28] Corresponding to the three main causes of premature mortality in Ireland of cardiovascular disease, cancer and accidents, they include smoking, alcohol, nutrition, cholesterol, hypertension, exercise and accidents. The target for smoking is to reduce the number of those who smoke by at least one percentage point per year so that more than 80 per cent of the population aged 15 years and over are non-smokers by the year 2000. The targets for alcohol misuse are to ensure that, before 1998, 75 per cent of the population aged 15 years and over knows and understands the recommended sensible limits for alcohol consumption, and to reduce substantially by 2004 the proportion of those who exceed the recommended sensible limits for alcohol consumption. Actions in the area of alcohol/substance misuse include education and training programmes and mass media initiatives that promote the avoidance of substance misuse.

The target for nutrition and diet is to encourage changes in the Irish diet by the year 2000 so as to include the recommended amount of essential nutrients and to provide the right levels of energy. The Nutrition Advisory Group to the Department of Health has published 'Recommendations for a food and nutrition policy for Ireland'.[29] The target for cholesterol is to achieve a reduction in mean serum cholesterol in the 35–63 year age group from 5.6 mmol/L to 5.2 mmol/L, and for blood pressure it is to achieve a situation where 75 per cent of the population in this age group have a blood pressure of less than 140/90mmHg, by 2005. A 30 per cent increase in the proportion of the population aged 15 years and over who engage in an accumulated 30 minutes of light physical exercise most days of the week and a 20 per cent increase in the proportion engaging in moderate exercise for 20 minutes three times per week are also sought. With regard to prevention of accidents a multisectoral approach is proposed with liaison at ministerial level to agree coordination in the accident reduction initiatives of the many agencies involved such as the National Safety Council and the Health and Safety Authority.

The Office of Health Gain, founded in 1995, is an initiative of the Chief Executive Officers of all health boards, supported by the Department of Health, to advance the Government's health strategy. Its aim is to facilitate joint action between health agencies, both public and voluntary, to achieve measurable health or social gain. It will collaborate with academic and professional institutions in appropriate areas, commission research and identify and disseminate information on good practice. It also plans to promote conferences, workshops, publications and reports related to its stated mission which is 'working together to achieve measurable health gain'. It publishes a quarterly journal 'The Journal of Health Gain', the first issue of which appeared in March 1997.[30]

To date the office has focused on smoking in young people, exercise and accidents as subjects for joint initiatives. The Smoking Target Action Group and the National Accident Forum are already in existence and a multidisciplinary group is currently drawing up a strategy for promotion of physical exercise. The recognition that small area data on the health status of the population was deficient has resulted in the establishment of an Irish Clearing House on Health Outcomes to organise systematic generation, collation and retrieval of data, building on the experience of the Health Information Unit of the Eastern Health Board which has produced a number of small area studies.[31-34] The Office of Health Gain is still in its development stage and success in promoting the health gain agenda will depend on adequate resources, effective leadership and cooperation and participation by the key players in the health and social services.

Future strategy

A wide-ranging review of the four year action plan is currently underway by the Department of Health & Children. A further strategy for health care for the years 2001–2010 is planned.

Women's health

A discussion document on women's health 'Developing a policy for women's health' was published in 1995.[35] It stated that future policy for women's health should have the following objectives:

- To ensure that women's health needs are identified and planned for in a comprehensive way.

- To promote the health and welfare of women.

- To ensure that women receive the health and welfare services they need at the right time and in a way which respects their dignity and individuality with ease of access and continuity of care.

- To promote greater consultation with women about their health and welfare needs at national, regional and local level.

- To promote within the health services greater participation by women both in the more senior service positions and the representative levels.

It has also been suggested that the improvement of women's health in the developing world would be an objective of this country's membership of WHO and of Irish aid to developing countries.[36-38]

Cancer strategy

The Department of Health published a cancer strategy document in November 1996,[27] followed by the announcement of an Action Plan for Cancer in 1997. The strategy document deals with all aspects of cancer services including reorganisation of treatment services, development of screening programmes, health promotion, palliative care and cancer research. The features of the action plan are:

- Development of regional and supra regional cancer services. Nine regional directors have been appointed, one in each health board and two in the more densely populated Eastern Health Board. The directors will coordinate all aspects of the service and will develop a plan for their regions.

- Appointment of a Cancer Forum with multidisciplinary representation including consumers.

- Establishment of expert bodies to implement national screening programmes for breast and cervical cancer.

The Minister for Health has also introduced legislation to facilitate the use of existing data sources to create population registers for screening programmes. A total age-sex population register is not available in Ireland at present. Additional funds for cancer research are to be made available through the Health Research Board, and an epidemiologist is to be recruited to the National Cancer Registry which was established in 1994. A total of £IR6 million was allotted to the development of cancer services in 1997, with further funding in 1998 and 1999.

National and regional initiatives

A number of initiatives have already been undertaken which will contribute to the achievement of strategy targets. They are summarised below.

The Patient's Charter[39] was introduced by the Department of Health in 1992 as a guideline for good practice for acute hospitals. Many of the recommendations within the charter have been adopted by acute hospitals, although it has not been enshrined in Irish law.

The Community Mothers' Programme was launched in Dublin in 1983; this is a child development and health promotion programme implemented by non-professionals who are successful experienced mothers, guided by family development nurses. Potential community mothers are identified by local public health nurses and once approved undergo a pre-service training course. Each community mother works under the guidance of a family development nurse who serves as a resource person, confidante and monitor, working in partnership with 15–20 community mothers. Each community mother aims at supporting 5–15 parents. A randomised controlled trial of delivery of the programme to disadvantaged first time mothers for children aged up to one year demonstrated a beneficial effect.[40]

The Substance Abuse Prevention Programme is a primary prevention programme run by secondary level schools on the dangers of substance misuse. The programme is delivered by teachers with specific training in the implementation and facilitation of the programme.

Smokebusters is a primary prevention programme implemented by teachers which aims to reduce the initiation of smoking among schoolchildren aged 7–11 years. Children are invited to join a Smokebusters club, where non-smoking is seen as the norm and knowledge of the health hazards of smoking is increased in an enjoyable and participative manner. Smokebusters has been introduced on a pilot basis in the Eastern Health Board with further extension proposed.

Needle Exchange and Methadone Maintenance Programmes have been introduced in Dublin in an attempt to curb the growing problem of drug-related illness. Both inner city and satellite clinics have been established to treat and counsel drug abusers.

In 1996, a new **primary immunisation scheme** was introduced, with all vaccinations delivered by GPs instead of in health board immunisation clinics and improvement in the notification and call/recall systems. Payment to general practitioners is on a fee-per-item basis, with a bonus payment where 95 per cent uptake level is achieved. This revised scheme was outlined in the strategy as part of a rationalisation of the National Immunisation Programme, with the aim of maximising the timely uptake of primary immunisation.

Dublin became a full member of the **Healthy Cities Project** in 1989. The Dublin Healthy Cities Project has been involved in a number of different activities including: the Rainbow Walking Challenge which aims to encourage people to walk on a regular basis; a restaurant campaign to request a minimum of 30 per cent table space to be non-smoking; the production of a new range of no smoking signs for the Dublin area; community-based pilot projects to promote community participation in health awareness and health action; and involvement in the 'Smokebusters' project.

Three hospitals are part of the **European Health Promoting Hospital Network**, two in the Republic of Ireland and one in Northern Ireland. In addition a National Network of Health Promoting Hospitals has been established in 1996, incorporating 48 hospitals to date.

General Practitioner Units have been established in each health board with GPs in practice employed on a part-time basis. The primary objective of these units is to facilitate, support and develop general practice as a whole. The work of each unit involves improving the interface between general practice, hospitals and other health services, supporting the provision of additional services within general practice and providing supports for all aspects of general practice with particular reference to improving standards, organisation and structure. Recent work of the General Practitioner Units includes pilot practice computerisation schemes with development of epidemiological information systems, and development of protocols at local level between hospitals and general practitioners regarding referrals, access to therapy and shared care.

The health, social and environmental problems faced by the travelling community have become priority areas for action. The perinatal and infant mortality rates of travellers in 1987 were 28.3/1,000 and 18.1/1,000[41] respectively compared with the national figures in 1987 of 10.4/1,000 and 7.9/1,000.[42] There is poor uptake of antenatal and postnatal services. The standardised mortality ratio of unhoused travellers for accidents is 843 and for housed travellers is 135, against an Irish SMR of 100.[41] Only 50–60 per cent of traveller children are located by the public health nursing service at the child's first birthday owing to the high mobility of the traveller community; immunisation uptake and attendance at developmental screening are less than 50 per cent.[43] There is low uptake of specialist child health services and poor continuity of care due to the high mobility of this group. Illiteracy is still a major barrier in allowing adult travellers to participate fully in society. While many travellers are now housed or use official serviced caravan sites, a considerable number persistently live in unofficial sites, on unused waste ground or on the roadside.[44]

Special initiatives have been introduced to attempt to redress some of the difficulties with the delivery of health services to the traveller community. Specialist out-reach clinics have been introduced in some parts of the country, either using a mobile or on-site clinic. Specialist public health nurses have been introduced also. Halting site inspections are now carried out in each health board, to ensure a standard level of service provision and safety. The community mothers' programme has been introduced to this group, with considerable success.[45]

Occupational health

The Safety, Health and Welfare Work Act 1989, which is closely in line with the EU Framework Directive, 1989, which it anticipated, has been a very significant piece of legislation. Prior to 1986 the law in relation to work was fragmented and piecemeal.[46] The Report of the Commission of Inquiry[47] highlighted deficiencies in occupational health and the majority of its concerns were addressed in the 1989 legislation. The Act established an independent national authority for health and safety at work, the Health and Safety Authority (HSA), and extended worker protection to all persons in employment as well as the self-employed and to persons who may be affected by work activities. Previous legislation only extended to about 25 per cent of the work force. It also obliges employers to provide a safety statement for the workplace and to consult with employees on matters of health and safety at work. The Safety, Health and Welfare at Work (General Application) Legislation, 1993 provides detail for the general principles set out in the 1989 Act.[48] The HSA provides information and advice on health and safety matters, arranges for enforcement of legislation through the industrial inspectorate and promotes positive preventive measures in the workplace. It also issues licences for certain operations, reviews and develops regulations and codes of practice in relation to health and safety standards and encourages and supports education and training in occupational health.

The HSA aims to provide a balanced approach to workplace health and safety through a combination of expert advice and support and, where necessary, enforcement of the law where serious contraventions occur. The philosophy of the organisation is well summarised in the Report of the Commission of Inquiry[47] which states that one of its aims is 'to provide a basis whereby employers and workers themselves, at the level of the undertaking, solve their working environment problems in cooperation with their representative organisations and under the supervision and guidance of the state in the person of the new Authority'.

Intersectoral cooperation

The Minister and Department of Health subscribe fully to the principle of multi-sectoral cooperation as enunciated in Target 18 of the WHO document 'Targets for Health for All'[49] and regular channels of communication with other government departments and interested institutions and groups are in existence. Some of these are in the form of standing committees/boards/councils and others take the form of ad hoc consultations when specific issues need consideration. At Dail (Parliament) level there exists, for example, a Public Accounts Committee, a Select Committee on Social Affairs, a Joint Committee on the Family and a Joint Committee on Women's Rights. All of these have all-party representation and would, inter alia, consider aspects of public health policy. At cabinet level there is a subcommittee on health promotion, established in 1988, which includes the Ministers for Health, Education, Agriculture and Environment. There is also a Minister for State at the Departments of Health, Justice and Education, with special responsibility for services under the Child Care Act, 1991, who chairs a committee of senior civil servants from these departments which has been very effective in developing policy for children in care.

The Department of Health has regular contact with other government departments on specific aspects of services, for example, with the Department of the Marine on the air-sea rescue service, with the Department of the Environment on accident prevention and major accident plans, with the Departments of Energy, Communication and Transport and Environment on ionising and non ionising radiation issues and with the Department of Justice on prison health. The department is also represented on a committee of the Department of Foreign Affairs which coordinates Irish aid abroad. The Departments of Health and Education regularly liaise on health promotion programmes for schools.

There are also many intersectoral boards/committees of major interest to public health on which the Department of Health is represented. A Road Safety Advisory Board has representatives from Health, Agriculture and the Marine as well as those from employer, trade union, health board, academic and consumer interests. A National AIDS Strategy Committee includes representatives from Health, Justice, Finance and Education. A large number of bodies also exist, representative of many interests, which have an advisory function to the Minister and Department of Health; examples of these would be Comhairle na n-Ospideal (the Hospital Council) which has a statutory role in regulating hospital appointments, the Irish Medicines Board and the Health Research Board. Membership of these bodies represent a range of intersectoral interests.

An exciting recent development has been the establishment of an All-Ireland Institute of Public Health, funded by the governments in Northern Ireland and the Republic of Ireland. A north-south implementation group is currently discussing organisational structures. It is envisaged that the Institute will coordinate cross-border cooperation and initiatives in the field of public health and the development has widespread support from all health personnel in Ireland.

Representatives from health personnel at all levels participate in European and international organisations such as WHO, the Council of Europe, United Nations Organisation, Food and Agriculture Organisation and the International Labour Office. They also participate in EC committees particularly those in DG V, Employment, Industrial Relations and Social Affairs and DG XII, Science Research and Development. The public health community particularly welcomes Article 129 of the Maastricht Treaty which strengthens the support by the European Commission for cooperation between Member States in community action towards disease prevention, research and health promotion. It is clear that Article 129 opens the door to EU-wide consultation on a wide range of public health issues and to multi-sectoral cooperation in actions directed towards the improvement of the public health throughout the Union.

Conclusion

In 1994, non-capital health expenditure in Ireland amounted to two and a quarter billion pounds, 8 per cent of GDP.[1] The National Strategy[1] identified strengths and weaknesses of the health system which need to be addressed. Strengths include high quality services with well qualified and committed staff, a strong voluntary sector which provides an integral part of the public system, a mix of public and private services which facilitates complementary roles, political consensus on the importance of an adequately funded service and a comprehensive planning framework from in-depth studies of the system in recent years. Weaknesses include lack of focus on specific targets with difficulty in assessing effectiveness, lack of adequate information systems, lower life expectancy than the EU average and the need to update organisational and management structures.

The national health strategy identified specific targets for action to achieve health gain and social gain.[1] Particular emphasis was laid on the provision of information on needs, activities, costs and outcomes in order that resources may be applied to achieve the greatest benefits to health. The implementation of the strategy has been subject to ongoing monitoring at health board and national level. The 1998 strategy statement further delineates current priorities and publicly states Governmental objectives for health care.[23]

The strategy represents a significant development in Irish public health policy.[1] The 1998 strategy statement reflects the recent policy of the Department of Health & Children to openly state priorities.[23] Substantial resource allocation, the continuing commitment of the Government and cooperation between those working in the health services at all levels will be needed to achieve the stated objectives.

References

1. Department of Health. *Shaping a Healthier Future. A Strategy for Effective Healthcare in the 1990s.* Dublin: Stationery Office, 1994.

2. Department of Health. *National Alcohol Policy.* Dublin: Stationery Office, 1996.

3. Report of a working party. *Community Medicine and Public Health. The future.* Dublin: Department of Health, 1990.

4. Commission on Itinerancy. Report. Dublin: Stationery Office, 1990.

5. Commission of Inquiry on Mental Handicap. Report. Dublin; Stationery Office, 1965.

6. Consultative Council on the General Hospital Services. *Outline of the Future Hospital System.* Dublin: Stationery Office, 1968.

7. Commission of Inquiry on Mental Illness. Report. Dublin: Stationery Office, 1996.

8. Study group appointed by Minister for Health. *The Child Health Services.* Dublin: Stationery Office, 1967.

9. Interdepartmental Committee. *The Care of the Aged.* Dublin: Stationery Office, 1968.

10. Working party established by Minister for Health. *Training and Employing the Handicapped.* Dublin: Stationery Office, 1978.

11. Working party on prescribing and dispensing in the General Medical Service. Report. Dublin: Stationery Office, 1975.

12. Task force on child care services. Final Report. Dublin: Stationery Office, 1980.

13. Report of the working party. *General Medical Services.* Dublin: Stationery Office, 1984.

14. Working party. *The Psychiatric Services Planning for the Future.* Dublin: Stationery Office, 1984.

15. Tussing AD. *Irish Medical Care Resources; an Economic Analysis.* Dublin: Economic and Social Research Institute, 1988.

16. Department of Health. *Health: the Wider Dimensions.* Dublin: Stationery Office, 1986.

17. Health Education Bureau. *Promoting Health Through Public Policy.* Dublin: Health Education Bureau, 1987.

18. Working party on services for the elderly. *The Years Ahead, a Policy for the Elderly.* Dublin: Stationery Office, 1988.

19. Commission for Health Funding. Report. Dublin: Stationery Office, 1989.

20. Review Group on Mental Handicap Services. *Needs and Abilities, a Policy for the Intellectually Disabled.* Dublin: Stationery Office, 1990.

21. Dublin hospital initiative group. Third report. Dublin: Department of Health, 1991.

22. National Council for the Elderly. *Health and Autonomy Among the Over-65s in Ireland.* Dublin: National Council for the Elderly, 1994.

23. Department of Health and Children. *Working for Health and Well-being.* Strategy

198   *Public Health Policies in the European Union*

Statement 1998–2001. Dublin: Department of Health and Children, 1998.

24. Department of Health. *Report of the Working Party on Tuberculosis.* Dublin: Stationery Office, 1996.

25. Eurocat. *Surveillance of Congenital Anomalies 1980–1990.* Brussels: Eurocat Central Registry, 1993.

26. Mayne PD, Mulhair P, O'Neill. (in press) 30 years of newborn screening in Ireland, 1966–1996. *Ir Med J Sci.* This is a paper given at a scientific meeting which is still in the process of being published.

27. Department of Health. *Cancer Services in Ireland: a National Strategy.* Dublin: Stationery Office, 1996 (in press).

28. Department of Health. *A Health Promotion Strategy Making the Healthier Choice the Easier Choice.* Dublin: Department of Health, 1995.

29. Nutrition Advisory Group. *Recommendations for a Food and Nutrition Policy for Ireland.* Dublin: Stationery Office, 1996.

30. Journal of Health Gain. *Sharing Information about Health Gain in Ireland.* Dublin: Office for Health Gain, 1997.

31. Johnson Z, Dack P. Small area mortality patterns. *IMJ.*1989;89:205–8.

32. Johnson Z, Jennings S, Fogarty J, Johnson H, Lyons R, Doorley P, Hynes M. Behavioural risk factors among young adults in small areas with high mortality versus those in low-mortality areas. *Int J Epid* 1991;20:989–96.

33. Johnson Z, Lyons R. Socio-economic factors and mortality in small areas. *IMJ* 1993;82:60–2.

34. Johnson Z, Dack P, Fogarty J. Small area analysis of low birthweight patterns in Dublin. *IMJ* 1994;87:176–7.

35. Department of Health. *Developing a Policy for Women's Health.* Dublin: Stationery Office, 1995.

36. Department of Health. *A Plan for Women's Health.* Dublin: Department of Health, 1997.

37. Department of Health. *A National Breastfeeding Policy for Ireland.* Dublin: Department of Health, 1994.

38. Department of Health. *Family Planning Guidelines.* Dublin: Department of Health, 1995.

39. Department of Health. *The Patient's Charter.* Dublin: Department of Health, 1992.

40. Johnson Z, Howell F, Molloy B. Community mothers' programme: randomised controlled trial of non-professional intervention in parenting. *BMJ* 1993;306:1449–52.

41. Barry J, Herity B, Solan J. *The Travellers' Health Status Study. Vital Statistics of Travelling People, 1987.* Dublin: Health Research Board, 1989.

42. Department of Health. *Report on Vital Statistics 1987.* Dublin: Stationery Office, 1990.

43. Task force on the travelling community. *Report of the Task force on the Travelling*

Community. Dublin: Stationery Office, 1995.

44. Barry J, Daly L. *The Travellers' Health Status Study. Census of Travelling People, November 1986.* Dublin: Health Research Board, 1988.

45. Fitzpatrick P, Molloy B, Johnson Z. *Community Mothers' Programme; Extension to the Travelling Community.* Dublin: Eastern Health Board, 1995.

46. Cusack D. Safety and health at work legislation. *Journal of the Irish College of General Practitioners* 1995;11(7):26–8.

47. Commission of Inquiry on Safety, Health and Welfare at Work. Report. Dublin: Stationery Office, 1983.

48. Cusack D. Health and hazards in the workplace. *Journal of the Irish College of General Practitioners* 1995;11(8):25–6.

49. World Health Organisation. *Targets for Health for All.* Copenhagen: WHO, 1995.

Appendix 1

Infectious Disease Regulations 1981
Notifiable Infectious Diseases

Acute Anterior Poliomyelitis

Acute Encephalitis

Acute Viral Meningitis

Anthrax

Bacillary Dysentery

Bacterial Meningitis (including meningococcal septicaemia)

Brucellosis

Cholera

Diphtheria

Food Poisoning (bacterial other than salmonella)

Gastro Enteritis (when contracted by children under 2 years of age)

Infectious Mononucleosis

Influenzal Pneumonia

Legionnaires Disease

Leptospirosis

Malaria

Measles

Mumps

Ornithosis

Plague

Rabies

Rubella

Salmonellosis (other than typhoid or paratyphoid)

Smallpox

Sexually Transmissible Diseases

syphilis	gonorrhoea
chancroid	lymphogranuloma venereum
granuloma inguinale	non-specific urethritis
chlamydia trachomatis	trichomoniasis
candidiasis	pediculosis pubis
ano-genital warts	molluscum contagiosum
genital herpes simplex	

Tetanus

Tuberculosis

Typhoid and Paratyphoid

Typhus

Viral Haemorrhagic Diseases (including lassa fever and marburg disease)

Viral Hepatitis

–   Type A

–   Type B

–   Type Unspecified

Whooping Cough

Yellow Fever

10

Public Health Policies in Italy

Alessandra Marinoni and Claudio Macchi

Introduction

Throughout this century Italy has witnessed great changes in the age structure of its population, as have the other countries in the European Union. The drop in the birth rate from 32.5 births per 1,000 inhabitants in 1900 to 10 in 1990 has brought about a considerable reduction in the number of young people.

At the beginning of the century about 40 per cent of the population was under 19 years of age, but by 1990 this percentage had dropped to 24.4 per cent. On the other hand, the reduction in the death rate has meant that the number of people over 60 years of age has more than doubled and is now 20 per cent or more, of whom almost 1/4 are more than 80 years old.

In the next few years these trends will be accentuated as there will be a further reduction in the number of young people and an increase in the number of the elderly, not only in percentage terms but also in absolute values (Table 1).

		0–19	20–59	>60–79	>80
Italy	1990	24.4	55.6	17.1	2.9
	1995 *	21.2	56.4	18.3	4.1
	2010	19.2	55.3	20.9	4.6
EU	1990	25.3	55.1	16.4	3.2
	1995 *	23.8	55.5	16.8	3.9
	2010	20.9	55.3	19.5	4.3

Table 1
Italy - Population distribution by age groups

Sources: Geddes M, 1995[1] based on * Eurostat. *Demographic Statistics*. Luxembourg: Eurostat, 1997.

Table 2

Percentage changes in avoidable deaths between 1995 and 1992 and rates per 100,000 inhabitants (1990-1992) standardised on the world population

Groups of avoidable mortality causes	Italy		EU	
	M	F	M	F
Group I: Primary Prevention*				
Decrease (%)	-7.9	36.1	-12.9	-28.4
Rate 1990–92 (per 100,000 inhabitants)	152.2	38.0	150.1	46.5
Group II: Early Diagnosis and Therapy**				
Decrease (%)	-67.4	-18.4	-61.1	-13.2
Rate 1990–92 (per 100,000 inhabitants)	1.4	26.2	1.4	27.6
Group III: Public Health and Care***				
Decrease (%)	-70.6	-82.6	-60.1	-71.6
Rate: 1990–92 (per 100,000 inhabitants)	70.4	22.4	92.2	30.7

Source: Geddes M, 1995.[1]

Notes:

* Group I: ICD IX
140–150,161 (malignant neoplasm of the lip, oral cavity, pharynx, oesophagus and larynx)
155 (malignant neoplasm of liver)
162 (malignant neoplasm trachea, bronchus and lung)
188 (malignant neoplasm of bladder)
430–438 (cardiovascular diseases)
571 (chronic liver disease and cirrhosis)
800–999 (violent deaths)

** Group II:
173 (malignant neoplasm of skin)
174 (malignant neoplasm of female breast)
180 (malignant neoplasm of cervix uteri 15–64 g.)
179,182 (malignant neoplasm of uterus)
186 (malignant neoplasm of testis)
201 (Hodgkin's disease 5–64 g.)

*** Group III
001–139 (infections and parasitic diseases)
204–208 (leukaemias)
393–398 (chronic rheumatic heart disease 5–44 g.)
401–405 (hypertension disease)
410–414 (ischaemic heart disease)
480–486 (acute pulmonary diseases)
531–534 (peptic ulcers)
540–543 (appendicitis)
550–553 (abdominal hernia)
574–575,1 (cholelithiasis and cholecystitis)
630–678 (complications of pregnancy, childbirth and puerperium)
745–747 (congenital cardiovascular anomalies)
770–779 (perinatal mortality)

This change is even more obvious when the two sexes are considered separately. The percentage of males over 65 rose from 8 to 12 per cent from 1950 to 1990 and is expected to rise to 19 per cent by 2025. For females it rose from 9 to 17 per cent and is expected to reach 26 per cent by 2025. Life expectancy in Italy is therefore high: it lies at 73.7 years for men and 80.6 years for women compared to the European average of 73 and 79.5 years respectively. In the next century, one fifth of the male population and one quarter of all females will be over 65.[1]

A consequence of this evolution is the increase in chronic illnesses, general disorders and illnesses leading to incapacity and therefore an increase in health expenditure.

Let us now present a synoptic outline of the health scene in Italy, the data for which comes from official statistics and from some ad hoc research. In the case of avoidable mortality, Italy has lower values than the European average in both men and women when all 27 causes of death are taken into account. Between 1955 and 1992 a 45.0 per cent decrease was recorded in males and 60.8 per cent in females, both of which are decidedly higher than the European average of 40.1 per cent and 48.8 per cent, respectively. The greatest decrease, found in those avoidable deaths that depended on sanitary conditions and health care, was most significant in women in whom cases of infectious diseases and tuberculosis dropped considerably between 1955 and 1992. By far the highest mortality rates are found in so-called 'Group I' which are influenced by primary prevention. In this group are tumours of the respiratory system, brain, liver, and violent deaths, which have a higher frequency in males. The fact that reduction in mortality has been so slight over the past twenty years shows how much remains to be done in terms of primary prevention (Table 2).

During the last 20 years, the avoidable death rate in males for conditions included in Group II (which are affected by early diagnosis and treatment) has practically disappeared. In females, however, it is still high in tumours of the reproductive system.

Whereas in the 1950s 2/3 of avoidable deaths were linked to sanitary conditions and health care, this figure has fallen to 1/3 for males and 1/5 for females in the 1990s.

Avoidable deaths linked to measures of primary prevention, which were introduced in Italy and Europe up to the 1970s, have been very slowly diminishing over the past 20 years. Taking into account all causes of death in Italy, the great mortality increase for all types of tumours in males should be emphasised. In that category, between 1955 and 1989 the Italian rate, standardised to the European population changed from 135 to 196 per 100,000 inhabitants with an increase of 142 per cent in the number of deaths compared to 91 per cent in Europe (Table 3 overleaf).

In women the mortality rate for Group II conditions has slightly decreased, from 103.8 to 102 per 100,000 but the absolute number of deaths has increased by 85 per cent compared to the European average of 59 per cent.

Between 1960 and 1989 there was a considerable increase in the mortality rate for lung cancer. It more than doubled in males (from 25 to 59 per 100,000 inhabitants) and

Table 3 Mortality from certain tumors in Italy and EU countries (rates per 100,000 inhabitants standardised on the world population).				
		Italy		*EU*	

		Italy M	Italy F	EU M	EU F
Total deaths	1955–59	35988	35056	242549	230713
	1985–89	86951	61143	463851	366639
% change (1985–89/1955–59)		+ 142	+ 85	+ 91	+ 59
All cancers	1960–64	151,2	106	167	106
	1985–89	196	102	189	107
	1960–64	25	3	37	3
Cancer of the:					
lung	1985–89	59	7	53	9
	1960–64	35	18	31	17
stomach	1985–89	19	9	15	17
	1960–64	13	10	17	14
intestine	1985–89	19	13	20	14
	1960–64	–	15	–	18
breast	1985–89	–	21	–	22

Source: Geddes M, 1995.[1]

females (from 3 to 7 per 100,000 inhabitants). An increase in cancer of the intestine, breast and oesophagus was also recorded whereas there was a drop in mortality from stomach cancer.

Taking into consideration the incidence of tumours, the estimated rate in 1990 was 250 per 100,000 inhabitants in males and 200 per 100,000 in females. For all cancers, Italy is similar to the average in the European Union, but is second for stomach tumours in males and females and fifth for lung cancer in males. It is, however, below the European average for cancers of the intestine, breast and oesophagus.

From these data some considerations emerge for the setting of priorities. The increase in tumours linked to the use of tobacco and alcohol shows the irrationality of human behaviour and, above all, the ineffectiveness of preventive measures in Italy. This is confirmed by the fact that between 1982 and 1993 the percentage of male smokers dropped in all EU countries except Italy, where it remained at 37–38 per cent.

A fundamental indicator of the level of health in a country is infant mortality. Italy unfortunately ranks poorly among the countries of the EU with a rate of 8.3 in 1992 behind Portugal, Greece and Luxembourg. Italy ranks first for mortality from diabetes in both sexes; second for males and third for females from bronchitis, emphysema and asthma; and third for cerebrovascular diseases. Italy is top of the list for homicides. Table 4 shows Italy's ranking vis-à-vis the EU with regard to a range of conditions.

Table 4

Avoidable deaths between 1955 and 1992 in Italy and EU

		Rates per 100,000 inhabitants standardised on the European population		Ranking in the EU countries	
		M	F	M	F
All causes	1955–59	1457.7	1167.0		
	1985–89	1033.6	606.7	7	6
Diabetes	1960–64	14.6	19.1		
	1985–89	22.3	26.4	10	1
Circulatory system	1960–64	596.9	471.6		
	1985–89	419.6	279.8	7	6
Ischaemic Heart Disease	1960–64	279.9	205.6		
	1985–89	144.0	65.9	6	5
Cerebrovascular Diseases	1960–64	180.9	141.1		
	1985–89	121.3	94.1	3	4
Respiratory system	1960–64	57.0	26.6		
	1985–89	81.8	30.6	7	penultimate
Bronchitis, emphysema, asthma	1960–64				
	1985–89	46.5	13.0	2	3
Accidents and poisoning	1960–64	83.9	29.3		
	1985–89	63.4	27.0	7	5
Road accidents	1960–64				
	1985–89	23.4	6.5	6	7
Suicides	1960–64				
	1985–89	11.4	3.9	penultimate	8
Homicides	1990	4.8	0.6	1	
	1960–64	–	8.2		
Maternal mortality	1985–89	–	0.3	penultimate	
	1960–64	–	14.3		3
Infant mortality	1992	–	8.3	3	

Source: Geddes M, 1995.[1]

While Italy has the lowest death rate from infectious diseases, the incidence of AIDS is high. In 1994, Italy ranked fourth for males and third for females among EU countries for AIDS deaths (Table 5). The most frequent incidence of transmission was among drug addicts (67 per cent)

Table 5			
Diffusion of AIDS in Italy (standardised rates per milion inhabitants)			
Incidence rate (1993)		*Ranking in the EU countries*	
M	F	M	F
123.5	37.1	4	3
Transmission categories:		European total	
Drug addiction	67%	8%	
Homosexuality	14%	9%	
Heterosexuality	10%	5%	
Transfusions	2%	21%	
Maternal/infant	2%	4%	
Undeclared	4%	53%	

Source: Geddes M, 1995.[1]

The health service, since 1992, has the highest number of doctors per capita and ranks second for the number of chemists, in the EU whereas there is a shortage of dentists and nurses (Table 6). An analysis of transplant data reveals a dramatic situation. Italy is at the bottom of the list for number of transplants provided and top for waiting list times.

Structure of public health

The Health Care Reform Act of 1978

Public Health operates in Italy in accordance with Act No 833, passed in 1978, which instituted the National Health Care Service.[2] Subsequently, between 1992 and 1993 Legislative Decrees Nos. 502 and 517 reorganised the economic and managerial aspects of the service.[3,4]

The 1978 Reform Act was the first fundamental step towards overcoming the existing dispersion of public health functions. Until then, the public health services had been split up into an infinite number of autonomous, hospital and health insurance bodies, those of general or specialised (e.g. psychiatric) interest and those concerned with checking and controlling hygiene and safety conditions in the living and working environment. In spite of difficulty in obtaining a reliable estimate of the number of these bodies, they were calculated to be about 40,000.

Table 6		
Provision of halth services in 1992		
	Per 1,000 inhabitants	*Ranking among the then 12 EU countries*
Health Personnel:		
Doctors	4.7	1
Chemists	0.9	2
Dentists	0.2	penultimate
Nurses	2.9	last but two
Hospital beds	7.2	7
Patient days per inhabitant per year	1.8	7
Transplants:		
Kidney:		
rate per 1,000,000	10.2	last
people on waiting list/transplants	11.8	first
Heart:		
rate per 1,000,000	4.2	6
people on waiting list/transplants	1.6	first
Lungs:		
rate	0.1	last
people on waiting list/transplants	1.6	first
Heart-lungs:		
rate	0.2	last
people on waiting list/transplants	3.5	2
Liver:		
rate	3.5	5
people on waiting list/transplants	0.7	2
Pancreas:		
rate	0.3	last
people on waiting list/transplants	3.5	first

Source: Geddes M, 1995.[1]

The Italian Constitution had already sanctioned the protection of health as a fundamental right of the individual and of public interest, which had to be assured as a mark of respect for the dignity and freedom of each individual. The 1978 Health Reform Act adhered to this principle.

The unit designated for this task was the National Health Care Service. The Service was charged with promoting, maintaining and restoring the physical and mental health of the whole population. It made no distinction between individual or social conditions and ensured that health care coverage was available to all citizens under conditions of equality. The State, Regions and local bodies throughout the country (municipal and provincial) were responsible for delivering the National Health Care Service and guaranteeing that it was available to each citizen.

Practically speaking, Italy moved away from a health care system that was mainly based on individual voluntary contributions (in which sickness benefit funds served certain categories of workers) or provided by the Municipal Authorities (which offered care to the socially-deprived). The new system foresaw that services would be provided free of charge to all citizens and would be financed, at least in part, by the State through tax revenues. Under the Health Care Reform Act, the National Health Care Service (including its regional and local authorities) was to be responsible for prevention, care and rehabilitation. Private health structures that had particular agreements with the National Health Care Service were assigned integrative functions in this Service. A well-defined plan involving all the competent organs at different levels was called for in order to set aims and quantify the costs involved.

The State (with some contribution from the Regions) planned the national economy and approved the national health plan, stipulating which health care services were to be guaranteed to all citizens. The standards were to serve as reference points for the Regions in order to achieve unification and standardisation of health care services throughout the country. The Regions, in turn, undertook planning and integrated regional health plans. The National Health Plan and regional health plans were valid for three years and stipulated:

- the general course of action to be taken

- aims

- the health care fund

- the allocation of the fund's resources

- planning of activities for collecting and managing the epidemiological, statistical and financial information that was necessary to judge results and to define the plan for the following three years.

In each Region, health management was assigned to legal bodies called Local Health Units. These Local Health Units were split into districts that were responsible for community health services which are often correlated to the social needs of the population. Following the indications of the regional health plan, the Local Health Units planned their own line of action and a three-year budget. The various bodies concerned with the management of the health care system (the State, Regions and Local Health Units) employed a finance system whereby health policy funds were allocated by the State to the Regions and by the Regions to the Local Health Units.

The problem of planning and defining health policy was addressed by the 1978 Health Reform Act and was closely linked to the social and economic problems of the country at national, regional and local levels. The latter were characterised by strong representation of the municipalities in the Local Health Units.

All the levels of the Health Care Service were to be managed by political administrators: the Minister of Health, Chairmen of the Regional Health Authorities and members of the administrative committees of the Local Health Units. It is therefore easy to see how these levels influenced and were influenced by politics in general.

A great deal of importance was thus given to political influence, to the citizens' say in health care choices and to the unification and standardisation of services throughout the country. The health care services were to be comprehensive, covering prevention, treatment and rehabilitation. The existence of a budget meant that decisions on expenditure would be rationalised and that criteria for evaluating the efficiency of services and effectiveness on the state of health of the population would be established. To accomplish this, an analysis of the relationship between aims, resources and results was made.

The implementation of the 1978 Health Reform Act immediately proved to be difficult for a number of reasons. First, there was a change in the political scene. A different political majority from that which had passed the Health Reform Act now occupied Parliament. Delays or defaults in national and regional legislation to implement the reform also contributed to the problems. Moreover, excessive importance was given to political decision-making. There was too much political intervention at some levels, particularly at the local level.

Another factor that hampered implementation was the launch of a public information campaign about the so-called 'Unhealthy Health System'. This was intended to exploit the disastrous functioning of the public health system as compared to the soundness of the private health sector.

Furthermore, there was a reluctance on the part of medical personnel to accept a process of reappointment that in some way questioned their medical role, authority and possibility of their working within private structures.

The continuous worsening of the general economic situation in the country also exacerbated the situation and led to indiscriminate, legally sanctioned general cuts in health funding (often ignored at a regional or local level).

Finally, failure in the planning system added to the unfavourable climate for reform. These difficulties began in the 1960s and continued through to the unsuccessful planning system described previously which decentralised planning power from national to local level. It is sufficient to observe that while the first national health plan was approved on 1 March 1994,[5] very few Regions have produced any regional plans (among the few are Piedmont, Veneto, Tuscany and Emilia Romagna).[6-9] Lombardy, which alone has a little under one fifth of the total population in Italy, is notable for its failure in this area.

The 1992–93 reorganisation

Between 1992 and 1993 a series of laws was passed to reorganise the National Health Care Service. These laws, which formed the basis for the planning system identified by the 1978 Reform Act, empowered State, regional and local units and for the first time foresaw that both the Local Health Units and the main hospitals could be turned into enterprises.

Under the new National Health Plan the State is responsible for (a) indicating which areas are to be given priority in the development of health services (the aim is eventually to achieve the standardisation of the state of health of the population), and (b) designating standard levels of health care on the basis of epidemiological and clinical data. The services to be guaranteed to each citizen must be specified and related to available financial resources.

According to this principle, a citizen no longer holds the 'absolute' right of access to health services (in accordance with the Constitutional principle of the protection of health as a primary benefit), but a 'relative' right in which the health services he/she is offered depend on the available resources of the National Health Care Service.

The Region has legislative and administrative responsibilities for general health and hospital care as set by national legislation. In particular, the region must oversee (a) organisation of services and activities concerned with the protection of public health and (b) criteria for the allocation of resources to Local Health Unit and hospital enterprises. The Region also directs the latter on management control and assessment of the quality of health services. If a Region decides that the per capita sum allocated to each citizen is insufficient or if additional services are required, it can impose a special tax to obtain extra funds.

The Local Health Units are enterprises with public legal status and organisational, administrative, patrimonial estate, accounting, managerial and technical autonomy. They ensure uniform levels of care in their own particular area, which usually corresponds to that of the provinces except for the mountain areas, small islands and large urban conglomerations. They can be delegated social health care responsibilities by the municipalities.

The hospitals are generally structures belonging to the Local Health Unit enterprises. There are certain cases in which hospitals can or must become enterprises with autonomous public legal status, for eaxmple, important multispecialty hospitals, hospitals directly administered by Universities or which are Centres for the clinical training of students enrolled at the Faculty of Medicine and, lastly, hospitals that are central operating headquarters for provincial emergency services.

Those hospitals which play an important role in the field of research are thus recognised as Research and Health Care Institutes and have specific norms.

A Director-General is responsible for the representation and management of each Local Health Unit and hospital enterprise. He or she is a manager who has experience in the management of public bodies or large private firms. (This is an obvious attempt to create top-management aimed at efficiency and not directly linked to the political environment.)

The Director-Generals are appointed by the Regions and have to choose an Administrative Director and a Medical Director (who must be a doctor) from candidates with suitable professional qualifications. The three Directors are tied to the Region or hospital enterprise by a private five-year contract that may be renewed or revoked for substantiated reasons.

It should be noted that the political decision-making power that each Regional Government embodies strongly influences the two kinds of enterprise. In fact, the Director-General's authority to decide, and his binding contractual agreement with the Region, means that the enterprise for which he is responsible is basically a specific expression of the Region itself.

Although existing legislation affirms the contrary, the link between local political and administrative authorities (i.e. municipal and provincial) and management of the enterprises is becoming increasingly weak.

In the new health reorganisation in Italy the role played by the municipalities is linked to the districts which are the most decentralised components of the National Health Care Service. These districts satisfy primary health care needs, community health services and certain ambulatory specialised care in a limited number of municipalities whose populations number in the tens of thousands.

As time goes by, it appears that local health planning choices are destined to elude municipal 'politics' and control more and more.

On 1 January 1995 another radical innovation concerning financing was introduced.[10] Local Health Units and hospitals' services are now classified according to the DRG (Diagnosis Related Groups) system which covers hospital admissions and day hospitals but does not, in fact, cover the whole range of health services. The traditional system of financing the cost of factors of production necessary for supplying services (personnel, materials used, necessary structures and equipment etc.) no longer exists.

Local politicians, usually urged on by health operators, were in the habit of exercising pressures to create new services and expand existing ones without worrying about the deficit in the health care system which the State usually settled through the Regions. This state of affairs worsened the general state of public finances.

Currently, an incremental-type logic (i.e. the addition of new services without discarding or converting what is no longer suitable or necessary) is no longer possible because of the competition between public and private structures to acquire 'customers' who can freely be admitted to either of them. The new situation means that health enterprises have to adopt management and economic criteria that take into consideration the costs and the predicted proceeds.

The previous Health Care Service was inflexible in the face of changing needs caused by new demographic and epidemiological developments such as the reduced birth-rate, ageing population, wider field of disabilities and chronic illnesses, reduction in many acute conditions and the rise of new ones like AIDS. The new service, which aimed to develop (a) a close link with the needs of the 'market' at a local level (which would influence the offer of services) and (b) a continual analysis of the relationship between supply, demand and the resources necessary for guaranteeing services within a balanced economic-business framework. The national and local authorities became technicalised.

Apart from its supervisory function, the State is responsible for fixing a per capita quota that is adequate for guaranteeing uniform levels of health care and that is compatible with other items in the Budget. This is the only aspect of State intervention that has any great effect on the Health Care Service.

The Regions, on the other hand, have a strong role in that they set up hospitals and health care enterprises, appoint their Director-Generals and lay down criteria for the organisation and financing of general health services. They also determine fees for hospital services based on the DRG classification system of hospital discharge diagnoses and regulate the public/private relationship by deciding which private structures shall be formally accredited. This last point has always been the subject of heated political discussion.

Since the Regions are free to make decisions regarding the reorganisation of the health care service, they have great discretionary powers in certain important spheres. For example:

*   centralised planning of structures (e.g. the reorganisation of the hospital network, or criteria and decisions regarding the accreditation of private structures) or a more liberal outlook whereby the market and other economic factors related to competition between public and private structures basically define the health scene.

*   the fixing of a fee-structure, which obviously affects the relationship between the public and private health sectors and influences the flow of patients towards one or the other. Access for patients coming from other Regions is also made easier or more difficult as the case may be.

*   control of the overall costs of the system and the decision to develop it further in spite of the limitations imposed by available financial resources. (These resources are the sum of the per capita quota for each resident plus an extra allowance paid by one Region to another, based on DRG tariffs, if one of its residents undergoes treatment outside his own particular Region).

*   an increase or reduction in the level of co-ordination between social and health care services. Social services are run by the municipalities but can be delegated to the health enterprises with their relative resources.

*   the setting up of a monitoring system for health care requests and needs and, if necessary, the use of the indicators pinpointed in the planning stage.

*   the planning, financing, discussion and approval of plans for the building of any health structures or acquisition of additional high technology equipment and systems.

- allocating authority to the Director-General of each Local Health Unit or hospital enterprise in planning and management decisions. This obviously affects the Director-General's freedom in decision-making but in any case he or she has to answer for all outcomes in the management of the enterprise.

As was to be expected, there were great differences among regions in terms of the definition of the geographic size of the Local Health Unit enterprises and the number of hospital enterprises to be created. This can be seen in Table 7, which presents data from all of the Regions in Italy.[11] There were also varying solutions proposed for the organisation of the health enterprises in the different Regions. These dictated, for example, how much decision-making and planning autonomy the enterprises were to have and how strong the link between social and health care services was to be.

It has also to be borne in mind that certain structures such as hospitals that are considered Health Care and Research Institutes, are partly outside the system described. Their scientific and research activities do not fall under the authority of regional planning and control.

Another reflection concerns the field of prevention. As a result of a people's referendum in 1994[12] activities for prevention, surveillance and control of the environment were no longer considered the duties and functions of the National Health Care Service but were delegated to the Ministry for the Environment and competent regional authorities.

Preventive health care measures are the responsibility of the Ministry of Health, which is supported by the Superior Institute of Health, the Superior Institute for Industrial Safety and Prevention and the Experimental Institutes for Prevention in Animals. The National Agency for the Protection of the Environment links to a corresponding agency to be set up in each Region. In the case of more specific health duties and functions the Region has to set up a prevention department in each local health enterprise offering, at minimum, the following services:

- public health and hygiene

- prevention and safety in the working environment

- nutrition and alimentary hygiene

- veterinary science, divided into the three areas that concern animal health: 1. hygiene in production, processing, commercialisation, storage and transport of all foodstuffs of animal origin and by-products, 2. hygiene in stock farms and 3. hygiene in zootechnical firms.

The critical point of the existing situation is that the general prevention sector has been split up. The National Health Care Reform Act of 1978 had, with great difficulty, created a single sector that came under the responsibility of the Local Health Unit but the 1994 referendum decided that the environment and health sectors should be separated. It stipulated, however, that this was to be done in such a way as to create a functional link between them.

Table 7 Local Health Unit and Hospital Enterprises and their catchment areas in each region

Regions	N° of Local Health Unit Enterprises (LHUE)	Thousand of inhabitants per (LHUE)	No. of LHUE per Province	No. of Hospital Enterprises (HE)	Thousand of inhabitants per HE	No. of HE per Province	HE/LHUE
Piedmont	22	196	2.7	7	615	0.9	0.32
Valle d'Aosta	1	118	1.0	-	-	-	-
Lombardy	44	202	4.0	16	556	1.5	0.36
Prov. Bolzano	4	112	4.0	-	-	-	-
Prov. Trento	1	457	1.0	-	-	-	-
Veneto	22	201	3.1	2	2208	0.3	0.09
Friuli Venezia Giulia	6	199	1.5	3	398	0.8	0.60
Liguria	5	333	1.3	3	554	0.8	0.60
Emilia Romagna	13	302	1.4	5	785	0.6	0.38
Tuscany	12	294	1.2	4	882	0.4	0.33
Umbria	5	164	2.5	2	410	1.0	0.40
The Marches	13	111	3.3	3	479	0.8	0.23
Lazio	12	432	2.4	3	1728	0.6	0.25
Abruzzo	6	210	1.5	-	-	-	-
Molise	4	83	2.0	1	332	0.5	0.25
Campania	13	439	2.6	7	816	1.4	0.54
Pugua	12	339	2.4	2	2033	0.4	0.17
Basilicata	5	122	2.5	1	611	0.5	0.20
Calabria	11	189	3.7	4	520	1.3	0.36
Sicily	9	558	1.0	17	295	1.9	1.89
Sardinia	8	207	2.0	1	1657	0.3	0.13
ITALY	228	251	2.3	81	705	0.8	0.36

Source: Authors' research.

Last but not least, there is the question of public and private health structures. Private structures may be accredited by the National Health Care Service and offer services under the same conditions as public structures.

The National Health Care Service does not cover any treatments carried out in non-accredited private nursing homes. It does not pay for pharmaceuticals that are not included in the National Pharmaceutical Manual, cosmetic surgery or extra services of a purely 'hotel-type' kind simply because a patient wants added comfort. No citizen is exempt from paying the amount due for these services.

Another case of services excluded from reimbursement is the so-called 'ticket'. This mechanism makes it compulsory for the patient to contribute towards the cost of certain services such as specialist check-ups, laboratory tests, X-rays and pharmaceuticals that are not considered essential for treating illnesses. Some citizens are, however, exempt from payment of the ticket and thus have access to the services free of charge. This group of people includes the elderly, those with a very low income and the chronically or seriously ill.

Anyone who requires urgent specialist treatment such as heart surgery and cannot be admitted in time to a public hospital has the right to be admitted to a non-accredited private nursing home or to be operated on abroad (even outside the EU) with almost total reimbursement of expenses.

Hierarchy and responsibilities for public health

This section looks at the hierarchy and staffing in public health and the responsibilities at each level concerning environmental, preventive and clinical services. This structure is illustrated in Figures 1 and 2 overleaf.

National level

The Ministry of Health's new organisation is based on departments, each of which has a Director-General appointed by the Ministry. He or she has generally had a career employed by the State but, within certain limits, may be hired from outside the government and appointed by a State Councillor or Ministerial Councillor. The departments are divided into (a) planning, (b) health personnel, technological resources and State-controlled health care, (c) prevention and pharmaceuticals, and (d) food, beverages and nutrition and veterinary science applied to the public health field. At the national level there are:

National Health Council, a body appointed by the Ministry of Health. It may advise or make proposals to the Government and plays a specific role in the drafting of the national health plan and the acquisition of technical advice to respond to legislation dealing with health matters.

Superior Institute for Health, which carries out research in the field of hygiene and

Figure 1
Decision-making in the National Health Care Service

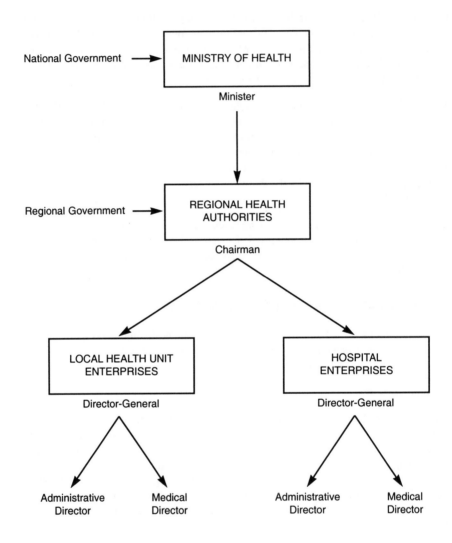

Figure 2
Bodies associated with the regional health system and their inter-relationaships

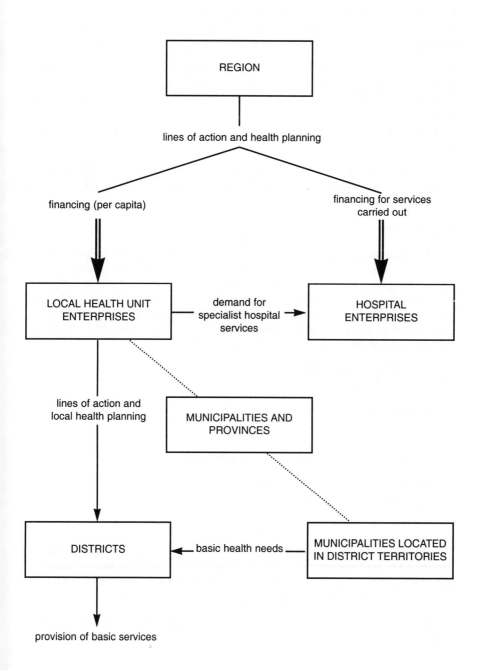

public health, collects the relative information and data and gives advice to the national, regional and local levels of the Health Care Service.

ISPESL, which carries out research in the fields of prevention, occupational disease, industrial accidents and safety in the work environment. It collects the relative data and information and acts as an advisory centre for all levels of the Health Care Service.

National Agency for the Environment, which has just been set up as a result of the 1994 Referendum. This Referendum stipulated that environmental problems of a more technical and less medical type (e.g. chemical, physical, geological etc.) were no longer to come under the auspices of the Health Care Service. The Agency is also responsible for the protection of the population and workers exposed to radiation and acts as an advisory centre.

Periodic exchanges of political viewpoints take place between the State and the Regions on health matters. The so-called State-Region Conference deals with general health questions and regulates the relationship between the State and Regions.

Regional level

The Regional Health Authorities each have a Chairman who is a member of the Regional Government. Each Health Authority is split into different services, most of which have greater or lesser specific functions concerning public health at a regional level. These functions include the study, planning and control of the Local Health Units and hospitals. The Authorities have the right to issue directives, decrees and ordinances on behalf of the Chairman of the Regional Government. The services that directly or indirectly concern public health are as follows:

• Public Health and Hygiene

• Veterinary Science

• Health Planning

• Hospitals

• Private Health Care Agencies with a specific agreement

• Primary care and community medicine

• Epidemiology and the Information System

• Financing

The executives of each service have come either from a career in the Regional Health Enterprises or have reached the top of their career as managers in the health enterprises and have been seconded. They are appointed by the Regional Government and have the power to act on behalf of the Chairman of the Regional Government.

The organisation of the Agency for the Environment and its related services is planned by the individual Regions.

Local level

A Medical Director, appointed by the Director-General, heads each Hospital and Local Health Unit enterprise. The Medical Director must meet qualifications of: length of service, specialisation, and a formative and professional curriculum either in the field of hygiene, epidemiology and public health or health services organisation.

The Medical Director, together with the Administrative Director, works side by side with the Director-General in any decision-making regarding the Hospital Enterprise. The Medical Director and the Director-General are responsible for outcomes regarding health, given available resources.

The organisation of the enterprises foresees a division into individual services or departments, such as Hygiene and Public Health, Prevention or Hospital Services. General responsibility for these services lies with doctors who have passed a national qualifying exam. Only doctors who possess the appropriate qualifications may take the examination.

The appointment of heads of the services or structures is made by the Director-General. His choice is based on an evaluation of all of the candidates made by a Medical Examining Board which represents the Medical Committee of the Enterprise. The appointed head is bound to the Enterprise by a personal, five-year, renewable contract.

The heads of the Preventive Services that are concerned with the area of the Local Health Unit enterprise have enormous responsibilities. Their functions include licensing the production and sale of any good that is subject to health and hygiene checks, giving permits in the building trade and in the environment, supervising the living and working environment and working towards prevention of infectious diseases. In these fields the heads of the Prevention Services have the power to intervene in any situation which compromises public health. They also act as judicial police in collaboration with the competent Judicial Authority.

The Medical Directors of the hospitals are responsible for hygiene in the hospital. They supervise: the preventive treatment of infectious diseases, cross infection, the protection of patients, visitors and workers against physical, chemical and mechanical risks, and the organisation of health services.

How does public health influence decision-making?

Through the collection and processing of data concerning the state of public health (including publication of periodic reports), the field contributes to political decision-making. Now, decisions are also subject to the regulations of the European Union. Regulated measures are those (a) concerning hygiene and safety regulations and (b) the production and sale of those products that are potentially dangerous to public health.

In Italy, legislation to implement EC Directives is slow and there are often delays in their practical application. The Local Health Units then have difficulty in enforcing the new norms and regulations; in addition, the firms, industries or services which are supposed to comply with the Directives offer strong resistance.

Health policy decisions are also affected by certain events that are 'blown up' and influence public opinion. The use of information campaigns (for example, the so-called 'Unhealthy Health System') have been very influential: these emotional appeals tend to influence health policy decisions and override the technical units' responsibility for decision-making.

Politicians and policy-makers do not always give enough weight to data, reports or research coming from the public health sector, particularly if the research is of an epidemiological nature. Politicians are often more influenced by the state of finances and tend to concentrate their efforts on matters that are of interest to professional sectors, rather than to the whole population. One recent important exception, however, concerns pharmaceuticals. This momentous decision followed corruption and bribery scandals at national level which directly involved the sector. While working to reduce the amount covered by the Health Care Service for each pharmaceutical product and increase the individual citizen's contribution, policy-makers completely revised the national pharmaceutical manual. The revisions in the manual led to the (a) inclusion of medicines of proven worth, (b) approval of a prescription charge (co-payment) known as a 'ticket' for those medicines of lesser importance, and (c) elimination of medicines of little or no proven effectiveness. In this reform the political decision was in harmony with the proposal put forward by the Technical Committee for Pharmaceuticals, which is an example of effective centralised decision-making upheld by scientific research.

Bearing in mind the above, the State, Regions and Local bodies resort to various initiatives, such as the publication of annual state-of-health reports. The most significant initiatives are reported below. It should noted, however, that whereas reports at a national level are published regularly and deal with certain topics year after year (making comparisons possible), regional and local levels have not followed suit, creating difficulties in planning and decision-making.

National level data

At a national level there are various sources of data. These include statistics from ISTAT (Central Statistics Institute), annual reports on the state of health published by the National Health Council, data from the Central Service for Health Planning at the Ministry of Health and data on infectious diseases from the Superior Institute of Health.

The data published by ISTAT and the National Health Council are not always complete and tend to be unreliable. Those from the Ministry of Health concerning mortality, data on public health structures and private data are usually a few years out-of-date and are also not always reliable. Data on infectious diseases, particularly morbidity-mortality from AIDS, published by the Superior Institute of Health are often incomplete. Further details concerning the data produced at a national level can be found in Annex 1.

Regional data

At a regional level, statistics and reports on the state of public health and its associated social and environmental aspects are published periodically. The care and assiduousness with which each Region fulfils this task is variable. Generally speaking the Regions in the North and some of the Central Regions meet their commitments adequately. Many of the Regions, however, show little or absolutely no interest.

There are various kinds of data collection regarding hospital activities. One is the more traditional type of data collection with its reports on indicators of available hospital wards and services, hospital beds and the activities and efficiency in hospitals. Over the past two years the more active Regions have organised data collection based on the classification of treated conditions according to DRG with the processing of hospital admission and discharge records.

The data assessment compares local and regional activities by DRG in order to analyse hospital performance in each particular specialty. Analyses are also made of the way in which hospital admission and discharge records are compiled with the intention of improving and standardising them. The cost/returns relationship in hospitals is also assessed on the basis of the tariffs attributed per DRG.

Local level data

As has already been said, the publication of health reports on the state of the local population, environmental problems and the performance of health structures, especially hospitals, varies considerably from one area to another. It should be pointed out that where local information systems exist they produce higher quality up-to-date information than the other levels. This is extremely useful for monitoring the state of public health. In reality, the Local Health Units and hospitals rarely respect their duty to present annual reports.

Clinicians have a tendency to project their own particular viewpoints in strong terms on diagnostic and therapeutic issues. This means that more attention is paid to clinical as opposed to general data on the management and organisation of public health.

How are health policy decisions and priorities made?

General health policy decisions are made at national and regional levels when their respective health plans are drafted. The plans specify aims, priorities and courses of action but, as discussed earlier, they are not issued very frequently. Furthermore, they must also be approved by law, which decreases the possibility that they will be enacted.

As a general aim, the 1994 Plan foresaw the achievement of uniform levels of health care. Uniform levels of health care are concerned with:

(a) Collective health care in the living and working environment, which directly concerns problems of prevention.

(b) Primary health care and community medicine.

(c) Day-time specialist health care centres throughout the country. This includes maternity and infant care and family-planning and is carried out at a district level by multi-specialty teams in mother and infant care advisory centres.

(d) Hospital care and assistance.

(e) Health care in institutions for permanent long-term patients and those who are not self-sufficient:

- psychiatric care for the mentally ill

- old people's homes offering health care

- health care for drug-addicts in therapeutic communities

- assistance for the mentally and physically disabled and those with nervous disorders both in Homes and in special Rehabilitation Centres.

In its aim to achieve uniform levels of care delivered by the Regions, the National Health Plan sets down priorities in certain fields:

Primary Health Care and Community Medicine Districts: integration of the district activities of the GP, polyclinics, specialist clinics and hospitals – creating an efficient and effective diagnostic and therapeutic fusion for the optimisation of health.

Emergency Structures and Services: Operating Centres for dealing with provincial emergency health calls, made by dialling '118'.

Suitable means of transport and equipment for medical assistance.

Integrated system of admission and emergency health services in which different hospitals have different levels of emergency services i.e. hospitals with a normal casualty department and those with units providing more intensive care.

Rehabilitation activities graded according to their complexity. These range from rehabilitation units for maintenance to those for rehabilitation after serious traumatic or pathological events.

Experimentation with new managerial theories: for example, public-private mix, etc.

Evaluation and control systems of health activities at various levels with the definition of an appropriate set of indicators that refer to:

- demand for and accessibility of the services

- resources used in the production and supply of services

- activities carried out

- results obtained

• quality of the services

Planned actions and project-specific aims

Priorities are summed up in projects, specific aims and planned actions which target a well coordinated use of allocated resources. A planned action is a plan of operations in a specific health sector that co-ordinates the activities of various health care services that have different duties and functions. Project specific aims are actions for health protection that are not limited to the Health Care System but involve competent authorities from other fields. The various bodies work together to achieve a comprehensive solution. Annex 2 at the end of this paper illustrates an example of a planned action and a project-specific aim.

Regional planning

Regional planning has the task of pinpointing courses of action, projects and specific aims that are to be achieved in the Region according to specific local requirements.

In the general plans or, as past experience has shown, more often in those regarding specific sectors, the Region intervenes in decisions concerning the development of new services and the expansion or closure of existing ones.

A series of Legislative measures including Act No 595[13] passed in October 1985, Act No 412[14] in December 1991 and Act No 724[10] in December 1994 (steps for the rationalisation of public expenditure) systematically have made the Regions adopt a plan for the reorganisation of the regional hospital network. The plan is seen as the initial and fundamental opportunity for rationalising the supply of hospital beds and activities and for adjusting to new requirements arising from the different health needs of the population. The correlation between how many services are offered, relative costs and available resources will affect the plan.

Whenever it is necessary to plan courses of action for particular age-groups (pathologies in children and the elderly) or for chronic conditions, it is obvious that planning must also take into account the relationship between hospital and community health services in general and social care services.

Even if, as often happens, there is no regional health programme expressed in an actual health care or hospital plan, decisions regarding the setting-up, expansion or reduction of services is in the hands of the Region. In fact, the Region has the power to respond to requests coming from the hospitals or local health enterprises and authorise the allocation of resources to a specific service or sector of activity.

However, in the face of general hostility towards adopting a real programme for regulating the supply of health care services, there has been a widespread tendency in the past to resort to legislative measures for resolving individual health problems as and when they arise. Examples of this are:

Act No 180/1978[15] abolished mental asylums and introduced various guarantees for the mentally-ill, such as voluntary admission, except in exceptional circumstances. This Act also brought psychiatric activities back into the realm of the health care system with the emphasis on assistance outside the hospital.

Act No 67/1988[16,17] provided for a ten-year plan for the health infrastructure, particularly for hospitals, and encouraged the Regions to plan the construction, extension or reconstruction of hospitals and health structures in general. This naturally implied a choice in the establishment or building up of services. So far, the implementation of this Act has been greatly affected by the complexity of procedures, uncertainty over available resources and a basic disregard on the part of most of the Regions concerned.

Act No 135/1990[18] planned a series of urgent measures for the prevention and fight against AIDS. These were mainly focused on the construction and reconstruction of hospital wards for infectious diseases (2,100 million Italian liras were allocated), followed by a series of guidelines and standards on how they were to be carried out. Up till now most Italian Regions have still not reached the approval stage of plans for the works they intended to carry out.

Public-private mix

Lastly, mention must be made of the public-private mix, which is a critical point in the health system and often underlies political conflicts and discussions. Until 31 December 1994, private structures under contract with the National Health Care Service were integrated with public ones. Since 1 January 1995 public and private structures have been on a par in the National Health Care Service and are thus both free to offer hospital services for in-patients under the same conditions.

Table 8 shows the number of beds in 1994 in each Region per 1,000 inhabitants taking into account public hospitals, private hospitals (which, under contract with the National Health Care Service, offer free medical treatment) and other private hospitals (where the patient has to pay for the medical care).[19–20]

Considerable differences exist among Regions. The greatest number of beds in public hospitals is in the Veneto Regions in north-east Italy and for private nursing homes under contract with the National Health Care Service in central Italy (in particular the Lazio Region). Public hospitals in the north, centre and south of Italy provide a total of 6.13, 5.64 and 5.34 beds per thousand population with occupancy rates of 75.66 per cent, 76.96 per cent and 69.81 per cent respectively.[21] In private hospitals the number of beds allocated are 1.40, 2.13 and 1.39 per thousand population in the north, centre and south of Italy, respectively. Of these 1.00, 1.73 and 1.19 are in private structures under contract with the National Health Care Service and the percentage of beds occupied is 87.76 per cent, 78.63 per cent and 75.43 per cent respectively.

Bed availability in the public sector was therefore (and still is) at its highest in the north of Italy, thus satisfying the majority of requests for hospital admission. Numerous patients are accepted from the other Regions too, especially the south. Totally private

Table 8

**Total number of beds per 1,000 inhabitants in each Region in 1994
(including Day Care Units).**

Regions	Public hospitals	Private hospitals under contract with NHCS	Public and Private hospitals under contract with NHCS	% private hospitals under contract	Private hospitals without contract
Piedmont	5.11	0.87	5.99	14.6	0.42
Valle d'Aosta	5.11	–	5.11	–	–
Lombardy	5.59	1.41	7.00	20.2	0.50
Prov. Bolzano	5.27	0.73	6.00	12.2	0.88
Prov. Trento	7.48	1.43	8.90	16.0	0.28
Veneto	7.11	0.56	7.67	7.3	0.22
Friuli Venezia Giulia	7.44	0.79	8.23	9.6	0.20
Liguria	8.09	0.44	8.54	5.2	0.39
Emilia Romagna	5.83	0.99	6.82	14.5	0.52
Tuscany	5.74	0.83	6.57	12.6	0.12
Umbria	6.12	0.50	7.62	7.5	0.10
The Marches	6.58	1.21	7.79	15.5	0.28
Lazio	5.08	3.25	8.34	39.0	0.58
Abruzzo	6.96	1.62	8.59	18.9	0.17
Molise	5.25	0.49	5.74	8.6	0.17
Cmpania	4.28	1.42	5.70	25.0	0.32
Puglia	6.83	0.91	7.74	11.8	0.06
Basilicata	5.25	1.91	7.16	26.7	0.03
Calabria	4.76	1.52	6.28	24.2	0.39
Sicily	5.05	0.92	5.97	15.3	0.17
Sardinia	5.70	0.97	6.67	14.5	0.17
ITALY	5.71	1.26	6.97	18.0	0.33

Data processed from Ministery of Health Planning Department figures, based on the population of 31 December 1993.[19]

hospital activity is highest in the north and in the centre (0.40 beds per thousand population compared to 0.20 in the south). This can be explained by the greater number of well-off patients in the north and centre who either pay for their own medical care or are covered by private insurance.

In the centre and south of Italy capacity in the public sector (5.46 beds per thousand population) is lower than in the north but in private hospital structures under contract with the National Health Care Service it is higher (1.41 beds per thousand population). In totally private structures capacity is low (0.29 beds per thousand population).

The difference between Regions in terms of public-private mix greatly affects choice in health policy. Private nursing homes and their own 'trade' unions form strong pressure groups that obviously influence the balance of available financial resources and planning strategies to their advantage. These pressure groups tend to go along with the more liberal ideas on health policy that prevail in certain important Regions like Lombardy.

Health personnel and doctors in particular form another strong pressure group. Unemployment is present in the south of Italy. Here, the Civil Service has become a sort of safety-net and jobs have often been granted in return for political favours. Some Regions like Puglia tend to adopt planning policies that favour the preservation of a large public sector in their attempt to maintain direct control of public health services. However, at the same time they try to adapt the provision of specialised services to suit the health needs of the population.

There are also considerable differences between one Region and another in terms of the number of staff. For example, in Lombardy the overall number of staff in the regional health system is 11.21 per thousand population. The number of beds in public hospitals is 5.59 per thousand population and on average 76.89 per cent are occupied.

In Puglia, on the other hand, there are fewer staff (9.81 per thousand population) but more beds in public hospitals (6.83 per thousand population). Only 71.32 per cent of beds are occupied and the average length of stay is longer (10.10 days versus 9.69 in Lombardy). At present both Regions have centre-right wing regional governments but have completely different planning policies. In Lombardy, no effective decisions have as yet been approved but planning policy appears to be oriented towards transferring financial resources to the private sector without an overall increase in expenditure. This sector is considered to be more efficient and a large increase in the number of beds in accredited private structures is foreseen. This means that there will be an increase in the overall number of services to be financed by the National Health Care Service.

The Region will only be able to curb expenditure by a reduction in tariffs that is proportional to the increase in services but there is a risk of reducing the quality of the services offered. Close collaboration between the public and private sector has been proposed for the province of Milan in particular as it is the core of the health system in Lombardy. The private sector is planned to have a predominant decision-making role in the running of the health structures.

In Puglia cuts are foreseen in the private sector. The Region will reduce the number of beds in private by accredited structures and cut DRG tariffs when the services provided are the same as in public hospitals.

When deciding on planning policies each Region has its own policy on coordination between the health and social services that are within the competence of the Local Health Unit Enterprise. Regional legislation in Veneto, for example, has instituted a strong link between the two with the setting up of a local enterprise that combines health and social services under the direction of a social director and the administrative and medical directors. In the Lazio region, on the other hand, the link between the two services is weak. Here, social services are carried out by the Local Health Unit enterprises only if they are delegated to do so by the municipalities and the services are only organised at a district level. Lombardy is considering the transfer of the responsibility for social services to the Local Health Unit enterprises but only if the individual municipalities decide to delegate this task to them and transfer the necessary funds.

The role played by the districts in the organisation and activities of the Local Health Unit enterprises also varies considerably from one Region to another. In certain Regions like Piedmont, Veneto, Emilia Romagna and Campagna, the districts are considered so important that they have their own budget whereas in others their role is not so well-defined.

A last difference among the Regions concerns the relative importance given to hospital enterprises and other services. Regions such as Lazio and Veneto, are on a par while others like Lombardy are considering making a radical distinction between hospital activities and primary health care. Each province is to have one Local Health Unit enterprise and one hospital enterprise. The hospital enterprise is intended to group together all the hospitals in the province and provide the specialist services commissioned by the Local Health Unit enterprise. The latter thus becomes a purchaser of hospital services and specialist out-patient services provided by the hospital enterprise, and it pays for these services and controls the quantity of services and their appropriateness.

Who decides on priorities for the individual patient?

The individual patient is entrusted either to a general practitioner (GP) or, in the case of young children, to a paediatrician who is chosen by the patient or his or her family from among doctors practising in the district where the patient lives. Each doctor is under contract with the National Health Service for primary care and community health services and may be changed for another GP in the same district if the patient so wishes. The chosen doctor is responsible for the health care of the patient either in the surgery or at the patient's home and if the need arises, and may decide on specialist out-patient care or admission to hospital. A GP may have his or her own private practice or work in private structures but cannot carry out other duties in the National Health Care Service apart from those as GP because the contract is binding. In theory, the GP should not direct patients to his or her own private practice but some in fact do so.

In order to have access to hospitals and specialist out-patient services, the individual citizen is given the legal right to choose freely between a public structure and a private one which has been formally accredited by the National Health Care Service. This choice may or may not be upheld by the patient's GP.

This free choice is considered a fundamental right of the citizen and is the essential prerequisite for free competition between public and private accredited structures. The latter are paid directly by the National Health Care Service for the services they have provided and both sectors are subject to the same Tariffs. Possible criticisms are that:

- in economic terms the local health enterprises, which receive the annual per capita quota for each person resident in the area under their jurisdiction, do not have the opportunity to negotiate with the public and private structures (that are offering services in comparative systems) for quality and cost of services. In fact, the individual's access to public or private structures cannot be controlled, not even in the case of services that are not emergencies. Thus the local health enterprise has very little contractual power.

- choices in therapy to be followed by the individual patient may not coincide with the indications made by his/her GP. This reduces the GP's opportunity to be more actively involved in the patient's diagnosis and treatment and leads to difficulty in setting up systematic contacts with specialists. Patients also frequently bypass their GPs and go directly to specialists and/or hospitals.

At hospital level, the doctor on duty determines the priorities for each patient who enters. The doctor decides whether, and to which ward, the patient is to be admitted. Once in the ward the patient is under the care and responsibility of the chief physician and the medical staff who provide appropriate diagnosis and therapy and subsequently decide on the date of discharge and the necessary follow up.

Local versus central political input into health policy decisions

Important health policy and public health decisions are generally the result of long debates carried on at the central level by the Italian government and Parliament.

The important Health Care Reform Acts in 1978 and 1992–93 involved choices that were basically made in the political and parliamentary environment. The 1978 Reform Act was the culmination of ten years of pressure from trade-unions and left-wing political parties. The 1992-93 Reform Act, on the other hand, was the outcome of more moderate points of view despite the fact that they were expressed by members of different political parties and involved differences of opinion in the medical field. This Reform was a result of persistent economic difficulties in Italy and answered the need to take measures to control the cost of health care. The well-to-do citizen was increasingly required to contribute to expenses for his/her health care.

The 1992–93 Reform Act also resulted from a growing liberal point of view to aim to achieve efficiency and quality in the health services. The goal was the creation of a health care system based on competition between one public structure and another, or between public and private enterprises. It was hoped that such a system would enable the services market to select the enterprises offering the best mix between costs and quality with a fee-structure fixed by the institutions. The Local Health Unit enterprises are responsible for authorising and controlling the running of health care activities.

A further stimulus to the Reform came from an emphasis on the concept of risk assumption, which became the responsibility of the enterprise. Formerly, it had been a feature of private enterprises but its application to public ones provided an alternative to the much disliked 'political' power existing in the local management of health care bodies. At this point the managers, who came from technical backgrounds, would be the guarantors and promoters of business-like efficiency in the enterprises.

Since the health care system is, on the whole, incapable of devising a planning method because of the various negotiations between the State, the Regions and the health enterprises, the Region ends up making health policy decisions. It has direct political control, appoints the Directors of the individual Local Health Unit enterprises and controls their activities. These local health enterprises are increasingly being taken away from municipal control and pressures.

However, at a local level a great number of organisational decisions are made although there is a tendency for medical staff to lobby or try to get the upper hand. Pressure groups, which mainly consist of clinicians, often exert a strong influence on local decision-making. Their success depends on how influential the individual clinicians are and how highly they are esteemed by the general public. They influence public opinion by underscoring (and sometimes exaggerating) the risks and dangers that could be involved for the well-being of patients if their proposals are not accepted by the Local Health Unit Hospital Enterprises. In reality they are often more interested in their own power and prestige and find support in the mass media. It must be pointed out that public health administrators tend to be less influential than clinicians.

The clinicians who belong to the various medical trade unions and to the scientific organisations that represent the different specialties are successful in exerting pressure on regional and local decision-making. The major national trade unions, on the other hand, are less influential in determining health policy.

Those Regions that have a regional health care plan for the organisation and function of hospital and local health care enterprises are able to make informed decisions. In these regions the reports written by enterprises become real operative local plans that consider the impact of regional planning decisions.

In other Regions where planning methods are poor, local proposals and decisions tend to be less analytical and do not fit easily into a systematic framework. This does not mean there is no room for local decision-making. On the contrary, the decision-making power of the Local Health Unit and hospital enterprises is strengthened as a result of the lack of regional planning restrictions but it is uncoordinated, which reduces the effectiveness of the health care system.

Decision-making is obviously more effective in Regions with health plans In these plans the Director-General possesses a great deal of freedom to make decisions concerning the running of enterprises. The presence of joint projects involving other enterprises also means that there is a general improvement in health care.

As well as regional contradictions in health planning there are other causes for concern.

A continuing atmosphere of uncertainty exists concerning the directorship of local health and hospital enterprises in certain Regions like Lombardy and Piedmont where the appointment of the Director-Generals has been contested in court. This certainly contributes to planning problems.

Italy has a high litigation rate, which affects decision-making effectiveness in the public health care field. This is a long standing problem and is still typical of public administration in Italy where a particular type of law known as 'administrative law' predominates. This is exactly the opposite of the situation in the private sector where civil law prevails and where a respect for formal regulations does not exist. Formal regulations aim at guaranteeing the legitimacy of formal administrative decisions before they are put into action. Therefore formality prevails over substance in the efficiency and effectiveness of decisions, speed of decision-making, carrying out of decisions and flexibility in the use of resources. All this serves no purpose in outcomes control in terms of costs and quality of the services used.

Poor and tardy decision-making often leads to lawsuits by individual employees or opportunistic third-parties. This is a typically Italian situation and does not seem to have any equivalent in Europe, at least as far as the public health service is concerned. This problem, which is only typical of public institutions and local health and hospital enterprises, has now worsened as a result of the competition between public and private structures. The latter are not subject to any of the above-mentioned legal complications that concern the public sector.

Decision-making in the public health field is also greatly hindered by restrictions, slowness in procedures and uncertainties over the possibility of obtaining funds for carrying out works and investments. All of these factors are conditioned by excessive bureaucracy at the regional level and (in the case of more important decisions) by ministerial authorisations involving more than one ministry.

These restrictions, together with recent changes in the management of Local Health Unit and hospital enterprises, cause enormous delays in the building of health structures. This is particularly true in the case of hospitals, which require a number of years of planning, allocating finances and building the structures. Bureaucratic delays have caused costs to escalate such that a budget allocated 10–15 years before construction is insufficient and hospital and outpatient structures remain only partly built.

Are there any underlying principles?

As has been explained, the Health Care Reform Act of 1978 laid down a series of fundamental principles taken up by the Italian Constitution and included in Article 1 of the Act itself:

> 'The Republic protects health as a fundamental right of the individual and of common concern by means of the National Health Care Service.'

and

'The protection of physical and mental health must respect the dignity and freedom of the individual.'

By the 1992–93 Reform Act the National Health Plan was to guarantee the best health care possible using the annual available resources. The Health Care System may, if the need arises, deal with Social Services if the Municipalities that usually have this task agree to delegate their responsibility to the System itself and provide the appropriate funds. The National Health Plan aims at a uniform level of health in the whole population and establishes standard levels of health care based on epidemiological and clinical data which, in turn, must specify the services to be guaranteed to each citizen depending on available funds.

If the Region so decides, additional levels of care that supplement the standard ones (which represent a sort of guaranteed minimum) are possible. This obviously contravenes the principle of equality of the citizen provided by the Constitution and requires the Region to levy extra taxation on its residents to finance operations. Further possibilities for obtaining services, in addition to those offered by the National Health Care Service, are available through integrative health funds which originate from:

- contracts and collective agreements, even businesses

- agreements among self-employed workers or professionals

- regulations in firms, bodies, public bodies or various associations.

As can be seen, in practice the Sickness-Insurance System (which was at its height before the 1978 Reform Act) returned to the scene with the 1992–93 Reform.

Availability of information for setting priorities and monitoring outcomes

Beyond the current statistics and periodical reports already mentioned, the following sources of information also contribute to priority setting and outcomes monitoring:

(a) A system of indicators for each specific geographical area in accordance with Legislative Decree 502, Article 10, 'Contents and modalities for the use of efficiency and quality indicators in the National Health Care System.'

(b) Data collection at all levels regarding the new classification system for normal admission or day-hospital according to DRG and related tariffs. The data refer to admission by DRG for each hospital and ward and whether a patient is within or exceeds the foreseen length of stay in hospital. They also take into account the cost/returns relationship per hospital, ward etc.

(c) Data collection regarding environmental pollution parameters such as:

- the recording of atmospheric pollution indicators: sulphur dioxide, nitric oxides, hydrocarbons, carbon-monoxide, particulates etc.

- the recording of pollution indicators for ground water destined for human consumption: non-specific parameters (nitrates, sulphates, chlorides, total hardness etc.) and specific pollutants (solvents, heavy metals, pesticides etc.)

- the recording of pollution indicators for surface water: non-specific parameters (BOD, pH, temperature, colour, solids in suspension and solids that can be sedimented etc.), specific pollutants (heavy metals, mineral oils, solvents, pesticides etc.) and micro-organisms.

Those hospitals that also function as research institutes produce annual reports on the services they have provided, whereas Out-patient Departments and services that operate outside the hospitals make periodic reports on their activities. These reports expose great differences in frequency and reliability between one area and another.

It should be emphasised that a great deal of ad hoc research is carried out at national, regional and local levels. Although a significant amount of data is produced, much of it is uncoordinated and of little use for epidemiological purposes. The main reason for the poor quality of these data lies in the fact that they are often produced by people who decide quite of their own accord to carry out a research programme and often do not have sufficient knowledge or grounding for doing so.

Occasionally, organised research is carried out at the national level by official bodies such as the Superior Institute of Health and at regional and local levels by technical bodies set up by the Regional government or by those University departments that are part of the Faculties of Medicine or Economics. In addition to these public bodies the Mario Negri Pharmacological Research Institute in Milan also contributes to the work. This is a private cum public foundation that carries out rigorous research on the effectiveness of pharmaceuticals and, in more recent years, has undertaken epidemiological studies and evaluated health services.

As researchers in the assessment field, we are in fact aware of the contradiction that exists between the soundness of the evidence of certain research and the fact that only by pure chance do those who decide on health care policies occasionally take our research into consideration. Moreover, 'the decider' seems to be more interested in assessing 'how much' is produced. The work loads and service costs seem to be more important than what problems exist and what the outcome is.

Conclusions

If one takes epidemiology into account then primary prevention has only brought about a slight decrease in conditions that are targets of primary prevention. Tumours have proved a particular problem as there has been an increase in lung cancer and cancer of the intestine.

The increase in tumours linked to the use of tobacco and alcohol shows the irrationality of human behaviour and above all the ineffectiveness of preventive measures in Italy.

The number of smokers is on the increase. Infant mortality remains high as do cases of diabetes, bronchitis, emphysema and asthma. Italy has a very high rate of violent deaths, many of which are homicides.

In terms of the provision of care, it is worth noting that in the European Union Italy has the highest number of doctors and lowest number of dentists together with the longest waiting times for transplants. There is a much greater disparity in health care provision between one region and another in Italy than between other European countries. The situation in Italy is traditionally one in which prevention is ineffective and health care is costly and inefficient.

Two radical attempts at reforming the system have been made. The first was in 1978 with the passage of Art. N. 833 which provided for the identification of all National Health Service activities and their assignment to the Local Health Units. The second was the reorganisation of the system in the years 1992–1993 which converted the Local Health Units and the more important hospitals into enterprises. In the latter case the intention was to promote a new kind of management aimed at efficiency without direct political interference. The enterprises aim to provide uniform levels of health care and reach a break-even point between costs and returns for services provided.

At present the regions vary greatly in the ways in which they carry out the directives laid down by the 1992–1993 Reform and many of the Regions still have not managed to propose a Regional plan. In spite of this the Reform has achieved good results as far as expenses are concerned. This partly is due to the fact that the regions have been 'advised' not to overspend their funds because their populations will be forced to pay regional taxes to cover the extra expenditure. Many Regions in the south of Italy, on the other hand, have been unable to curb excess expenditure in certain health care sectors and improve existing inadequacies in health care. For this reason there is a high flow of patients from the south to the north of Italy for medical care. It is thus safe to say that the reforms have triggered an improvement in the Italian health care system with positive results in terms of efficiency and expenditure control. However the process is still not finished and since the reform is being carried out and interpreted in so many different ways by the individual regions the political debate on the future of health care in Italy remains open.

References

1.   Geddes M. *Rapporto sulla salute in Europa. Roma:* EDIESSE, 1995.

2.   Legge 23 dicembre 1978, n. 833 'Istituzione del Servizio Sanitario Nazionale'.

3.   Decreto Legislativo 30 dicembre 1972, n. 502 'Riordino della disciplina in materia sanitaria, a norma dell'articolo. 1 della Legge 23 ottobre 1972, n. 421'.

4.   Decreto Legislativo 7 dicembre 1993, n. 517 'Modificazioni al decreto legislativo 30 dicembre 1992, n. 502, recante riordino della disciplina in materia sanitaria, a norma dell'articolo. 1 della Legge 23 ottobre 1992, n. 421'.

5. Decreto del Presidente della Repubblica 1 marzo 1994 'Approvazione del Piano sanitario nazionale per il triennio 1994–1996'.

6. Regione Veneto. Legge regionale 20 luglio 1989, n. 21 'Piano socio-sanitario regionale 1989–1991'.

7. Regione Emilia-Romagna. Legge regionale 9 marzo 1990, n. 15 'Piano Sanitario Regionale per il triennio 1990–1992'.

8. Regione Piemonte. Legge regionale 23 aprile 1990, n. 37 'Norme per la programmazione socio-sanitaria regionale e per il Piano Socio-Sanitario Regionale per il triennio 1990–1992'.

9. Regione Toscana. Legge regionale 2 gennaio 1995, n. 1 'Disciplina sull'organizzazione e funzionamento delle Unita Sanitarie Locali e delle Aziende Ospedaliere ai sensi degli artt. 3 e 4 del D.L. 30/12/1992, n. 502 e successive modificazioni'.

10. Legge 23 dicembre 1994, n. 724 'Misure di razionalizzazione della finanza pubblica'.

11. Ragioneria generale dello Stato. *Relazione generale sulla situazione economica nel Paese nel 1995.* 1996.

12. Decreto Legge 4 dicembre 1993, n. 496 'Disposizioni urgenti sulla riorganizzazione dei controlli ambientali e istituzione della Agenzia nazionale per la protezione dell'ambiente', convertito in Legge 21 gennaio 1994, n. 61.

13. Legge 23 ottobre 1985, n. 595 'Norme per la programmazione sanitaria e per il piano sanitario triennale 1986–1988'.

14. Legge 30 dicembre 1991, n. 412 'Disposizioni in materia di finanza pubblica'.

15. Legge 13 maggio 1978, n. 180 'Accertamenti e trattamenti sanitari volontarie obbligatori'.

16. Legge 11 marzo 1988, n. 67 'Formazione del bilancio annuale e pluriennale dello Stato'.

17. Decreto Ministeriale 29 agosto 1989, n. 321 'Regolamento recante criteri generali per la programmazione degli interventi e il coordinamento tra enti competenti nel settore dell'edilizia sanitaria in riferimento al piano pluriennale d'investimenti'.

18. Legge 5 giugno 1990, n. 135 'Programma di interventi urgenti per la prevenzione e la lotta dell'AIDS'.

19. Ministero della Sanita – Dipartimento della Programmazione. Attivita gestionali ed economiche della U.S.L. *Annuario statistico del Sistema Sanitario Nazionale.* 1996.

20. Istituto Nazionale di Statistica. *Le Regioni in cifre.* Roma, 1995.

21. Ministero della Sanita – Servizio centrale della programmazione sanitaria. Flussi informativi delle unita sanitarie locali. Roma, 1996.

Annex 1 – Data on public health produced at a national level

Statistics from ISTAT (Central Statistics Institute) on:

Demographic population trends

Deaths by causes per municipality

Data regarding bed density and utilisation and personnel employed by Health Structures

Specific psychiatric data, data on spontaneous abortions and abortions

Economic and financial data on the management of hospitals and Local Health Units

ISTAT research into families (random and periodic)

Report on the state of health in Italy

Published annually by the National Health Council (the Technical-Consultative Organ of the Ministry of Health) on:

Demographic aspects of the population including mortality by causes

Social condition of the population and relative indicators

Infectious and degenerative diseases

Hospital nosology

Accidents, industrial accidents and suicides

Living habits (health education and health promotion, food and nutrition, alcoholism, nicotine addiction, drug-taking)

Environmental health (protection of the living environment, food hygiene and safety)

Activities of the central health organs

Activities of the Local Health Unit enterprises and other public and private structures operating in the social and health care field

Planning, resources policy and control (the carrying out of the health care plan at its various levels, the National Health Care Finance System, the health care information system, the pharmaceutical industry, the quality of health care)

Development and carrying out of research programmes

Personnel policy

Mortality survey split up for each Local Health Unit

This survey is published by the Central Service for Health Planning of the Ministry of Health and is based on the data-processing of the death certificates compiled by all doctors certifying death. The published data are usually four or five years old. Similar surveys are published periodically by some Regions, as for example, Lombardy, Veneto and Emilia Romagna but they too use data that are a few years out-of-date.

Private data and data regarding public health structures

These are produced and published by the Health Information System of the Central Service for Health Planning at the Ministry of Health. They are based on the processing of the administrative data from the Local Health Unit enterprises, which are systematically collected from special returns from every hospital. For each Local Health Unit these data show how many hospitals there are, what specialised operative units exist for each specialty, the distribution of hospital beds and day hospitals, the availability of high quality therapeutic and diagnostic equipment and the hospital personnel by speciality and grade for each hospital. In this case, too, the data available are always considerably overdue and the quality is mediocre.

Data on infectious diseases and in particular morbidity-mortality from AIDS

These data derive from the compulsory declarations of infectious diseases made by general practitioners. At the Superior Institute of Health there is an epidemiological department for infectious diseases which collects the data from all the Local health Units.

The completeness of the data varies considerably.

Annex 2 – Example of a planned action and two projects-specific aims

Prevention and treatment of oncological illness

PLANNED ACTIONS

put forward at a national level,

- organ transplants for the three years from 1994–96
- care of chronic kidney (renal) patients

Example:

PLANNED ACTION 'CARE OF CHRONIC RENAL PATIENTS'

* Epidemiological pinpointing of specific health care needs and the provision of dialysis services and kidney transplants

* Definition of a precise strategy for allocating the best possible care in compliance with present technological developments at the lowest financial and social cost

- setting priorities
- the promotion of activities for the prevention and early diagnosis of kidney diseases
- diffusion of renal advice centres and out-patients departments throughout the country
- diffusion of operative nephrology units
- organisation of the regional network integrated with services for dialysis
- functional link between ambulatory health care and dialysis centres and nephrology departments in hospitals which are to be considered reference or assessment points for each catchment area
- intensification of kidney transplant activities (in connection with the other planned action
- organ transplant)

* Pinpointing the steps to be taken in order to carry out the planned aims:

- setting up a network with operative units and out-patient nephrology departments
- involvement of primary care and Community Health services in actions concerning risk factors (e.g. hereditary, occupational etc.)
- organisation of the dialysis service network at four different levels:

- Hospital Centres with highly qualified assistance (Reference Centres)

- Centres for dialysis dispersed to other hospitals

- Centres for dialysis offering limited care

- Activities for domiciliary dialysis

- fixing of a standard number of personnel in relation to the number of patients undergoing treatment

- transport organisation for patients who are not self-sufficient

- provision of dialytic and nephrological facilities in Health Care Homes for the elderly linked to the Hospital Reference Centre

- promoting of information on the importance of organ donations and the boosting of the transplant service network

- training and refresher courses for health operators in the sector

PROJECT-SPECIFIC AIMS

These were promoted on a national level to particular groups of the population, such as mothers and infants and the elderly, for the three years from 1994–96.

Example:

PROJECT-SPECIFIC AIM 'MOTHER AND INFANT CARE'

Aim: to reduce further the perinatal death rate to at least 10 per cent in the regions where it is higher:

* Operational strategies

- prevention and health care education

- contributions in the field of education in collaboration with school authorities and other institutions involved in aspects of childhood and adolescence

- promotion of responsible family-planning and special care for pregnancies at risk

- prevention and control of genetic conditions

- rendering health care services less impersonal

- setting up of round-the-clock emergency services

- appropriate planning of services throughout the country concerned with the most important emerging maternal and infant diseases.

* Measures to be taken during the three years of the plan:

- setting up of mother and infant care departments to integrate social and health care aspects. This involves the conversion of paediatric and obstetric facilities existing in large hospitals into paediatric pluri-specialised complexes together with an increase in out-patient and day-hospital services

- pinpointing of specialised regional centres for pregnancies at risk

- increase in advice centres and community paediatrics with the conversion of little-used paediatric and obstetric hospital facilities into daytime rehabilitation and out-patient services

- increased and improved distribution of intensive and semi-intensive therapy and organisation of emergency transport for new-born infants

- various activities in the field of prevention, public information and health care promotion

* the setting up of national epidemiological registers at the Superior Institute of Health which contain all the data collected in the regional registers.

11

The Health System and Health Policy in Luxembourg

Danielle Hansen-Koenig and Mady Roulleaux

Introduction to the health system

The main characteristic of the Luxembourg health system is a split in the provision and financing of prevention and care and treatment. Prevention comes under the responsibility of the Ministry of Health, with interventions provided by a few public services and by private non-profit associations, financed by the State. The competence for care and treatment is shared by the Ministry of Health, which supervises the organisation of health services and subsidises the hospital sector, and by the Ministry of Social Security which is responsible for the sickness insurance system. Services, including primary care, are provided by doctors (general practitioners, specialists) and other health professionals in independent practice and by hospitals (public, semi-public, private). They are financed through the statutory sickness insurance system and the State budget. Recent developments have led to the integration of some preventive measures into the sickness insurance scheme, thus moving prevention into independent medical practice.

Various other government departments are involved in health-related areas, such as the Ministry of Environment (air and water pollution, waste, noise), the Ministry of Family Welfare (homes for elderly people including nursing care, home aid services, handicapped), the Ministry of Labour (safety at work), the Ministry of Housing (housing projects, subsidies for individual homes), the Ministry of Education (training of health professionals, health education in schools, the 'Healthy Schools' project) and the Ministry of Transport (traffic safety). Owing to the small size of the country, planning, supervision and control are highly centralised. The various responsibilities for health in Luxembourg are illustrated in Figure 1 overleaf.

Figure 1 Luxembourg: health-related responsibilities

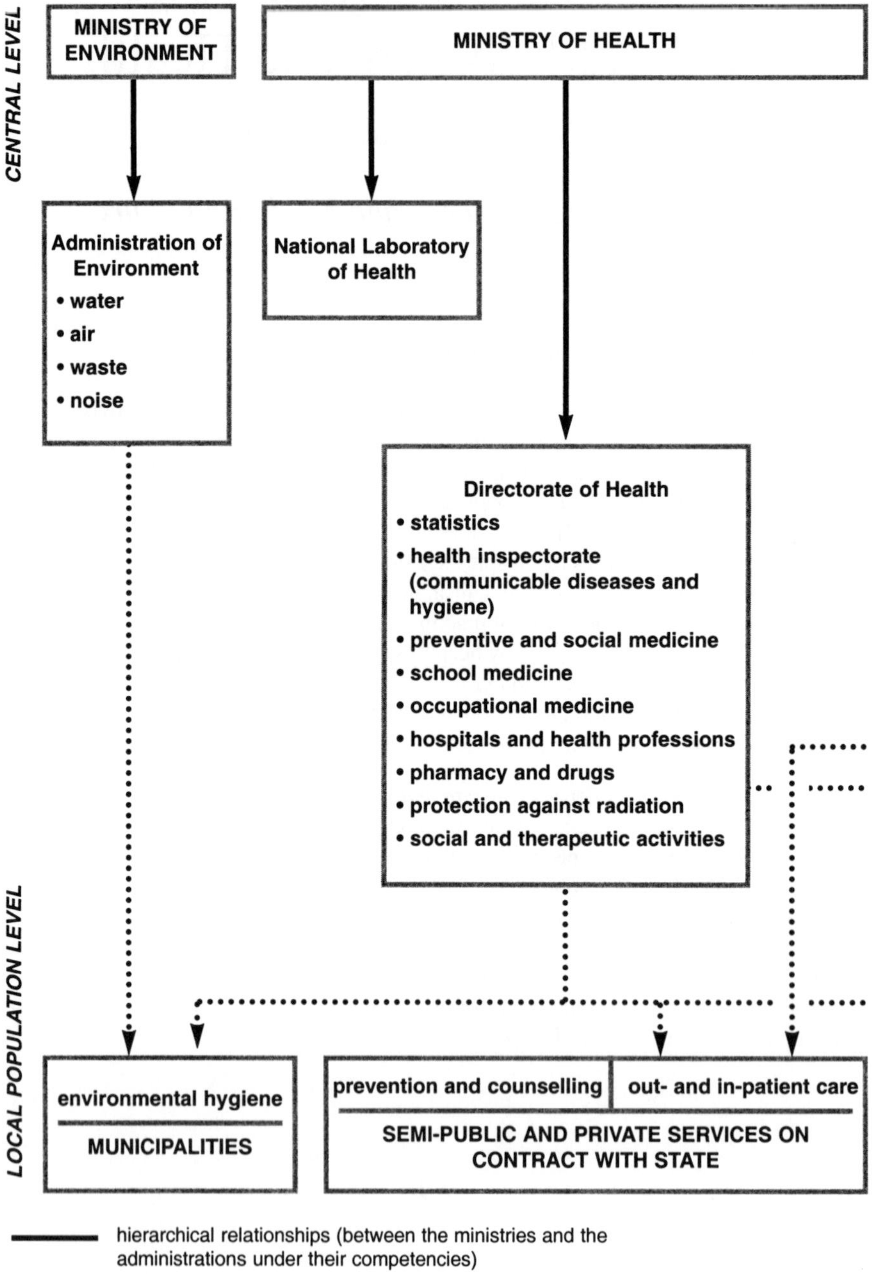

hierarchical relationships (between the ministries and the administrations under their competencies)

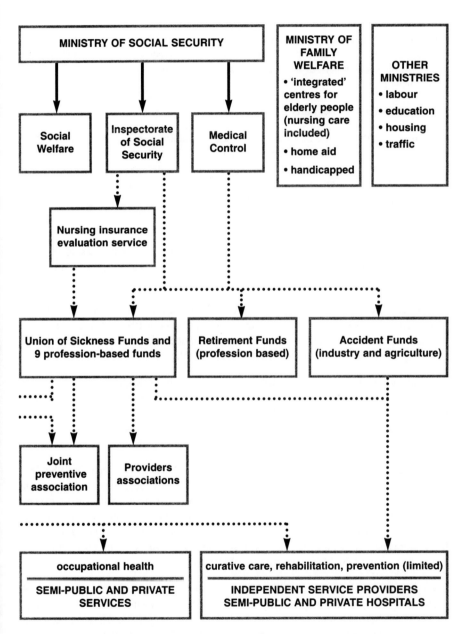

.... non-hierarchical relationships which differ according to responsibilities
(supervisory, partnership, negotiation, financing)

Health status

Life expectancy

Life expectancy has risen from 68 years (in 1976/78) to 72.6 (in 1990/92) in men and from 75.1 to 79.1 years in women.[1,2] The difference between men and women slightly decreased during this period: the average for men rising by 4.6 years compared with 4 years for women.

Infant and perinatal mortality

Over the past 25 years, the infant mortality rate has fallen from 24.9/1,000 to less than 5/1,000 live births. Perinatal mortality fell from 24.7/1,000 to around 5/1,000 total births.[1,3] The most important decline was registered in children born to mothers belonging to groups at risk after the introduction of preventative measures during pregnancy; this is likely to have contributed to the overall improvement.

Mortality[1]

Cardiovascular disease, mainly coronary heart and cerebrovascular diseases, cancer and accidents make the greatest contribution to overall mortality. The causes of death varies according to age group.

In children aged 1–14 years, accidents are the leading cause of death (in 1986/90 they accounted for 47 per cent) followed by cancer (12 per cent in 1986–90) and congenital anomalies (9 per cent in 1986–90). Annual total numbers of deaths in this age group range from 7 to 19 in 1986-90 and from 4 to 22 in 1991/95.[4]

In the age group 15–24, accidents account for 66 per cent of deaths (1986–90). By far the most common are deaths from motor vehicle accidents. Although the general mortality rate from road traffic accidents has decreased over the last 20 years, there has been a slight increase in this age group in both men and women. Suicide accounts for 10 per cent of deaths (1986–90) and this is an increasing trend.

In the age group 35–64, cancer is the main cause of death (36 per cent in 1986–90) followed by circulatory disease (28 per cent in 1986–90), accidents (8 per cent in 1986–90) and suicide (5 per cent in 1986–90). The most frequent causes of cancer deaths are cancer of the lung, colon and rectum and cancer of the prostate in men, and in women cancer of the breast, colon, rectum and the lungs. The percentage of deaths from lung cancer in women has increased over the last 20 years (from 3 per cent of all cancer deaths in 1968–70 to 7 per cent in 1988–90).

Surveys carried out between 1987, 1993 and 1998 demonstrate that smoking has declined in men and increased slightly in women and adolescents aged between 11 and 18 years. In men, the number of regular smokers has fallen from 41 to 32 per cent, whereas the rate in women has increased from 25 to 26 per cent and, in adolescents, from 10 per cent in 1990 to 11 per cent in 1998.[5]

For cancer mortality in women, the percentage of deaths from cancer of the cervix has fallen from 4 per cent (1968–70) to 2 per cent (1988–90), the percentage of deaths from breast cancer increased from 17 per cent (1968–70) to 21 per cent (1988–90). In 1964, a specialised public screening service was established and cervical smears are strongly recommended. The national screening programme for breast cancer started in 1992.

Over the past 15 years, there has been an important decline in death rates for coronary heart and cerebrovascular disease in both men and women. It is most substantial in the age group 55–64: for coronary heart disease the death rate has fallen by 38 per cent in men and 41.9 per cent in women, and for cerebrovascular disease by 17.9 per cent in men and 14.5 per cent in women.

As no information is available on the prevalence of these diseases in the population, developments in mortality cannot be related either to prevention or to improvements in treatment.

Over the last 30 years, decreasing trends have been registered for road traffic and occupational accidents. There is, however, an upward trend in the death rate from suicide.

Excessive alcohol consumption is a significant problem. Despite a decline over several years, the death rate from liver cirrhosis remains high and excessive drinking comes second in risk factors related to deaths from road traffic accidents.[6] Measuring alcohol consumption by sales statistics is not accurate as cross-border shopping is quite significant in Luxembourg.

In the age group 65 and over, circulatory diseases (54 per cent in 1986–90) and cancer (22 per cent in 1986–90) are the main causes of death. In women the death rate for cerebrovascular disease is nearly double that of coronary heart diseases.

The increasing number of older people who are unable to care for themselves because of chronic illnesses, physical disabilities and mental disorders is a major concern in health and social policy.

HIV/AIDS

At the end of 1997, a cumulative total of 127 AIDS cases had been reported of whom 74 had died. Homo/bisexual contact is the predominant transmission mode (51.2 per cent), heterosexual contact comes second (18.9 per cent) followed by intravenous drug use (15.7 per cent). More than 20,000 HIV tests are carried out in the population per year.[7]

Administration[8]

The Minister of Health is responsible for defining and implementing health policy within the Government's programme, for controlling the application of the laws and rules on health and health services and for the supervision of health institutions and services. These tasks are carried out by:

The Directorate of Health and its specific divisions:

The Division of Health Inspection (or Health Inspectorate) dealing with public hygiene, communicable diseases and environmental medicine.

The Division of Preventive and Social Medicine working in prevention and health promotion.

The Division of Curative Medicine responsible for the planning and control of hospital care, quality control in laboratories and the supervision of the practice of health professions.

The Division of School Medicine supervising school health services and providing services in secondary schools.

The Division of Occupational Health responsible for the planning and control of occupational health services.

The Division of Pharmacy responsible for licensing medicines and supervising the practice of the profession of pharmacist.

The Division for Protection Against Ionising and Non-ionising Radiation.

The Service for Social and Therapeutic Activities is responsible for supervising services dealing with handicaps, mental illness, drug addiction, home nursing services and nursing homes for the elderly.

The Directorate of Health organises services for the early detection of sight and hearing deficiencies in infants, for delivering equipment for hearing defects and for counselling patients.

Public institution for nursing homes

The National Laboratory of Health has been established by law and has several specific divisions: bacteriology and parasitology, virology, immunology and cytogenetics, pathological anatomy, clinical cytology, haematology, biochemistry and endocrinology, toxicology and pharmaceutics and food control. It carries out laboratory work related to health and hygiene for public authorities or private persons and epidemiological studies and research within its various specialties.

With the passage of Law 23 December 1999, all former state nusing homes, while remaining public institutions, were given financial and administrative automony. They are now managed in accordance with civil law but with the supervision of the Ministry of Health.

Formal relations between the Ministry of Health and the semi-public and private sector

The Ministry of Health appoints the following posts:

- representatives to the board of administrators of various public hospitals and institutions managed according to private law;

- representatives to the board of administrators of private organisations of public utility whose services are partly funded by the State: Luxembourg League of Medico-social Prevention and Welfare, and the Luxembourg Red Cross;

A law introducing agreement and supervision of services, and providing a legal basis for contracts between the State and private associations was passed in July 1998. The law provides for two committees; one dealing with questions related to contracts, the financing of services and planning, and the other advising, more generally, on the conditions for the coordination of services and on the need for new services.

Formal collaboration

Collaboration has been introduced by law in the following areas:

- Between the Ministry of Health and the Ministry of Social Security for hospital planning. The Permanent Commission for the Hospital Sector, presided over by the Director General of Health is an advisory body to both ministers for all questions related to the hospital programme, hospitals and financial contributions of the State to this sector (Law on hospitals, 1998).

- Between the Ministries of Health, Labour and Social Security within the Council for Health and Safety at Work. The Council, presided over by the Director General of Health, is an advisory body to the ministers for defining priorities for health protection in various industries, establishing safety standards, measuring the outcome of occupational health interventions and designing information and education programmes for employers and workers (Law on occupational health, 1994).

- Between the Directorate of Health and the Union of Sickness Funds for carrying out prevention programmes (Law on health insurance and health reform, 1992). The collaboration is based on contracts between both public administrations. The proposals for programmes are forwarded by the Directorate of Health.

- Between the Ministry of Health and the Ministry of Education for training of health professionals and approval of professional qualifications from abroad (Law on re-organisation of nurses' schools, 1995).

- A mandate for collaboration is given by law to the Division of Occupational Health and the Inspectorate of Work which falls under the Ministry of Labour, supervising safety at the work place (Law on occupational health services, 1994), and to the

Division of School Health and psychological services under the Ministry of Education (Law on school medicine, 1987).

Cooperation between governmental departments, public administrations and the private sector takes place within public institutions (prevention of drug abuse), national committees (AIDS) and councils (which are advisory bodies to a minister on specific topics, e.g. hygiene, education, youth, handicap etc.) or working groups (nosocomial infections, diabetes, care during pregnancy).

Intersectoral cooperation is a basic guideline of the 'Health for All' (HFA) strategy of the Ministry of Health for its future activities.

Legal framework for health and health-related areas

The legal framework includes a range of laws and rules in various areas, e.g. control of communicable diseases, protection of the environment and against radiation, housing, safety at work, traffic safety, product and food safety, pharmaceuticals and medical devices, training and practice of health professions, hospital planning and funding, prevention and health promotion, school health, occupational health, restriction of publicity for tobacco and prohibition of smoking in different places, prevention of drug abuse. The legislation was largely developed following EU directives.

Preventive interventions during pregnancy and early childhood, introduced in 1977, are provided in private medical practice with no contribution to doctor's fees, but with financial incentives for mothers/parents; participation is a condition for the granting of birth allowances. These are administered by a public institution under the Ministry of Family Welfare, whereas preventive interventions are covered by the sickness insurance.

School health services were reorganised in 1987. Frequency and content of examinations are determined by regulation.

A law on *occupational health* services was passed in 1994. It aims to protect the health of workers at the workplace and to prevent accidents and occupational diseases.

A public institution for the *prevention of drug abuse*, which is supervised by the government and financed by the Ministry of Education, was created by law in 1994. This centre is responsible for coordinating preventive activities in the field of drug addiction. Emphasis is given to preventive activities in schools. The head of the Division of Preventive Medicine at the Directorate of Health is a member of the board of administrators.

A new law on *hospitals* was passed in July 1998. It succeeds the previous laws on hospital planning (1976) and development of hospital services according to the needs of the country (1990). The previous legislation had introduced a basic plan for hospitals, health professionals and equipment, and financial contributions by the State for investment programmes. The new legislation now makes contributions for public and private hospitals 50 or 80 per cent according to the type of investment. A government commissioner is in charge of the financial control of State subsidies. The new law also introduces coordination of hospitals and hospital departments, standards and guidelines for their organisation and functioning and it defines the rights of patients.

The *national hospital programme* (1994) will be updated following a detailed inventory of the current situation.

The criteria for *emergency medical aid* were set out by law in 1988.

Administration and organisation of the sickness insurance system[9]

The sickness insurance system is under the responsibility of the Ministry of Social Security. The Ministry's supervision and control are operated by two administrations: the General Inspectorate of Social Security which supervises legal, regulatory, statutory, contractual and financial operations, and the Office of Medical Control which deals with disability at work, authorisations for reimbursement (including treatments abroad), medical profiles, supervision of out-patient care, and abuse of health care by patients.

Insurance is jointly managed by public institutions, the Union of Sickness Funds and the various occupationally-based funds. The boards of the Union and the funds are mixed elected bodies. The president of the executive committee and the staff of the Union and sickness funds are civil servants or employed by the State. All funds cover the same provisions, except income support which is limited to the workers' scheme.

The fees of health care providers and the prices of supplies are negotiated between the Union of Sickness Funds and the professional associations of the different providers in independent practice or commerce.

Services and supplies eligible for reimbursement are registered on lists of items (nomenclatures) adopted jointly by the Ministers of Health and Social Security on the advice of a special committee. This advisory body is composed by representatives of both governmental departments, the Union of Sickness Funds and health care providers. Medicines have to be on the official list of the Ministry of Health.

The hospital sector is highly privatised as even public hospitals are managed according to private company law. Hospital legislation and reimbursements of sickness funds are equally applicable to public and private hospitals. Hospital budgets are negotiated by the Union of Sickness Funds with each hospital taking into account developments for the next two years. Budgets encompass investments in movable assets (equipment etc.) and immovable assets (land, buildings etc.) up to the amount which is not covered by State contributions. Investments have to be authorised by the Minister of Health according to existing legislation. Hospital budgets can be adjusted in line with actual developments. A special committee rules on disagreements. The results of the negotiations with all providers have to be agreed by the Minister of Social Security.

As a rule, patients pay for services and are reimbursed by their sickness funds. Reimbursements range from lump sums to a rate of 100 per cent of the negotiated tariffs. Reimbursement rates for doctors' fees are 80 per cent (95 per cent if there is more than one visit within 28 days) and 100 per cent during hospitalisation. Rates for dentists' fees are 80 per cent. Dental prostheses are covered at a rate of 80 per cent, or 100 per cent of the agreed tariffs if the patient has an annual check-up. The agreements with doctors and dentists provide for additional fees to be covered by the patient. These can be charged for first-class hospitalisation, personal services, dental prostheses and services beyond what is regarded as necessary and useful.

Medicines included in the official list and issued on prescription are reimbursed at a rate of 80 per cent of the price, as fixed by the Minister of Economy. A preferential rate of 100 per cent is applied to products with a precise therapeutic purpose and to all products used for the treatment of a long-term and costly illness. A reduced rate of 40 per cent is applicable for products with limited therapeutic purpose. Non-essential products or those prescribed for preventive purpose are not reimbursed. Laboratory analyses and blood products supplied by the Red Cross are covered at a rate of 100 per cent of the agreed tariffs.

Most supplies are reimbursed at a rate of 100 per cent of the agreed tariffs, based on reference prices. A flat-rate amount is applicable for spectacles. Services and supplies which are not eligible for reimbursement are determined by the statutes of the Union of Sickness Funds.

The sickness insurance covers the day-rate of a second class room in hospital. A fixed daily contribution is charged to the patient. Insurance does not cover subsistence costs if a patient only needs nursing care.

Direct payment by sickness insurance is made for hospitals, pharmacies, laboratories, blood supplies, the national screening programme for breast cancer and the hepatitis B immunisation programme.

The law on sickness insurance and health reforms stipulates that health care services have to be limited to those which are necessary and useful. The volume of services is subject to different control mechanisms; authorisation by the Office of Medical Control is required for predetermined services, and limitations are set on the number of visits to a practitioner per week, sessions of physiotherapy, ultrasound scans during pregnancy, medicines issued on one prescription and so on.

A supervisory committee headed by the Director of the Office of Medical Control, composed of delegates from the board of the Union of Sickness Funds and the professional groups representing providers, may ask for accounts from a provider whose professional activities appear to justify this.

The Union of Sickness Funds is responsible for the budget of the sickness insurance system. State participation is determined by law. It is equivalent to 10 per cent of the contributions of people in work and 250 per cent of contributions of retired people; it must not exceed 40 per cent of total contributions.

A committee composed of representatives of the Ministers of Social Security, Health and Finance, of professional organisations of employees and employers and of health care providers is convened annually by the Minister of Social Security to supervise the total annual income and expenditure of the sickness insurance system. An 'alarm' device signals the need for specific actions, either additional levies, increase of patients' contributions, or regulation of the volume of consultations and services.

Sickness insurance does not cover prevention, except preventive dental examinations, preventive interventions during pregnancy and early childhood (based on law), screening for breast cancer and part of the hepatitis B vaccine programme (joint programmes based on contracts with the Ministry of Health).

The 1992 law on sickness insurance and health reform introduces three formal links between health authorities and the insurance system:

1) Contracts between the Directorate of Health and the Union of Sickness Funds for prevention programmes.

2) Delegations of the Ministry of Health and the Directorate of Health at the permanent committee for the hospital sector.

3) Delegations of the Ministry of Health and the Directorate of Health at the concerted action committee for cost regulation.

In June 1998, long-term care insurance was introduced by law. Provisions include home and institutional nursing care, rehabilitation, home aid, nursing appliances, alterations to homes, counselling and support. An individual care plan is designed for each patient. Benefits will be paid from January 1999.

The role of local authorities

Public health problems legally belong to the municipal councils. The Director-General of Health or a delegated public health officer is the mandatory advisor to the local authorities. In fact, their responsibility has become limited to environmental problems such as distribution of drinking water, sewage, waste disposal, housing and local traffic rather than to preventive medicine and health promotion. Only a few larger towns organise school health services. Most municipalities rely on the comprehensive medico-social service set up by private associations and funded by the Ministry of Health. Standing committees in the municipal councils cover environmental and social problems rather than health.

Although local authorities share responsibility for the health of the population, activities in the field of prevention and health promotion are left to the national health authorities. Presently, the Division of Preventive Medicine of the Directorate of Health is trying to introduce the WHO 'Healthy Cities' programme, in which the country has not yet participated.

Services

Environmental services

Protection of the environment (air pollution, water and sanitation, waste disposal etc.) comes under the responsibility of the Ministry of Environment via the National Administration of Environment and municipalities. Some municipalities have established environmental services which act as consultants to the local administrations and the population.

Information services available to the population of the whole country are organised by private non-profit associations, subsidised by the Ministry of Environment and the Ministry of Health. There is close collaboration between the administration of environment and private associations.

An environmental medicine service has been set up in the Health Inspection Division of the Directorate of Health. It carries out analyses on request in cases of suspected environmental hazards for the health of individuals in their homes. Various private associations act as pressure groups for more specific problems related to the protection of the environment and they get some support from the public. There is much public debate on environmental problems.

Prevention and preventive services

The priorities of the Ministry of Health cover the following areas:

- Hospital planning.
- Reform of psychiatric services with decentralisation and development of outpatient clinics with a view to secondary and tertiary prevention.
- Development of nursing care for elderly people: home nursing services and nursing homes.
- Implementing the 'Health For All' strategy of the World Health Organisation.

A 'Health For All' paper was prepared by the Directorate of Health and published by the Ministry of Health in 1994.[1] It is a first attempt at a comprehensive description of health problems based on mortality statistics, and integrates European programmes (EU and WHO) into a national strategy for prevention and health promotion. Emphasis is given to a multisectoral approach to health problems. The HFA strategy sets priorities in the following areas:

Cardiovascular diseases by promoting healthy nutrition and physical activity, by reducing alcohol consumption and detecting risk factors.

Cancer: prevention of lung cancer through an overall anti-tobacco policy and promotion of screening for breast and cervical cancer.

Diabetes: a national programme for diabetes in line with the St Vincent Declaration has been drawn up. It focuses on early detection of non-insulin dependent diabetes in order to prevent complications.

Accidents: prevention campaigns for road traffic accidents have had no impact on young people in the age group 15–24 years hence they are to be the first target group.

Registration of communicable diseases will be revised, immunisation coverage will be determined and the official immunisation programme will be up-dated. Immunisation against haemophilus influenzae B and hepatitis B has been introduced in the meantime and a strategy for the surveillance and prevention of nosocomial infections has been designed.

A comprehensive programme for *prevention and detection of HIV infections and care of AIDS patients* is to be carried out under the supervision of the AIDS Surveillance Committee.

The HFA paper outlines the objectives of *occupational health* services and legislation was passed in 1994.

A service for *environmental medicine* was created at the Directorate of Health to introduce a medical approach to environmental problems, complementary to the technical approach of the administration of environment.

Protection against radiation has been extended to non-ionising radiation and led to a specific programme including measurement of UV-rays, control of solariums and education of personnel and a public awareness programme.

There is an urgent need to collect data and set up a *health information system* in order to monitor the outcome of the HFA strategy.

The 'Health For All' strategy requires action by other ministries. However, coordination and monitoring by the Ministry of Health is not yet operational. The budget for health promotion and preventive services is part of the budget of the Ministry of Health and is subject to the legal consultation and decision process.

The Division of Preventive and Social Medicine

The Division of Preventive and Social Medicine of the Directorate of Health is involved in planning and organising prevention programmes and health promotion campaigns. It undertakes projects on its own behalf and collaborates systematically with schools, health professionals, medico-social/social services and private associations.

Major health problems are subjects of continuing activities. They include cancer, nutrition, smoking, alcohol abuse, HIV, and accident prevention. Some new initiatives or approaches are:

Cancer prevention focusing on the hazards of sun and UV-ray exposure. This is a multi-annual programme set up by the Division of Preventive Medicine and the Division of Radioprotection. Activities include:

- technical controls on appliances and information to personnel in public swimming baths and solariums,

- seminars for professionals in beauty parlours with the collaboration of the professional federation,

- information campaigns in the media and public events, posters, leaflets and booklets for public distribution.

Smoking: Promoting non-smoking is carried out in partnership with the Luxembourg Cancer Foundation which has set up an exhibition to be shown in schools on the hazards of smoking. It also runs the Smoke Busters Club for children. Emphasis is given to World Anti-Tobacco Day with widespread publicity in the media and to specific targets chosen according to the theme for special action. Pubs, restaurants and hotels have been recent targets. A comprehensive analysis of the application of the law restricting publicity for tobacco and prohibiting smoking in different places has been carried out by the Directorate of Health and steps have been made to enforce the law.

Alcohol and traffic accidents: the Road Safety Association and the Division of Preventive Medicine joined in a media campaign for young drivers encouraging them not to drink when driving. Recent campaigns by the Ministry of Transport also focused on this area. The 'Health For All' document provides evidence, however, that mortality from traffic accidents is still increasing in young people aged under 25.

Nutrition: healthy nutrition is the main subject of an ongoing public information campaign aimed at everyone, from children to the elderly.

Great importance is given to *health education for children and adolescents.* The Division of Preventive Medicine produces health magazines several times a year on specific topics. These are distributed in primary and secondary schools.

The National Committee Against Alcohol Abuse is in charge of anti-alcohol health policy including epidemiology, treatment of abusers, counselling of their families and health education campaigns.

Maternal and child health

Medical supervision during pregnancy and early childhood. Preventive services during pregnancy and early childhood are provided by law. Antenatal and postnatal care for mothers is given by private obstetricians and by midwives. Preventive medical examinations of children are performed by (private) paediatricians in maternity hospitals/services and in independent practices or at the child health clinics of the Red Cross (free of charge). Preventive services for children between 2 and 4 years are carried out in private practice. Preventive dental examinations for children of this age group are carried out by private dentists.

Preventive services during pregnancy and early childhood are reimbursed by sickness funds or by the Ministry of Health if there is no compulsory or voluntary insurance.

Special screenings in infants: Children are screened for metabolic disorders at birth, for vision defects between 6 months and 4 years and for hearing defects at the ages of 6 months and 30 months. These screenings are performed by specialised services belonging to the Directorate of Health and are free of charge.

Immunisation is not compulsory but recommended to parents who are invited to have their children immunised. Paediatricians encourage immunisation. The vaccines of the official vaccination programme are delivered free of charge by the Ministry of Health.

There is no current registration of immunisation in children. Surveys carried out within the school health services do not give up-to-date information. In 1996, the Division of Preventive Medicine carried out, with the collaboration of a public health school of a university of a neighbour country, a survey in children aged 2 to investigate their immunisation status and the reasons for non-immunisation in order to improve information to parents and to counter opposition. Immunisation coverage is very high.[10]

The inclusion of immunisation against hepatitis B in the official immunisation programme has been adopted as a joint initiative of the Union of Sickness Funds and the Directorate of Health, the costs of vaccines being shared by both. Thus, for the first time, sickness funds participated in vaccine costs and in promoting immunisation.

Information campaigns aimed at mothers-to-be and young parents are carried out by the Division of Preventive and Social Medicine. A 'pregnancy calendar' and a comprehensive booklet on 'the health of the child' have been published recently to support information given by obstetricians, paediatricians and other health professionals.

Promoting quality of perinatal care: Following a debate on people-centred prenatal and delivery care, convened by the professional association of midwives, the Minister of Health established a mixed working group to make proposals for promoting the quality of perinatal care. A resolution to up-date the national perinatal programme was agreed in the Chamber of Deputies. The mandate for the work was given to the former working group composed of representatives of the professional associations of gynaecologists-obstetricians, paediatricians, midwives and of the Ministry and the Directorate of Health.

School health services: Preventive services for children at school (from the age of 4 onwards) is provided by law. Full-time school health services are organised by a few municipalities but most of the school health services are part of the comprehensive medico-social and social service jointly organised by the Luxembourg League of Prevention and Social Welfare and the Luxembourg Red Cross.

The school health service in secondary schools is operated by the Division of School Medicine at the Directorate of Health, which is also responsible for planning and coordinating school health services. The Healthy Schools Project comes under the responsibility of the Ministry of Education.

Preventive dental examinations in pre-school and primary education are performed by the school dental service of the Division of School Medicine at the Directorate of Health.

Occupational health services were introduced by law only in 1994. The law establishes a national occupational health service open to all employers who do not organise their own service or participate in an inter-company service. Occupational health services are organised by one or a group of industrial companies.

Supervision, coordination and control of services belong to the Division of Occupational Health at the Directorate of Health. Collaboration with the administration for safety at work is required by law. The Division of Occupational Health works closely with occupational health services of companies and assists them to find solutions to specific problems. General problems arising from the implementation of the law are discussed with trade unions and information sessions are held for workers' delegations of industrial companies. Field studies have been undertaken with other divisions/services of the Directorate of Health, particularly the Division of Health Inspection, the Service of Environmental Medicine and the relevant administration of the Ministry of Labour.

Screening programmes A specialised cervical cancer screening service at the National Laboratory of Health carries out cytological examinations free of charge. Women have the smears at their private gynaecologists' or practitioners and at family planning clinics. No formal programme has been introduced. Coverage among younger women is good because of the use of contraception, which requires medical supervision. Mortality from cervical cancer has dropped sharply. It can be assumed that the uptake in women in the age group 50–65 will increase as a preventive medical examination is part of the breast cancer screening programme. The number of smears sent to the specialised service at the National Laboratory of Health has increased.

The National Programme for *Breast Cancer Screening* in women in the age group 50–65 is a joint programme of the Directorate of Health, the Union of Sickness Funds and the Luxembourg Cancer Foundation. The programme is carried out in private medical practice and the radiological services of hospitals. The coordination centre is located at the Division of Preventive Medicine of the Directorate of Health. Emphasis is given to continuing quality control, evaluation of the programme and continuous education of professionals cooperating in the programme. Supervision is carried out by a steering committee with representatives of the three organisers, the various professionals participating in the programme and the federation of hospitals. Representatives of the medical profession have called for closer collaboration with the coordination centre and are included in a management group.

A survey carried out at the end of 1995 of women belonging to the target group shows that a more active role for general practitioners is likely to increase acceptance of the programme. A project for continuous education of general practitioners has been developed with their professional association. Information in the media and sessions with women's associations are carried out.

Following the St Vincent Declaration, a programme for *early detection of diabetes* and prevention of complications was developed at the Directorate of Health by a working group composed of the Director General of Health, delegates of the Division of Preventive Medicine, and specialists working in diabetes care and with the diabetes patient association. No agreement could be reached with the Union of Sickness Funds for a joint programme.

AIDS prevention The AIDS surveillance committee set up by the Minister of Health coordinates all activities in prevention and care and collaborates closely with international organisations such as WHO, the Council of Europe and the European Union. Activities in prevention and care are carried out by the Division of Preventive Medicine and private non-profit associations which are represented at the committee.

Prevention measures include:

*   Information campaigns aimed at the general public and more specifically at young people in public locations, by radio and TV commercials, posters, street stalls, information files for secondary schools, information for health professionals etc. Information is provided with the distribution of condoms whenever possible.

*   Specific action for risk groups: *Prostitutes* – promoting use of condoms, HIV detection and immunisation against hepatitis B on a voluntary basis. *Detainees* – individual information is provided by members of a self-help organisation, and HIV tests are offered on a voluntary basis by the medical service in prison. *Drug addicts* – a private non-profit association working with drug addicts contributes to AIDS prevention by working on the exchange and disposal of syringes (issued with information on AIDS prevention) and by participating in the methadone substitution programme. The number of drug addicts admitted to the programme has doubled and it is planned to extend the programme. Moreover, the methadone substitution programme has been regionalised: an increasing number of private general practitioners and psychiatrists are participating in the programme and methadone is distributed by an increasing number of pharmacies, hospitals and psycho-social services.

HIV tests associated with counselling are offered free of charge on a voluntary basis. They are performed anonymously on request.

Clinical services

The independent practice of the medical profession has been an obstacle to establishing clinical services. This sector is limited to: clinics for respiratory diseases (former tuberculosis clinics) and child health clinics – both have a long tradition and are part of the preventive services of the comprehensive medico-social service organised by the League for Prevention and Medico-social Welfare and the Luxembourg Red Cross. In addition there are mental health clinics and family planning clinics. These are managed by private not-for-profit associations and funded by the State. Mental health clinics have formal contracts with the Ministry of Health and family planning clinics have contracts with the Ministry of Family Welfare.

Mental health. A report on psychiatry in Luxembourg, funded by the Minister of Health was produced by foreign consultants. The report was submitted to a working group of representatives of all services and associations working in mental health to make proposals for a programme on reform of psychiatry. The report was widely debated and special attention was given to the issue by the standing committee on health in the Chamber of Deputies.

Family planning. Contraception is mainly dealt with in private medical practice as all contraceptives (except condoms) are delivered on medical prescription only. Contraceptives are not reimbursed by sickness insurance. Publicity follow the same rules as that for medicines. Contraceptives are delivered free of charge in the family planning centres to young people and to people who cannot afford them.

The family planning centres offer sex education sessions for secondary schools on a voluntary basis with teachers and the psycho-social services of the schools. They also offer marital and psychological counselling to individuals and couples, abortion counselling and help for rape victims and sexually abused children. This issue has been adopted as a priority by the Ministry of Family Welfare.

Equity in health is an implicit concern of health and social policies. Thus preventive services are either free of charge or covered by the State if a person is not insured (e.g. medical services during pregnancy). The minimum income guaranteed by the State to people with very low or no income provides for sickness insurance in the workers' scheme. Conditions for voluntary insurance have been extended and contributions can be paid by the welfare system. The coverage of the population is about 99 per cent. A national service for immigrants at the Ministry of Family Welfare is responsible for coordinating and providing help for immigrants and refugees.

Health policy decisions and priority setting

Public health policy decisions and priority setting are left to the health authorities at the central level. Municipalities cope with environmental and social problems rather than with issues related to prevention and health promotion. Priority setting includes the political options of the Minister of Health or the Council of Ministers and proposals of the various departments of the Ministry of Health taking into account:

(1) Major health problems.

(2) WHO and EU programmes: these programmes provide an impetus for action at the

national level.

(3) Proposals of private health services and health professionals. The mixed advisory committees with representatives of the state (several ministries) and from private, non-profit associations which run services are effective mechanisms for concerted proposals and action.

The Council of Hygiene, which is an advisory body to the Minister of Health, has the main influence in its specific field.

Legislative and consultative process

The process of decision-making in health is illustrated in Figure 2 overleaf. Before being submitted to a vote at the Chamber of Deputies, which has a standing committee for health and social affairs, draft laws undergo a mandatory consulting process through the Council of State (members are appointed by the Grand-Duke to advise on proposed legislation and amendments and give their opinion on every question referred to them by the Government or by law) and the professional chambers (elected by the working population according to professional status, employers and self-employed). If health services and health professions are concerned, the mandatory consulting process is extended to the Medical Board (with representatives of doctors, dentists and pharmacists), the Council of other Health Professions (which brings together all health professions not represented at the Medical Board) and, if relevant, the Permanent Committee for Hospitals.

The comments and proposals of these advisory bodies come before the Chamber of Deputies and the Council of State.

Trade unions, the various associations of health professionals, the Union of Hospitals, and other private associations contribute to the legislative procedure through the advisory bodies where they are represented or, in some cases, directly to the Minister of Health and to the Members of the Chamber of Deputies.

The Economic and Social Council, composed of representatives of industries, trade unions, government departments and public institutions is an advisory body to the Government. Every year, the Council issues a position on economic, financial and social matters relevant for the country. In recent years, special attention has been given to the financing of sickness insurance, selective investments in the hospital sector and adequate planning at national level. Occupational health, safety at the workplace, protection of the environment and nursing insurance have been specific topics of discussion [11] A position paper on public health was issued in 1973.[12] However, a background paper on health has not been finalised because a consensus between delegates of trade unions and employers could not be reached.

The various advisory bodies mainly act at the request of the Government despite a right to take the initiative which has turned out to be rather inefficient.

Figure 2 Luxembourg: decision-making in health

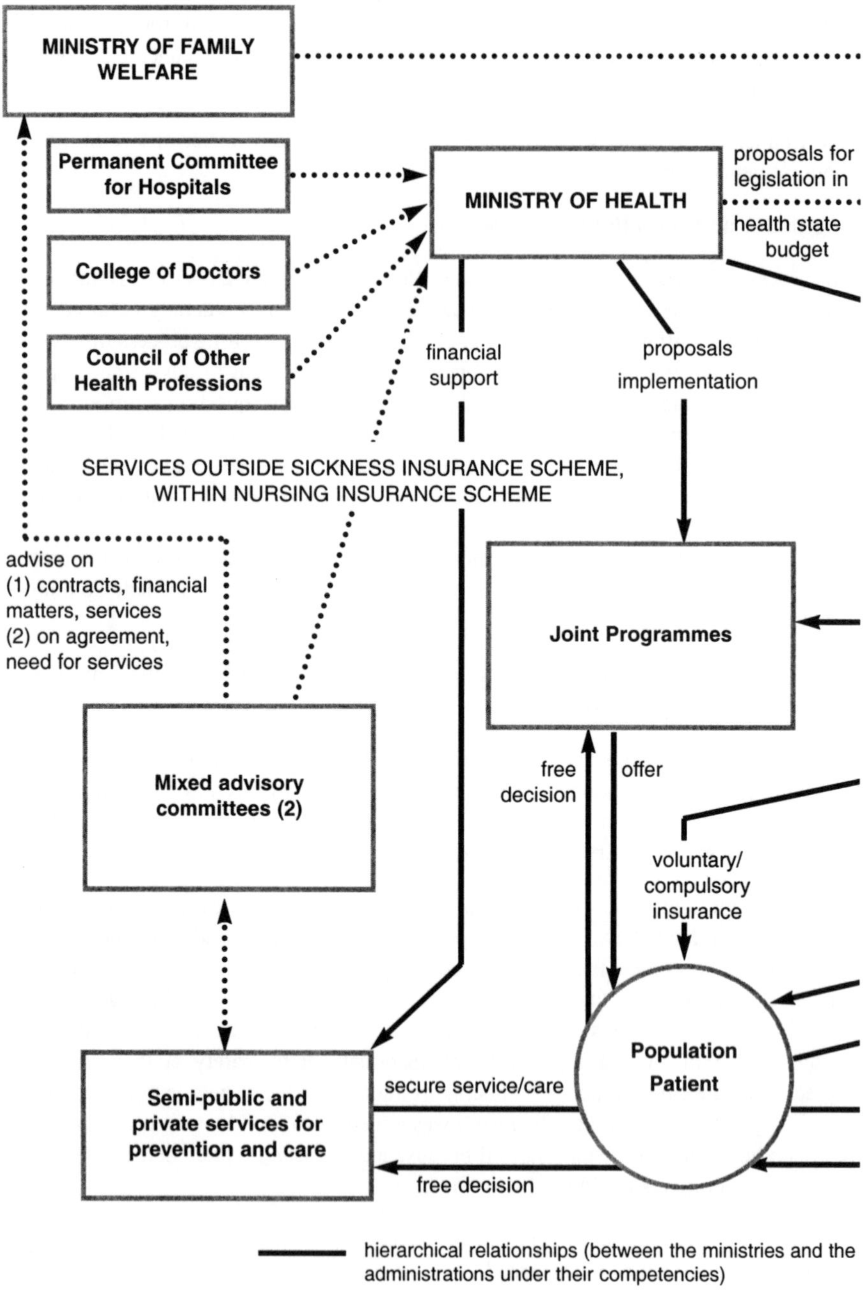

MINISTRY OF FAMILY WELFARE

Permanent Committee for Hospitals

College of Doctors

Council of Other Health Professions

MINISTRY OF HEALTH

proposals for legislation in

health state budget

financial support

proposals implementation

SERVICES OUTSIDE SICKNESS INSURANCE SCHEME, WITHIN NURSING INSURANCE SCHEME

advise on
(1) contracts, financial matters, services
(2) on agreement, need for services

Joint Programmes

Mixed advisory committees (2)

free decision   offer

voluntary/ compulsory insurance

Population Patient

secure service/care

Semi-public and private services for prevention and care

free decision

—— hierarchical relationships (between the ministries and the administrations under their competencies)

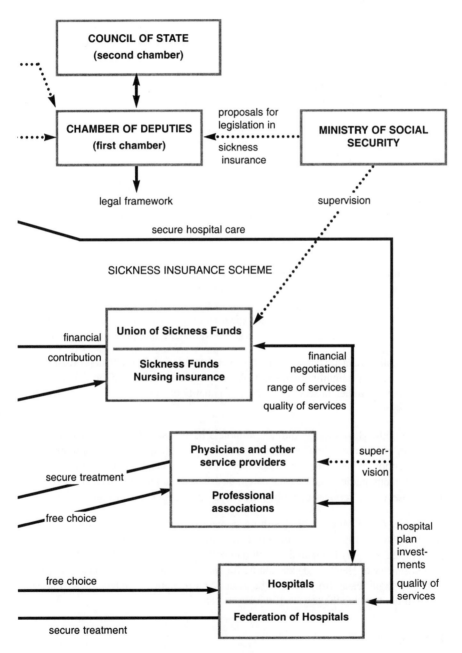

COUNCIL OF STATE
(second chamber)

CHAMBER OF DEPUTIES
(first chamber)

proposals for
legislation in
sickness
insurance

MINISTRY OF SOCIAL
SECURITY

legal framework

supervision

secure hospital care

SICKNESS INSURANCE SCHEME

financial
contribution

Union of Sickness Funds

Sickness Funds
Nursing insurance

financial
negotiations
range of services
quality of services

secure treatment

free choice

Physicians and other
service providers

Professional
associations

super-
vision

free choice

secure treatment

Hospitals

Federation of Hospitals

hospital
plan
invest-
ments

quality of
services

••••••• non-hierarchical relationships which differ according to responsibilities
(supervisory, partnership, negotiation, financing)

Information available

Traditionally, mortality statistics, statistics on transmittable diseases, occupational diseases, occupational accidents and road traffic accidents have been the only available data.

Currently, a small amount of data is recorded for the environment on concentration levels of some air pollutants, ozone and radiation levels.

Having previously used foreign consultants for reports on specific problems (e.g. perinatal mortality, hospitals, mental health) or relied on foreign data, efforts are now being made towards creating a more systematic national approach.

Surveys have been or are presently being carried out on drug addiction, smoking habits, nutrition, immunisation coverage, needs and demands of women during pregnancy and delivery and attitudes towards screening for breast cancer. Until now, the National Screening Programme for breast cancer has been unique in integrating formal quality control into a prevention programme.

In 1987, a public research centre in health was created by law. It is financed by the Ministry of Education (responsible for research) and the Ministry of Health. The new service plan provides for more involvement of the research centre in public health by creating resource centres for epidemiological studies, biostatistics and quality of care assessment. A cancer registry was set up at the National Laboratory of Health in 1987.

Efforts to collect data are hampered by the liberal practice of the medical profession and, more generally, by a highly privatised health sector. Developments in the sickness insurance system and in health services focusing on quality of care are likely to improve data on morbidity.

Introducing the HFA strategy did not promote a basic discussion on prevention versus treatment, even though the Government committed itself explicitly to health promotion and prevention by adopting the strategy. However, in general, public and professional debate is about medical and hospital care rather than about prevention and only specific, limited preventive services could be introduced into the sickness insurance scheme.

The budget of the Ministry of Health for preventive services increased by 30 per cent between 1989 to 1992, but the ratio of expenditure for prevention and care remains at 1:15 (1992). Roughly compared, the ratio of expenditure for prevention in the accounts of the Ministry of Health and expenditure for care of the sickness insurance was 1:65 in 1992.[13,14] Significant efforts have to be made to reorientate the budget towards prevention in order to reach the targets of the HFA strategy.

References

1.   Ministère de la Santé. *Santé pour tous.* Luxembourg, 1994.

2. STATEC-CEPS/INSTEAD-IGSS. *Bulletin d'informations démographiques et sociales.* Luxembourg, 1996;2.

3. Ministère de la Santé. *Rapports d'activité 1996.* Luxembourg, 1990 and 1996.

4. Direction de la Santé. Service des statistiques sanitaires. *Statistiques des causes de décès.* Luxembourg, 1986 and 1995.

5. Fondation Luxembourgeoise Contre le Cancer. ILReS. *Enquete sur le Tabagisme dans la Vie des Jeunes.* 1998.

6. Ministère des Transports. *Bilan des accidents de la route.* Luxembourg, 1996.

7. Comité de surveilance du SIDA. *Rapport d'activité.* Luxembourg, 1997.

8. Service Central de Législation. *Annuaire officiel d'administration et de législation.* Luxembourg, 1995.

9. Ministère de la Sécurité Sociale. Inspection générale de la sécurité sociale. *Aperçu sur la législation de la sécurité sociale.* Luxembourg, 1995.

10. Direction de la Santé – Division de la Medecine Preventive et Sociale. Ligue Luxembourgeoise de Prevention et d'Action Medicosociales. Croix Rouge Luxembourgeoise. Ecole de Santé Publique de l'Universite Libre de Bruxelles. *Enquete de Couverture Vaccinale au Grande-Duché Luxembourg.* Internal government document, 1996.

11. Conseil Economique et Social. *Avis sur la situation économique, financière et sociale du pays. Période 1991-1995.* Luxembourg.

12. Conseil Economique et Social. *La santé publique. Avis.* Luxembourg, 1973.

13. Ministère de la Sécurité Sociale. Inspection générale de la sécurité sociale. *Rapport général sur la sécurité sociale au Grand-Duché de Luxembourg 1993.* Les différents types de soins de santé, 1994:102. Luxembourg, 1994.

14. Service Central de la Statistique et des Etudes Economiques (STATEC). *Annuaire statistique du Luxembourg 1995. Crédits budgétaires du pouvoir central dans l'intérêt de la santé publique par sous-fonction. 1996.* Luxembourg, 1996.

12

Public Health and Health Policy in the Netherlands

Louise J Gunning-Schepers

Introduction

The Netherlands is a relatively small, but densely populated country with 15 million inhabitants. It has an average life expectancy of 74 years for men and 80 years for women.[1] Other indicators of health all point in the direction of good overall health status even if compared with other northern or western European countries. Contrary to other European countries, however, the post-war baby boom lasted for 30 years but with a very abrupt reduction in the number of births between 1969 and 1975. The resulting instability in the age structure of the population means that the Netherlands still has one of the lowest percentages of over 65's in the population but will move by 2030 to a position of having the oldest population. This very rapid ageing will have a major impact on health and health care needs in the future and its financial consequences are already an important issue in health policy.

In this chapter we will describe the current public health structures but we shall also address some of the policy issues generated by this demographic shift in health needs. We shall use the common definition of public health as: 'the science and art of preventing disease, prolonging life and promoting health through organised efforts of society'. In the Dutch medical specialty of public health medicine (still under the old name of social medicine) prevention, policy and management are included. That is why we shall not only address the organisation of preventive services (public health per se) but also pay attention to some of the policy issues concerning health care provision and, perhaps more importantly, health care reforms. But we will do so only in as far as it illustrates the specific efforts of society to improve the health of the population.

Responsibility for Dutch public health policy

Article 22.1 of the Dutch constitution states that the Government is responsible for measures to safeguard the health of the population. To implement this, the Government has a Minister of Health who proposes policies to Parliament that will either directly affect the determinants of health or will enable the population to have access to effective health services.

The Ministry of Health is not itself in charge of the provision, organisation or financing of health services as there is no national health service funded by taxation. A mixed social and private insurance system finances a mostly private, non-profit, system of health services. Government is, however, closely involved both in decisions concerning the total budget and the services to be provided. The reason for this is that the insurance premiums are, for a large part, income-dependent and paid for by employers and employees and, as such, are important elements in social and economic policy-making. An exception is the public health services, which fall under the direct responsibility of local government.

The ministry itself is directly responsible for the allocation of funds through which the municipalities organise preventive services, setting guidelines for the distribution of financial resources over the different institutions of health care, monitoring the health status of the population and proposing policies to improve it, even if that involves measures to be taken by other ministries. It does so by publishing policy documents[2] to Parliament in the course of one cabinet period (four years) and, to accompany the yearly budget, a policy document in which the distribution of resources is described and documented. This last document, the *Financieel Overzicht Zorg* (FOZ – Financial Overview of Care[3]) has over the years become more and more of a directive in a policy arena where the most important decision-makers are the purchasers (sickness funds or private insurance companies) and the providers (representatives of doctors, hospitals and other institutions).

In recent years, the ministry has actively encouraged patient or consumer organisations to participate as a third party in the negotiations. Patient representatives are included in many of the decision-making bodies, and consumer organisations are funded to investigate and compare different packages offered by insurers, the information given to consumers concerning drugs, and other aspects of health care where individuals can make a choice. For the services covered by social insurance (about 70 per cent of the total budget) national councils, on which all of the above parties are represented, are entitled to negotiate binding agreements concerning, for example, services covered (*Ziekenfondsraad*, which determines in great detail both the services covered and the criteria for eligibility), tariffs for remuneration of services (*Centraal Overlegorgaan Tarieven Gezondheidszorg*) and the procedure for the allocation of services, such as that for admission to a nursing home (*Commissie Indicatie Stelling*).

In these negotiations the partners have to stay within the legal and financial boundaries set by Government. Although the minister is not able to control directly either the services provided or the budget allocated, he or she sets the rules and through a complex web of advisory and representative bodies the different partners negotiate within the margins set by national government. It means, however, that these same partners have to cooperate if any type of health reform is proposed by the Government and approved by Parliament. Some of the partners have the power to veto reform, but none has the power by itself to effect change. It is this complex interdependency that makes it so difficult for outsiders to understand why perfectly reasonable and apparently rational policy initiatives of successive ministers have not been implemented. The network of partners involved in public health policy is illustrated diagrammatically in Figure 1.

Figure 1
Network of partners involved in public health policy

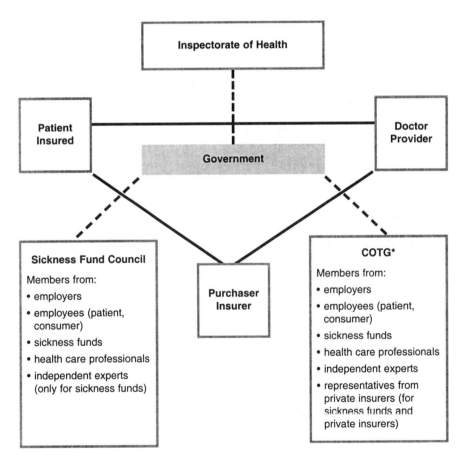

* *Central Overlegorgaan Tarieven Gezondneidszorg*
  (determines tariff for renumeration of services)

In the current structure, most of the health care policy decisions are made at a national level. However, some specific elements of health policy have been devolved to a local level. These include all preventive or public health services (including some environmental tasks) and many of the special services for the elderly and the handicapped. Budgets for these services are distributed to the municipal budget on a per capita basis, but not always earmarked for specific services. Occupational health services are completely privatised and some operate at a national level while others are active regionally.

The National Institute for Public Health and Environmental Issues (RIVM) has an important role in some areas of research such as vaccination, and in monitoring health indicators (prevalence of cardiovascular risk factors etc.) and environmental indicators (air quality, water pollution etc.). It also provides regular overviews of the nation's health and environmental status as basic information for policy purposes. In these documents, data collected by the Central Bureau of Statistics (population, mortality and health interview data) and by the Centre for Health Care Information (registration of health care utilisation data) are presented as well as an overview of related research done in research institutes in the Netherlands.[1]

At the beginning of this century the Government had already set up an independent Inspectorate of Public Health in order to report on the population's health and the quality of the health care system. This Inspectorate contains regional departments. It has always had important powers to protect the health of citizens and can investigate individual practitioners and health care institutions. As such, it serves as an independent quality assurance system.

The Dutch health care system

The current Dutch health care system has evolved over time mostly through private initiatives but almost always non-profit-making and without any clear structure or plan. It was organised along the lines of the church denominations, as were so many of the social institutions in the Netherlands. This element has become less important over time, enabling many relatively small institutions to merge. In the period 1980–1992 the number of hospitals decreased from 231 to 157, but the number of beds per 1,000 inhabitants decreased only from 5.2 to 4.2, illustrating both a trend to larger hospitals and shorter hospital stays. Similarly, the number of sickness funds decreased from 53 in 1985 to 26 in 1993.[4]

In those years, attempts were made by Government to achieve a more balanced geographic distribution of physicians and services. Since the Netherlands is such a small and densely populated country, distances to most services are very short. However, some regional distribution has been achieved for very highly specialised services. This is possible because for these so called *artikel 18* technologies, (named after the article giving the minister far-reaching powers over the dissemination of new technologies) the ministry has the right to decide on the volume and the location of services offered. It usually involves procedures that necessitate large investments in infrastructure or training or are only required by limited numbers of patients. Examples are transplants, open heart surgery and certain procedures in neurosurgery, radiotherapy and neo-natal intensive care. Centralising these services increases effectiveness by concentrating knowledge and experience, and increases efficiency by limiting the number of institutions making the necessary investments. Occasionally it involves services that are still considered experimental and can be offered only in a strictly controlled scientific setting.

The health care system can be described in different levels:

The public health system: targeting the total population in a certain geographical area and primarily responsible for preventive services such as infectious disease control, health education, vaccinations, screening, environmental services, etc.

The primary care system: those general health services that are directly accessible to individuals. The most important being the general practitioner with whom individual patients are registered and who is the gate keeper to more specialised services.

The secondary care system: comprising all specialised services such as specialist physicians, hospitals and nursing homes.

There are approximately 37,500 physicians in the Netherlands, half of whom are clinical specialists; 7,900 are general practitioners; and between 5,000 and 6,000 work in the field of public health. The number of medical students admitted each year is limited by the Government.

Health care financing

Total health care costs in the Netherlands are close to 60 billion Guilders, which is around 9 per cent of GDP.[2] This percentage stabilised in the early 1980s. Of this budget, 33 per cent is spent on hospital care, 18 per cent on primary care, 9 per cent on nursing homes and 9 per cent on homes for the elderly, 7 per cent on mental health care, 9 per cent on care for the handicapped, 10.4 per cent on medication and medical devices, 1.4 per cent on preventive services and slightly more than 5 per cent on administrative costs.

These costs are paid for by social insurance (69 per cent), private insurance (14 per cent), Government subsidies (10 per cent) and other sources, mostly direct payments by individual users (8 per cent).

The Netherlands does not have a national tax funded health service. It has a mixed public and private system of health insurance in which an individual's income level determines whether he/she is compulsorily insured with a sickness fund, for which income-related premiums are collected through employers and employees, or whether one can choose freely with which private company one is insured. In this case the premium is not income-related but, increasingly, risk-adjusted. Although insurance is not compulsory over the sickness fund income level, very few individuals are not insured. For long-term care and other crises everybody is insured through a social insurance (AWBZ) for which an income-related premium is collected.

Most treatment services are paid for either by the sickness fund (social insurance) or the private insurance system. These two systems not only differ in the way they raise funds but also in the ways money is allocated, services are reimbursed and in the influence of Government in deciding the package of benefits covered and delivery allowed. For all services (including physicians' fees) tariffs are determined at a national level which are binding for all partners. For sickness fund patients no payments are required at the time of service delivery; institutions or doctors are reimbursed directly according to pre-agreed mechanisms (for instance, capitation fee for GPs, fee for service for hospital specialists, and fee for service within a pre-set budget for hospitals). For the privately insured, there is wider differentiation in terms of co-payments and services covered (for instance, including homeopathic medicine or excluding certain elements, such as drug costs, from the insurance coverage).

Obviously, the different choices have consequences for the premium paid, as increasingly do age and other factors differentiating risks. The conditions can be negotiated at the time of entry into the insurance system. Sometimes options are no longer open to individuals when they reach a certain age. Most private insurance coverage requires the patient first to pay the doctor or hospital and then ask for reimbursement from the insurance company.

The choice of coverage by sickness fund or private insurance is determined each year by the Government and is dependent on level of income. This can have great consequences for income since the sickness fund premium is not only income-related, but covers all family members, while private insurance requires separate premium payments for each individual. It depends on individual circumstances whether sickness fund or private insurance coverage is preferred. Virtually nobody covered by the sickness fund also takes on private insurance except to cover additional services such as dental care which was recently excluded from the sickness fund for adults.

In recent years there has been much discussion about the position of the over 65s. They have been transferred to the private insurance schemes but the Government has reached agreement with private insurers to offer them a standard package of services with a fixed premium which does not differ too much from the contribution they made to the sickness fund coverage before they drew their pension. The loss made on this category of insured is redistributed among all insurers. However, their position remains an issue for health policy.

In 1987, an expert committee chaired by a former Philips executive, Mr Dekker, proposed a fundamental reform of the Dutch health care system. The most important aims of the reform were to make a basic (but limited) insurance package for every citizen with a partly income-related premium and the introduction of competitive elements into the field of insurers and providers of health care. The reforms that were proposed by the Dekker committee,[5] and later adapted by the State Secretary Simons, have not been fully implemented partly because they failed to gain the full support of all the parties involved both in Parliament and in the health care field. In the retrospective analysis as to why different parties could not agree on certain elements of the reform while at the same time voicing great support, much was made of the fact that most parties involved, as well as the general public, failed to see what the problems were with the existing system that warranted such a fundamental reform. However, despite the failure to implement the proposal fully, some steps were taken, such as abolishing the requirement that sickness funds must offer a contract to all practising physicians. In addition, much has changed recently in anticipation of the reforms, such as in the insurance world where the distinction between sickness funds and private insurance companies seems to be becoming blurred.

In the recent past, although there was a difference at the level of the individual insured and the related rules and regulations, the organisation of services was never dependent on the type of insurance. There were no sickness fund hospitals or physicians who would treat only privately insured patients. All services are basically accessible to everybody, priorities are strictly determined by need. This also applies to institutionalised care for the elderly, handicapped and to home care. In some areas where there are many immigrant groups, services will often have access to interpreters to help identify needs and many of the institutions try to employ representatives of the minority groups living in the area they serve.

Contribution of health services to public health

Although the health care system is mostly devoted to diagnosis and treatment of individual patients, some of the services have a direct responsibility for prevention. Many of them are confronted increasingly with financial constraints and thus have to make policy decisions about the allocation of funds to different types of services or to the selection of patients from waiting lists. For each level of care we will briefly outline current practice and then discuss the policy issues or current concerns in public health policy.

Public health services

Facts: In 1990, the '*Wet Collectieve Preventie Volksgezondheid*' (Collective Prevention Act[6]) was passed in Parliament and implemented. It stipulates that all local municipalities must have access to a '*Gemeentelijke Gezondheidsdienst, GGD*' (Municipal Health Department). Most larger cities already had such a department, but many of the smaller local authorities joined forces and created a GGD which had a more regional character. It may thus serve more than one municipality, but its geographical area is not one of fixed regional borders. Increasingly smaller GGDs are merging. In 1998 there were 54 GGDs.

By law, they must provide the following services: infectious disease control, school health services, advice to local government on health matters and assistance and medical care in case of disaster. They must have access to expertise in the following fields: epidemiology, health education, public mental health, and provide assistance to the national screening programmes. Additional services can include ambulance services, selection of patients for nursing home admission, services for the homeless, methadone and other drug-related services, and selection of patients who are entitled to services for the handicapped. These additional services are not necessary in all communities and therefore are not mandatory. Infant clinics for the under fives (including vaccinations) are traditionally not organised by the GGD, with the exception of Amsterdam, but by a non-profit organisation, the *Kruisorganisatie* (Cross organisation) which is also the organisation responsible for home nursing.

Preventive programmes offered to the general public include:

Infectious disease services including, for example, clinics for sexually transmitted diseases and tuberculosis control.

Vaccination services including childhood vaccinations against diphtheria, tetanus, polio, pertussis, rubella, measles, mumps and, since 1993, Haemophilus Influenzae B. Special additional vaccinations are offered for high risk groups, such as hepatitis, BCG, influenza, etc.

Screening: Phenylketonuria and Congenital Hip Dislocation screening of all newborn, cervical screening (all women aged 30–60 years are screened every five years), breast cancer screening (all women aged 50–69 years are invited every two years), and a series of screening tests are done for all children at the regular (between 10 to 14) visits to the infant clinics and later at school.

Health education: Many programmes are specifically developed for local populations, but there are programmes everywhere offered through primary and secondary schools as one of the elements of the basic curriculum, and disseminated through mass media such as television and radio and in specific campaigns. These address smoking, AIDS and other sexually transmitted disease prevention, information about drugs and alcohol, traffic accident prevention and, more recently for example, folic acid intake to prevent neural tube defects.

All of these services are provided for all citizens. Doctors working in these organisations are registered public health physicians (either in maternal and child health or community medicine), who have completed their public health training of two and a half years after becoming physicians. In future years their training will become a four-year programme in community medicine.[7]

The other specialisation in public health medicine is that of occupational medicine. These physicians work in the occupational health departments. By law[8] almost every company must have access to an occupational health physician (on average 1 per 2,000-2,500 employees) who is responsible for the preventive policy of the company, does regular check ups and is responsible for policies concerning work absenteeism and disability claims. These occupational health departments are commercial for-profit organisations, which have to compete. As a result, currently, a lot of pressure is put on occupational health physicians to keep companies satisfied. This does not always make their task in the field of preventive interventions easier.

Policy issues: Public health services (collective preventive services) are responsible for a geographical area, defined by municipalities which at the local level have the power to set policies and determine the budget of these services. This means yearly negotiations about the budget level and the services to be offered. In cases where a GGD serves more than one municipality, it also means more than one partner is involved in these negotiations.

The money allocated to prevention at a national level is transferred for that purpose to the local budget, but not earmarked, and as local budgets have been under heavy pressure lately, the money spent on prevention is less than was originally intended. Policy-making was also decentralised to the local level, originally with the intent of stimulating intersectoral action and allowing a more active input of the population in the priority setting process. A recent evaluation of the WCPV[9] assessed the extent to which the objectives of a decentralised public health network were being achieved and had rather negative findings. Municipalities do not seem to take the opportunities afforded by the law to achieve an integrated health policy. Health is not very high on the political agenda of local government, especially at a time when budgets are overstretched. In the large cities there has been an unprecedented dismantling of the traditional municipal health departments, as local governments try to achieve greater efficiency of services by privatising some parts of the service and cutting some services not legally required. There is currently great concern as to what these cuts will mean for the ability of the municipal health departments to maintain coverage of some hard to reach sub-populations. Traditionally these preventive services have always been used by the whole population, and they have been able to achieve a reasonably equitable distribution of their services, even if that meant more input of resources and energy in targeting deprived populations.

However, there are also more positive developments such as the integrated public policy efforts in some municipalities involved in the Healthy Cities movement and the attention given to deprived neighbourhoods with the renewed policy interest in social inequalities in health. In these intersectoral programmes social services, housing departments, employment and educational services as well as the municipal health department and often general practitioners (GPs) work together to improve the living conditions in certain areas of the city or in certain sub-populations, such as recent immigrants or ethnic minorities.

Primary care

In 1990, there were approximately 7,900 GPs working in the Netherlands with an average patient population of 2,500. Half of these work in some form of group practice. They are paid through a capitation fee for the sickness fund patients and through a fee for service for the privately insured patients, but with nationally negotiated fees. GPs traditionally have a responsibility for some preventive programmes, which include contact with individual patients. They carry out the smear tests for the cervical screening programme, are encouraged to register the most important risk factors for cardiovascular disease among their adult patients, and are actively involved in the influenza vaccination of elderly and high risk patients. Obviously, they can make an important contribution to health education if questions concerning contraception, smoking, alcohol, physical activity and diet are asked. In recent years there have been several experimental programmes to see what conditions in GP practice (such as availability of computers or additional training for the doctors' assistant) encourage the active participation of GPs in health promotion programmes. A prevention guide was published that looked specifically at the scientific evidence base for the preventive services to be provided by GPs, midwives and school doctors.[10] For their contributions in specific collective prevention programmes such as cervical screening, they have negotiated additional remuneration. Important other care providers (with a preventive aspect) in primary care are:

The midwife: who in the Netherlands provides prenatal and obstetric care to most normal deliveries (30 per cent of which are still done at home). She is often very successful in helping women adopt a healthier lifestyle during pregnancy.

The pharmacist: who in the Netherlands is responsible for the delivery of all prescription drugs. With their completely computerised system they are able to monitor prescriptions at an individual level and play an important role in preventing adverse combinations of drugs.

The dentist: until very recently dental care was partly covered by the sickness fund provided that the individuals went for a dental check-up every six months (about 5 per cent of total health care costs were spent on dental care). A deliberate effort has been made in the last 25 years to provide regular check-ups and dental health information to all school children either through the school health service or through special dental hygiene programmes. Since 1995, most dental care is no longer covered by the sickness fund for all adults (over 18 years of age). Unless individuals want to pay the costs of dental care directly (which some do) it has to be privately insured. Every year approximately 75 per cent of the population visit a dentist, both sickness fund and privately insured patients.[2]

The home nursing service: as explained above, in many communities this service still provides the under-five clinics, but it also provides health education in a large number of other fields such as the prevention of sleeping problems, weight reduction classes, accident prevention programmes etc.

Policy issues: The most difficult issues here concern the role of the GP versus the public health departments in their responsibility for specific preventive programmes. When the cervical screening programme was transferred to the GPs it was thought that the closer contact between patient and GP would increase the attendance of women in the screening programme and would also prevent a large number of additional smears being requested by GPs who are unaware of the programme. Similarly, there has been a tendency to include GPs in many other prevention programmes, again assuming that their contact with individual patients might improve the effectiveness of some health education messages and improve the uptake of specific programmes such as influenza vaccination for the elderly. In general, a large number of additional tasks concerning either prevention or allocation decisions have been suggested for GPs because of their unique position as gate keepers. Increasingly, however, GPs have indicated that these additional tasks need to be remunerated at a certain level and municipal health departments have claimed that by giving extra attention to the individual, the population-wide perspective necessary for effective programmes is reduced.

Secondary care

Most specialised care is organised in institutions. Specialist doctors work in hospitals even for their out-patient care. Hospitals are allocated a fixed budget and reimbursed for the patient care provided according to nationally negotiated tariffs, up to the limit of that budget. For certain highly specialised forms of treatment (*artikel 18*), the total number of patients to be treated is fixed at a national level by the central government, a number which can not be exceeded in any given year. Increasingly, there are waiting lists that develop as the budgetary constraints become more severe. Specialists, however, are not yet officially part of the hospital budget. In most cases they are still paid through a fee for service system for both their outpatient services and for the services given to patients admitted to hospital. Access to specialist care and hospital services (including emergency services) is only through referral, primarily from the GP. Increasingly, hospitals provide day admissions for minor surgery, etc. These experiments are encouraged by providing special subsidies.

An important element in specialised care is the nursing homes. There were 53,000 nursing home beds in 1993 of which approximately half were for psycho-geriatric care. Nursing home physicians have evolved into a separate medical specialty with their own training and medical register. To be admitted to a nursing home an 'indication' must be given by an independent committee. However, everybody is covered for nursing home care through the social insurance. There are waiting lists for admission, which differ by region. Sometimes, delays in admission to nursing homes can keep hospital beds occupied longer than strictly necessary. This happens mostly for stroke patients. There are often very intensive forms of cooperation between hospitals, nursing homes and home care departments in a specific region to facilitate the transfer of patients. Many of these innovative projects were financed with special funding provided to improve the continuity of care for chronic patients.

Policy issues: Most of the policy issues here concern the high burden of costs created by institutionalised care, both in hospitals and other institutions. A percentage which will undoubtedly increase as the ageing of the population increases demand. The hospital budget has done much to increase efficiency. However, the traditional separation of hospital budgets and the specialists fees in the financing of in-patient care especially, has long been a major hurdle in rational cost containment policies in the secondary care sector. After all, it is often a doctor's decision to admit and treat a specific patient thereby generating costs to be paid from the hospital budget. As long as the doctor is not employed by the hospital, it is difficult for a hospital manager to set priorities.

Following a report by the Biesheuvel committee[11] experiments were started to include specialists fees in the hospital budget. These will provide further tools for prioritising resource allocation. However, as the length of waiting times start to increase, waiting lists are being used as pressure instruments to claim additional resources for certain specialties or institutions. There is an inherent problem in a system whereby an insurance policy (even if it is a social insurance) gives individuals the right to certain services and the financial constraints limit the availability of such services. Occasionally, individuals have been given the opportunity to obtain services abroad (open heart surgery) or families have battled in court to have patients admitted to institutions for the mentally handicapped.

The most recent policy issue concerns the request for priority treatment for employees. This is the result of the recent privatisation of sickness benefits. This law requires employers to pay the salaries of their employees for the duration of their sickness leave for up to one year. Previously this was collectively insured, now many companies have taken out private insurance to cover sickness benefits. However, the insurance companies offer risk differentiated premiums based on the number of days of work missed in the past. So suddenly employers have an incentive to get their employees back to work as soon as possible and are trying to negotiate deals with providers or institutions to bypass existing allocation mechanisms and waiting lists for earlier treatment. Since selection from waiting lists is traditionally based on the health needs of the patient or on the eligibility of the patient (for instance in the case of a tissue match in organ transplants) this claim for priority treatment has created a lot of discussion. The Government has reached an agreement with employers and unions to avoid such priority treatment.

Policy-making in the Netherlands

For the first 25 years after the second world war, health policy-making focused on increasing the supply of health services to meet the rapidly expanding demand for services generated by the universal financial access through the social insurance system (the sickness funds) and the increasing effectiveness of medicine. Only in the mid-1970s was there time to reconsider both the organisation of the health care system and the increasing percentage of GDP spent on health. In that period there were a number of policy documents[12,13] trying to rationalise the very fragmented system of these basically private institutions into some coherent system, including a distinction between primary care and secondary care, restating the importance of the GP as the gate keeper to the more specialised services in hospitals and elsewhere, and reintroducing a public health service at a regional level, later to be driven and financed by municipalities. As costs continued to rise and the oil crisis of 1973 put the Dutch economy under severe strain, cost containment became an important policy issue. The most important determinants in health were reviewed to see whether the population's health could be better served. At the same time a series of policy documents looked at health care reforms in order to increase the efficiency of the health care system.

This reorientation back to the population's health as the goal of health policy and its broader determinants, coincided with the World Health Organization's 'Health for All' campaign[14] and the *Targets* document of the WHO European office[15] in 1985. This provided the basis for an important policy paper in 1986, the *Nota 2000* ,[16] in which for the first time in many years Government policy was set out again in relation to the health status of the population with priorities set in terms of health goals. This policy document provided an epidemiological overview of the health status of the population, its determinants and possible interventions for primary prevention. These were later made explicit in quantified health goals and targets, widely discussed at a number of meetings with all the parties in the health field to create the necessary support. Unfortunately, a change of Government meant that the document was never sent to Parliament. The impact of the paper was felt, however, with the decentralisation of the preventive services with the WCPV,[6] in which municipal health departments are required to conduct health needs assessment, and with renewed attention to social inequalities in health. It also firmly brought back the idea of a periodic report on the population's health. Since then, this area of health policy-making has evolved into a health-oriented policy document at the start of each cabinet period based on a more comprehensive four yearly report on the population's health status by the RIVM, as discussed earlier.

An important element in the health policy debate in recent years has been the question of 'essential health services'; which services should remain accessible to all and therefore financed through the social insurance system. In 1991, the Dunning Committee published its report 'Choices in Health'.[17] It advocated a community approach to prioritising health services and specifically exempted the long-term care services such as institutions for the mentally handicapped or psycho-geriatric care from the prioritising system. It then proposed to screen services covered by the sickness funds according to the following criteria:

- Are they necessary services?
- Are they effective?
- Are they cost-effective or efficient?
- Could they be paid for by individuals?

Following publication of the report, the Ministry of Health commissioned a large number of projects to discuss the proposals of the committee with health care professionals and the general public. These projects often confirmed support for the criteria put forward by the report, especially concerning effectiveness and efficiency. This further strengthened the technology assessment programmes funded by the sickness fund council and the development of clinical guidelines and GP standards for care based on scientific evidence. In some medical schools, discussing treatment and allocation decisions along the lines of the Dunning criteria has become part of the regular curriculum.

However, applying these criteria to select those services for which continued collective responsibility would be guaranteed proved more difficult than expected. Although effectiveness and cost effectiveness could be established fairly easily, it proved exceedingly difficult to define what necessary care is or at what point individuals could be expected to be financially responsible. This was illustrated when the current Minister of Health proposed at the beginning of the previous cabinet period to take oral contraceptives out of the services covered by the sickness funds. Although it concerned only services to women aged over 21 and after the first visit, and although the price of a month's supply of pills hardly exceeds the price of one packet of cigarettes, the opposition from women's groups was such that the plans were abandoned.

Social inequalities in health have recently received a lot of attention in health policy. In 1988 the Scientific Council for Government Policy convened a restricted meeting to explore the issue.[18,19] Very few data on the Dutch situation were available, but on the basis of reports of local differences in health in Amsterdam the expectation was that such differences might also exist throughout the Netherlands.[20] Since then, a five-year research programme has identified health inequalities by socioeconomic groups for nearly every indicator of health. Following the final report of the research programme (its general findings are described by Mackenbach[21]), a second research programme has started which looks specifically at the effectiveness of interventions to reduce inequalities. The interventions to be looked at in the first part of the programme concern specially designed health promotion programmes to redress unequal distribution of risk factors, programmes aimed at a more equal utilisation of existing health services, and also some on occupational exposure.

Table 1

Major Dutch health policy documents

Year	Policy Document	Aims
1974	Stuctuurnota Gezonheidszorg[12]	Regionalisation of health services, separation of primary and secondary health care, introduction of public health services in all municipalities.
1982	Wet Voozieningen Gezondheidszorg[13]	Decentralised planning, never implemented.
1986	Nota 2000[16]	Dutch policy paper in response to WHO 'Health for All'.
1987	Committee on structure and finance of health care[5]	Dekker reforms, introducing limited competition and regulated market of social insurers, partially implemented.
1990	WCPV (collective prevention law)[17]	Decentralising responsibility for public health services to municipalities. Implemented.
1991	Choices in health care[17]	Dunning report on prioritising services, partially implemented.

Table 1 lists the major reforms and reports on health care policy. Of the health care policy documents produced to date, the most well known are obviously those of the Dekker reforms.[5]

In judging the importance of these policy documents one has to keep in mind, however, that the Netherlands does not have a national health service and therefore policy documents are not always accompanied by the power to implement the policy goals put forward and eloquently defended. Implementing such reforms in the Dutch policy context requires the commitment of the different partners involved, each of which has the power to veto change. This interdependency in policy-making makes abrupt reform unlikely, but does allow changes of the system without explicit parliamentary policy-making. Looking back, the Dekker reforms may not have been formally implemented, but they did create change especially in the functioning of the sickness funds and insurance companies. Sickness funds are encouraged to adopt a more market-oriented approach and have evolved in many cases from regional offices to large national corporations, often in close collaboration with private insurance companies.

Conclusions

Health is reported to be the most important thing in life for a large majority of the Dutch population, as is repeatedly shown in survey results. But when intersectoral policy options have to be weighed up, the health argument is not always given the attention one would expect given the above statement. This is illustrated by the difficulties of banning tobacco advertising and the recent political debate about the privatisation of the sick leave benefits insurance discussed earlier. In those cases, interests other than public health have prevailed. However, if one looks at the organised efforts of society to maintain and improve health, the Netherlands has not done badly. Effective preventive programmes have been implemented and offered to the total population, allowing for extra effort to be put into reaching hard to reach groups such as immigrants or deprived families, and health care services are accessible to all, including long-term care such as nursing homes, psychiatric care, home nursing and institutionalised care for the handicapped. Recent concerns about cost containment have lead to a greater focus on health technology assessment and efficiency measures in service delivery. The Dunning report has elicited the first comprehensive debate on essential services.[17]

However, minute cracks in the system are surfacing which under future pressures from the ageing of the population, innovative (diagnostic) technology and the expectations of the public, may well necessitate more explicit prioritising of the allocation of resources. Increasing waiting lists and the open discussion about giving priority to those who have to return to work indicates that the improvements in efficiency of the system may have achieved their maximum potential, so that health care reforms are unlikely to be the only answer to cost containment. It is in the coming political debate about how much money society is willing to be spent on maintaining and improving the population's health and on what that money is spent, that public health will have to provide rational arguments and prove its worth.

References

1. Ruwaard, D. en PG Kramers (eds). *RIVM, VolksgezondheidToekomstVerkenning. De gezondheidstoestand van de Nederlandse Bevolking in de Periode 1950–2010.* 's-Gravenhage: SDU, 1993.

2. Nota van het Ministerie van VWS. *Gezond en wel.* Rijswijk, 1994.

3. Ministerie VWS. *Financieel Overzicht Zorg 1995, Tweede Kamer, vergaderjaar 1994– 1995, 23904, nrs. 1-2.* 's-Gravenhage: Sdu Uitgeverij, 1994.

4. Maas v.d. PJ, Mackenbach JP (eds). *Volksgezondheid en Gezondheidszorg.* Utrecht: Bunge, 1995.

5. Commissie Structuur en Financiering Gezondheidszorg (Dekker committee). *Bereidheid tot verandering.* 's-Gravenhage: SDU, 1987.

6. *Wet op de Collectieve Preventie Volksgezondheid.* Staatsblad: The Hague, 1990:300.

7. *COCMO advies aan de dekaan van de NSPH.* Utrecht, 1994.

8. Arbeidomstandigheden wet (Arbowet). 's-Gravenhage: Staatsblad, 1988.

9. Inspectie voor de gezondheidszorg. *Gemeentelijke betrokkenheid bij collectieve preventie.* Rijswijk, 1995.

10. Schaapveld K, Hirasing RA. *Preventiegids, een praktisch overzicht van preventiepro- gramma's voor huisartsen, verloskundigen en medewerkers in de jeugdgezondheid- szorg.* Assen: van Gorcum, 1993.

11. Commissie Modernisering Curatieve Zorg (Commissie Biesheuvel). *Gedeelde zorg: betere zorg.* 's-Gravenhage: SDU, 1994.

12. Ministerie van Volksgezondheid en Milieuhygiene. *Struktuurnota Gezondheidszorg Tweede Kamer. vergaderjaar 1973–1974, 13 012.* 's-Gravenhage: Staatsuitgeverij, 1974.

13. *Wet Voorzieningen Gezondheidszorg WVG.* 's-Gravenhage: Staatsblad, 1982:563.

14. World Health Organization. *Health for all by the year 2000.* WHO Assembly, Geneva: Resolution 30.43, 1977.

15. World Health Organisation. *Targets for health for all: targets in support of the European regional strategy for health for all.* Copenhagen: WHO Regional Office for Europe, 1985.

16. Ministerie WVC. *Nota 2000. Over de ontwikkeling van gezondheidsbeleid: feiten, beschouwingen en beleidsvoornemens. Tweede Kamer, vergaderjaar 1985–1986, 19500.* 's-Gravenhage: Staatsuitgeverij, 1986.

17. Commissie Keuzen in de Zorg (Dunning committee). *Kiezen en delen.* Rijswijk: Ministry for Wellbeing, health and cultural affairs, 1991.

18. Wetenschappelijke Raad voor het Regeringsbeleid (Scientific Council for Government Policy). *Public Health Care. Report 52.* 's Gravenhage: Staatsuitgeverij, 1997.

19. Wetenschappelijke Raad voor het Regeringsbeleid. *De ongelijke verdeling van gezond- heid. V58, Voorstudies en achtergronden.* 's-Gravenhage: Staatsuitgeverij, 1987.

20. Maas v.d. PJ, et al. *Vergelijkend Buurtonderzoek Amsterdam II, naar sterfte en zieken-*

huisopnamen. Amsterdam: UvA/ISG, 1987.

21. Mackenbach JP. *Ongezonde verschillen: over stratificatie en gezondheid in Nederland*. Assen: van Gorcum, 1994.

13

Public Health and Health Policy in Austria

Engelbert Theurl

Introduction

The European healthcare systems differ widely in their epidemiological, ideological, political and organisational background and framework and so the task of public health faces quite different environments in different countries. This country report first provides an overview of the constitutional framework of Austrian health care policy and the role of public health in this country's Bismarck-model system.[1–2] This is very important because the degree of decentralisation of the political system in general marks the cornerstones for the structure of the decision process in the health care sector. Next, the report will illustrate the process of priority setting in Austria. The final part of the paper will pose some important open questions for the Austrian health care system.

The constitutional framework of Austrian health care policy

Constitutionally Austria is a federal state with a three-tier system of central (federal government), regional (provincial) and local (municipal) authorities. The distribution of responsibilities, spending authority and revenue authority is based partly on constitutional and partly on non-constitutional regulations. Such distribution can be described as moderately decentralised, even though decentralisation is mainly characterised by 'a decentralisation of law enforcement'. The distribution of revenue authority is greatly centralised. There is practically no revenue sovereignty (in particular tax sovereignty) at the provincial level, and at municipal level it is very limited.

In the distribution of responsibilities a distinction must be made between an area of sovereignty and an area of private enterprise administration. In the first area the state acts as an institution endowed with enforcement measures, whereas in the latter area the state acts like a private economic unit. The distribution of authority according to the Austrian Federal Constitution (Articles 10–15) exclusively applies to the area of sovereignty. Within the area of private enterprise administration, however, each regional and local authority can with certain restrictions – territorial ones, for example – act independently of the distribution of authority in the area of sovereignty. This also applies to activities in health care policy. The preconditions for such activities are the political will to perform these activities and adequate financing capabilities. Thus, the centralisation of tax sovereignty is an important barrier to local and regional health care initiatives within private economic administration (for example, the WHO 'Healthy Cities' projects).

Figure 1 shows the assignment of important authorities in the Austrian health care system and in adjoining fields between the federal government, the provinces and the municipalities for the sovereignity area, while Figure 2 overleaf describes the decision-making process in the health care system. It is basically accepted that all areas that are not regulated by the constitutional distribution of authority fall within the competence of the provinces. This implicit preference for federalist solutions has in the recent past repeatedly led to delays in restructuring at the federal level. This particularly applies to matters that had no political relevance at all at the time of the assignment of authority (1920) and, thus, remained unregulated. However, due to the economic developments since then, those matters have become extreme problem areas today. Environmental protection, in particular, must be mentioned in this context.

A prominent feature with far-reaching consequences is the fact that health care matters generally fall within the federal government's authority. The hospital sector is the responsibility of the federal government in areas of basic legislation (the fundamentals of the financing mechanism, minimum standards for regional density of capacity, hierarchy in the hospital sector), but the implemention and execution of legislation (supply of facilities, supervision, regulation) falls within the competence of the provinces. The federal legislation fixes the framework for the density of hospital, its function and the financing mechanism. Regarding the horizontal distribution at the federal level, the federal government's authority in health care is shared among the Ministry of Labour, Health and Social Affairs and the Ministry of Science, Transport and Arts. The federal government has basically a regulatory function in health care. The financing of the health care system is with some exceptions (hospital cooperation fund, medical research and education) not a task for the federal level. Medical care outside the hospital is organised and financed on a contract basis between the regional chambers of physicians and the social security system.

The regulatory function of the Ministry of Labour, Health and Social Affairs comprises the following fields in particular:

- The coordination of all matters in the field of public health (the prevention of and fight against infectious diseases, health care in schools, preventive health care, mental health, the market in medical products and contacts with international organisations);

Figure 1 The assignment of important functions in the Austrian health care system

Matter	Federal Government			Provinces			Municipalities	
	GG	*GGG*	*VZ*	*GG*	*AGG*	*VZ*	*ÜW*	*EW*
1 Health care (including nutrition, food quality control, but excluding (5)	x		x					
2 Labour law and social security system	x		x					
3 Private insurance system	x		x					
4 Scientific institutions of the federal government	x		x					
5 Sanatoria, hospitals and nursing homes		x			x	x		
6 Population policy (only equalisation of burdens on families)	x		x					
7 Population policy: maternity welfare, infant and young people's welfare, poor relief		x			x	x		
8 Transport (national)	x		x					
9 Environmental protection (emissions), air quality control (excluding heating systems), waste and hazardous material management	x		x					
10 Local sanitary police, ambulance service, mortal remains and interment							x	
11 Matters which are exclusively or mainly in the interest of the local municipalities								x

Key:
GG   Gesetzgebung (Legislation)
GGG Grundsatzgesetzgebung (Principle legislation)
AGG Ausführungsgesetzgebung (Implementing legislation)
VZ   Vollzug (Execution)
EW   Eigener Wirkungsbereich der Gemeinden (Municipalities' own sphere of action)
ÜW   Übertragener wirkungsbereich der Gemeinden (Sphere of action transferred to municipalities)

Figure 2 The decision-making process in the Austrian health care system

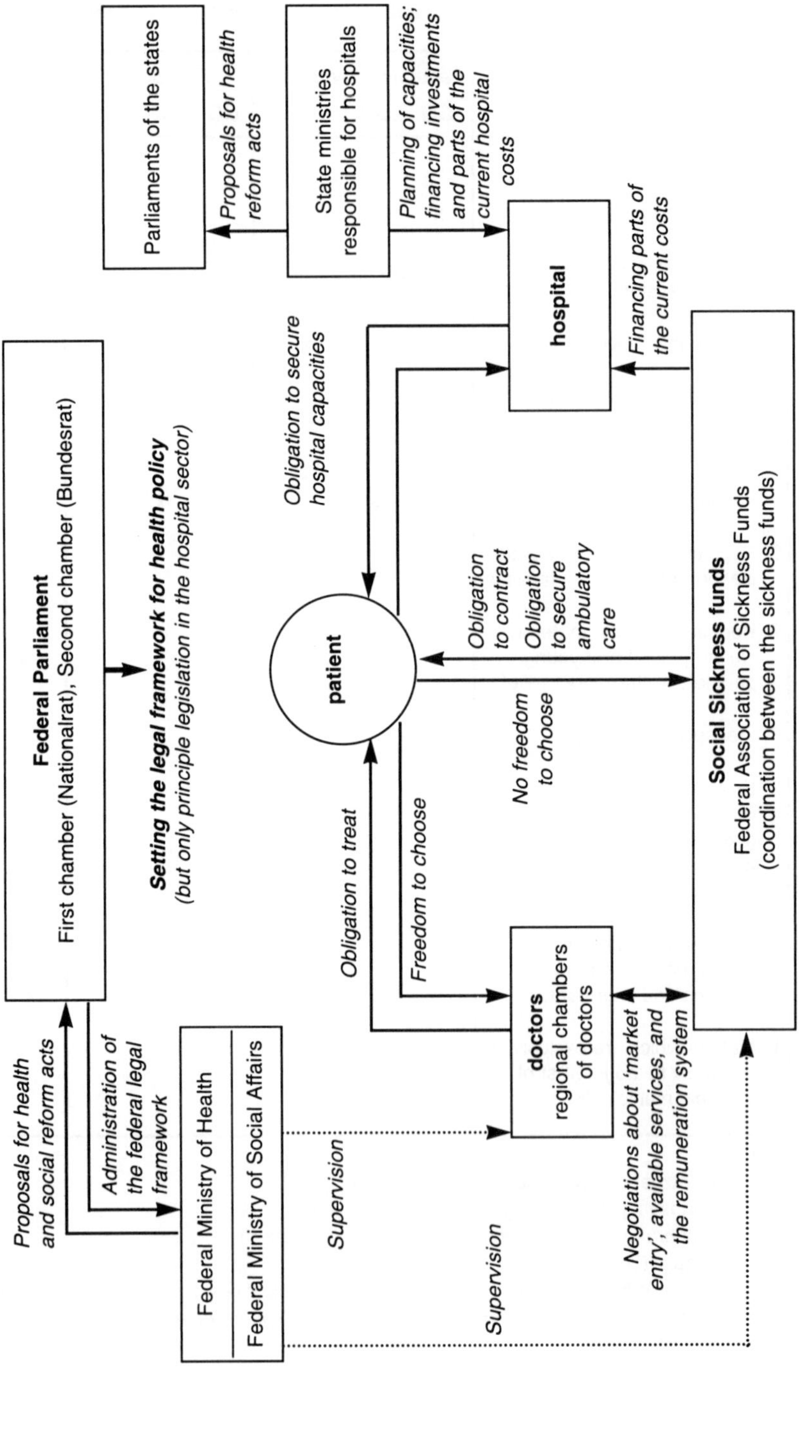

- Regulation of the market for pharmaceutical products;

- Food matters and veterinary administration;

- Health care training and research matters fall under the dominion of the Federal Ministry of Science, Arts and Transport;

- General social policy;

- Social security matters;

- Issues of labour law, among other things matters of occupational medicine and health care and the protection of labour;

- Matters of general and special welfare except for maternity and infant welfare;

This distribution of authority has significant consequences for Austrian health care policy:

At the federal level health care policy is largely characterised by regulatory control. Medical care provided by registered doctors is financed by social health insurance funds, while in-patient treatment is financed by social health insurance, federal and municipal funds. The compulsory social health insurance system is based on the individual's occupation and is financed by income-based contributions of employers and employees. Unemployed and retired people are also covered under this system. The influence of economic interest groups in influencing decisions in the social health insurance system is very high. The federal government's health care policy in the past was weakened by a largely *dysfunctional* distribution of authority between the Federal Ministry of Health and the Federal Ministry of Labour and Social Affairs. It was not until 1972 that a separate Federal Ministry of Health was established. However, so far this ministry has only been endowed with minimal authority. The task of regulating health care policy at an Austria-wide level could not be performed on this basis. Since 1997 the health care sector has been incorporated into the Federal Ministry of Labour, Health and Social Affairs.

In the relationship between federal government, provinces' and municipalities' health care policy is largely characterised by the fact that the responsibility for implementing legislation for hospitals falls within the competence of the provinces. Thus, an Austria-wide regulation of hospital capacities is only possible to a limited extent. In order to lessen the numerous regulatory deficiencies resulting from this fact, a central fund was set up in 1978 with the aim of, among other things, regulating hospital investments. However, for a number of reasons this fund has not fulfilled expectations.

As health spending was rising very rapidly in the early 1990s, part of the challenge facing those responsible for health policy was to find suitable ways of slowing this rate of increase of hospital costs. In an internal convention between the federal government and all provinces, January 1, 1997 marked the beginning of the implementation of a radical health reform. A flat rate per case payment method was introduced for hospital financing, so that hospitals were no longer financed on the basis of the length of stay of the patients but on the basis of the services provided. To calculate the rate, it is assumed that every patient constitutes a case, with the rate per case determined by the services provided and by the diagnoses made – corresponding to a number of points. The value of the individual case is determined in each province on the basis of the endowment of the respective provincial fund.

Instead of the Hospital Cooperation Fund (KRAZAF), a fund on the level of the province with extensive planning power has been set up to implement the new financing system. These funds are financed by the federal government, the provinces, the municipalities and the social insurance funds. The social insurance funds pay a block transfer to the provinces based on historical figures and related to the increase of their revenues. There exists no connection between the payment of the social insurance funds and the provision of services within the provinces.

As a part of the internal convention between the federal government and all the provinces a new Austrian Health Plan will be introduced. This plan consists of the Hospital Plan including a Major Medical-technical Equipment Plan, both of which are subject to ongoing review and further development. Other sub-plans, such as a Hospital Out-patient Department Plan, are in preparation. Many individual projects for internal quality assurance have been implemented in the hospitals. In a new model project entitled 'Quality in hospitals' launched in February 1998, strategies for solving selected problems arising in hospitals are being developed and specifically implemented in eleven hospitals.

This deficiency in the regulation of hospital capacities in the past were aggravated by the fact that hospital capacities and service functions outside the hospitals by registered doctors are planned and regulated separately. The regulation of hospital capacities is essentially the duty of regional and local authorities (especially provinces), whereas the regulation of capacities in out-patient treatment (registered doctors) is applied within the framework of long-term bilateral overall agreements between the Chamber of Physicians, which has regional competence, and the Main Association of Social Insurance Providers (the coordinating body for social security providers at the federal level).

As already mentioned, any deficiencies in the coordination of capacities in the health care sector in the future should be limited by several strategies. One is the introduction of an Austrian Health Plan, which will include in-patient and out-patient capacities. There also exists the political will to extend the diagnosis-related financing system to the out-patient capacities. In addition to this, measures have been discussed to manage the flow of patients through the health care facilities.

Important care institutions that may act as substitute health care institutions (social welfare facilities, nursing facilities, medical care for the aged, etc.) fall within the authority of the provinces and municipalities. This leads to many and diverse coordination problems between these services at regional level which are being particularly aggravated by the increasing proportion of old people in the total population and the multimorbidity associated with it.

The role of public health in Austrian health care policy

Public health and public health centres

The above analysis reveals that the strengthening of public health must be based on the existing institutional structure in Austria. The fact that health care policy at the federal level is mainly (only) regulatory and that the actual performance and financing of services is provided by subordinate regional and local authorities (provinces, munici-palities) and at the parafiscal level makes direct implementation of public health initia-tives difficult. Therefore, the Ministry for Labour, Health and Social Affairs at the federal level must, above all, be seen as a supplier of ideas and information and as a coordination and support institution for decentralised initiatives. As far as institutional authority is concerned, the starting point of these initiatives at the federal level is the area of 'public health'. This sphere of action is covered within the framework of indi-rect federal administration and within the framework of private enterprise administra-tion by regional sanitary headquarters at provincial level, by medical officers decentrally and by municipal organs within the framework of their local authority.

The organisational structure of this sphere of action is, especially at subordinate levels, based on a relatively traditional concept of public health and how to influence it.* The sphere of action of those administrative facilities is extremely heterogeneous and comprises both classical sovereignty tasks of public health and, increasingly, newer public health duties, such as health promotion.

In the sphere of 'public health' several problem areas may be identified which indicate a requirement for a more basic reform of this area from the public health standpoint. The requirements concerning profession and organisation are huge, particularly at subordi-nate levels. It is inevitable that the sovereignty function provided for by law frequently leads to deferring long-term tasks of public health care. This critical situation is made more difficult by a considerable shortage of medical and other personnel. Research and specialisation in the area of public medicine and public health are only partly available in Austria so there is no relevant scientific infrastructure to fall back on.

As early as 1991 a team of experts of the Federal Ministry of Health and Environmental Protection made a reform proposal for reorganisation, which is still relevant today. This concept sees the public health centres as considerably revalued hubs of a considerable revalued public health care. The following structure is suggested within the framework of that proposal:

---

* *The German-speaking countries have a long tradition in public health matters, which can be traced back to the population theory of mercantilism two centuries ago. The population theory of mercantilism has to be seen as a counterpart to the pessimistic view of the popu-lation school of Robert Malthus. The main goal of mercantilism is the prosperity of the national economy. International trade is seen as a zero-sum game. A healthy population, which is able to act as worker, consumer and soldier, is considered as an important basis of national prosperity.*

1. Departments for the tasks of sanitary authorities which concentrate on the area of health protection.

2. Departments for public health which are interdisciplinarily centred on social medicine, community medicine, epidemiology, health promotion, health management. These departments should fulfil public health tasks.

3. A department for medical check-ups and prophylaxis, health advice and education. This department would act as a link between the public health area and the curative areas of health care.

In all, this reform step should replace the hierarchical profile of public health departments by a service profile. These newly structured public health departments are also seen as service and support institutions for regional social and health districts and initiatives which are being established. However, the realisation of this scenario involves legal and organisational measures and financial expenditure and, despite some improvements, has yet not been achieved. But it appears to be the only meaningful model within the framework of a comprehensive health care policy.

In Austria, public health as a general objective and as a criteria for assessing any public policy is divided into separate areas. However, it cannot be said that there is a systematic orientation towards this aim. In principle all laws that are introduced into Parliament via the Council of Ministers require the approval of all ministers. Laws with negative effects on health could, at least theoretically, be blocked, even though in practice there are relatively tight political limits to this blocking. Furthermore, there is an extended procedure for assessing bills prior to parliamentary procedure which in particular involves different interest groups and the administrative institutions concerned (for example, provincial sanitary headquarters). To what extent changes can be made based on these revisions of laws depends on numerous factors. Moreover, there are consultations (for example, working groups) between federal ministries at civil service level in the law-making procedure in case of cross-sectional tasks. However, considerable success in establishing health-related interests has recently been achieved in the environmental field (for example, the introduction of the Environmental Impact Assessment, EIA).

To coordinate the activities in the fields of health promotion and primary preventive medicine, which authority legislation renders very diffuse, a forum called 'Healthy Austria' was founded in 1988 by important pillars of the Austrian health care system. This forum aims at establishing active health promotion as a third area of health care along with medical care and health protection. The following strategies of implementation are being applied:

- The improvement of the quality and quantity of health promotion services offered, with the foci of activities specifically fixed.

- The improvement of cooperation with the provinces and municipalities.

- Working out infrastructural and financing models for health promotion.

In the past, the activities of the forum were oriented towards early disease recognition programmes (1989: precautions against cancer; 1990: prevention of heart and circulatory diseases). With the restructuring in 1992 these foci were abandoned in favour of targets towards exercise, diet, smoking, healthy teeth, and the documentation of health promotion, evaluation, basic research or information service for groups acting at the grassroots level.

Health indicators in Austria

Although in past years Austria experienced a lower health status than other European countries, statistics from recent years have demonstrated an improvement. The average life expectancy for females rose from 80.2 years in 1996 to 80.5 years in 1997. Males saw an increase from 73.9 years to 74.1 years over the same period.[3]

Nearly all indicators show a positive development in the health status of the population over the last few years. There has been a significant decrease in perinatal mortality, perhaps as a result of several preventive measures that were introduced in 1970. Further trends in population health include:

- In 1995, 34,268 people in Austria developed cancer. This is an 11.3 per cent increase over the 1985 figure, which can be traced to the change in the average age of the population. With 88.7 new cases per 100,000 inhabitants, prostate cancer is the most frequent type of cancer of men, followed by lung cancer with 70.4 and intestinal cancer with 63.7 cases per 100,000. For women, breast cancer is by far the most common type with 89.8 cases per 100,000 inhabitants in 1995. Due to a significant increase in smoking, lung cancer among women increased in recent years.

- The trend in the development of infectious and contagious diseases can no longer be described as a general decline. The tuberculosis situation is quite stable, although the rate of 17.4 new infections per 100,000 inhabitants is slightly higher than the European Union average (14.4).

- The most striking and alarming result of school medical examinations is a high and rising number of abnormalities in posture. A similar trend can be seen in respect to allergies, while the development of teeth health is quite promising. The WHO target of not more than three teeth with cavities in twelve-years-olds was reached in 1994/95.

- The number of fatal accidents in road traffic is traditionally high in Austria, but was decreasing substantially in 1998.

Public health and social health insurance

In Austria, approximately 50 per cent of public health expenditure is covered by social health insurance, which makes it necessary to analyse the question of to what extent public health objectives have been included in the set of policy targets of social health insurance bodies in recent years. In the past the development of policy objectives was heavily influenced by the situation that prevailed when social health insurance was first introduced more than 100 years ago. From the beginnings of epidemic control in the medieval towns of Italy and Germany, the specific tasks of public health centres – particularly promoted by the population theory of mercantilism – developed in the following centuries.

Thus, measures of preventive health care – in particular those of a population level nature – were largely excluded from the set of policy targets of social health insurance bodies. For a long time the restoration of the state of health (primarily) to regain the ability to work was the basis of intervention as well as the basis of the financial commitment of social health insurance bodies. This emphasis can also be explained by the structure of decision-making in social health insurance bodies, namely the dominance of the representatives of employers' and employees' organisations. Non-improvable states of health continued to be excluded from the obligation of social health insurance bodies and depended on other compensation systems (for example, social welfare). Social welfare legislation has made a few basic corrections in the last few years that partly includes elements of the public health concept (following the expansion of the term 'health' itself):

- The introduction of a uniform state-financed need-based nursing allowance in 1993 took account of the changes in the age structure of the population and, thus, in risk structure as well as of the resultant overtaxing of other compensation institutions (i.e. social welfare). At the same time, the provinces were committed to building the infrastructure required for persons in need of care, for the information of and advice to the population and for the coordination of services until the year 2010.

- The existing deficiencies (for example, great regional differences due to the constitutional framework) in psychosocial care were taken account of by the legal regulation of the new medical profession of psychotherapy. In addition, a basic restructuring of this sector is planned for the nearer future which should strengthen the role of service institutions outside the hospital.[4] A comprehensive network of coverage of community-integrated basic care with a combination of social, psychiatric and psychological services has been developed in some provinces.

- The 50th Amendment to the General Social Security Law, i.e. the introduction of social health insurance as a standard insurance benefit, meant a considerable step towards a country-wide supply of psychotherapeutic services although some problems remain (for example, the remuneration of psychotherapists).

- Psychotherapeutic care in hospitals was embodied in an Amendment to the Hospital Law in 1993.

Basically, the prevailing opinion – particularly among representatives of social health insurance – is that prevention is a communal task due to the legally regulated division of labour in health care. The area of early disease recognition in particular is assigned to social health insurance, even though in the recent past some other measures have been taken – in particular, media campaigns – to prevent unhealthy behaviour. At present, two

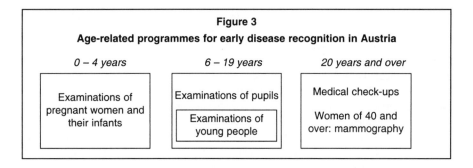

Figure 3

Age-related programmes for early disease recognition in Austria

0 – 4 years

Examinations of pregnant women and their infants

6 – 19 years

Examinations of pupils

Examinations of young people

20 years and over

Medical check-ups

Women of 40 and over: mammography

main programmes of early disease recognition are being offered within the framework of social health insurance. Figure 3 shows the medical check-ups currently offered to the total population.

Two-thirds of the expenditures for examinations of pregnant women and their infants are covered by the federal government, one third by social health insurance. This programme was introduced in 1974 with the aim of reducing an infant mortality rate which was previously comparatively high. The programme consists of five examinations of pregnant women, five examinations of their infants in their first years, including one orthopaedic, one ear, nose and throat and one ophthalmic examination, as well as further examinations of infants at the end of their second, third and fourth years. Since April 1992 the programme has also comprised one hepatitis examination of pregnant women as well as two optional ultrasound examinations of the infants' hips. In the past, nearly 100 per cent of pregnant women with their infants availed themselves of this programme, among other things because the payment of maternity benefit depended on the proof of the examinations undertaken.

The check-ups for school children and young people provide a standardised examination. They focus particularly on a check-up of the visual and hearing capabilities and of the locomotor and supporting apparatus.

Since 1974 medical check-ups are a compulsory task of social health insurance bodies. Explicit examination targets are as follows:

- Arteriosclerosis, heart and circulatory diseases, increased blood pressure

- Carcinomas (especially carcinomas of the intestines, carcinomas of the cervix) and malignant growth which are detectable by clinical methods at an early stage

- Diabetes

- Chronic respiratory diseases

Medical check-ups comprise a basic programme and an additional gynaecological programme for women. The latter includes taking the history, a gynaecological examination and a mammography for women aged 40 and over. The examination must also be accompanied by detailed medical advice, including elements of modern health promotion. Medical check-ups are mainly carried out by general practitioners. Persons aged 19 and over may avail themselves of medical check-ups, which are mainly carried out by registered doctors (mostly general practitioners, partly specialists). In 1996, participation in medical check-ups was 8.9 per cent Austria-wide; however, there are relatively great variations between the individual provinces. The regional differences in participation in the programme have not been fully explained. However, they are attributed for the most part to the social health insurance bodies' different policies when 'inviting' the population to take part in the programme, a different way of incorporating medical check-ups in regional health care programmes, different traditions of preventive health care and different remuneration schemes for medical check-ups. There are extremely wide regional differences in participation in the gynaecological examinations (Austria-wide: 3.4 per cent, approximately 25 per cent in Vorarlberg). Women more take advantage of medical checkups than men. The usefulness of those screening programmes is, on the whole, considered questionable (including the problem of reaching target groups, the epidemiological usefulness, etc.). There are still no comprehensive evaluation programmes available for these medical check-ups.

As early as 1948 the examination of young people was introduced as a standard benefit of social health insurance bodies. The target groups are young people who are already in work. The programme of this examination is basically screening-oriented. However, since the 1992 reform increasingly it includes elements of primary health preventive medicine. The programme is designed for young people between 16 and 19, with a yearly basic programme being complemented by particular focus programmes (for example, strain at workplace, additional gynaecological programme) in the following years. In 1996, 55 per cent of the target group participated in the examination; there were, however, distinct regional variations. The general opinion, when judged by the principles of general screenings, is that the medical examination part of the young people's examination has reached its target. On the other hand, it is thought that its counselling elements and the health promotion components should be expanded. Only a limited scientific evaluation of the results of these medical check-ups is available at the moment. Especially no evaluation of the effectiveness and of cost-benefit ratios of this programme is available.

Setting priorities in Austrian health care

The previous two sections contain important information relevant to this issue. Austria's social health insurance-based health care system is both functionally and geographically very segregated. The main function of the federal government is a regulatory one. The delivery of services is effected by subordinate regional and local authorities and via performance contracts of social insurance with providers. The overall health care budget and also the structure of the budget (curative care, preventive services) is therefore not determined on a federal level but is the result of quite independent decisions on the different levels of the health care system. Thus, total regulation of health care by the federal government, according to the priorities of health care policy, is only possible to a very modest extent. No national establishment of priorities which are centred on output-related criteria (for example, economic cost of diseases) has been made. In addition, this setting of priorities is aggravated by the fact that treatment by registered doctors outside the hospital is distinctively separated from in-patient treatment. This is also the case for the planning of the capacities in these two sectors. So an overall planning of priorities, which includes the whole range of services, is not possible at present. The different types of financing and financing institutions in the two sectors make it impossible to compare accurately between output and prices and, thus, are a hindrance to an optimum division of the labour of these two sectors. Health care policy in the last 25 years has been essentially characterised by the attempt to achieve an Austria-wide coordination of capacities, especially in the in-patient sector. For this purpose, the Hospital Cooperation Fund was established at the federal level with the aims of regulating capacities. There is general agreement that this goal has not been reached. The change in the finance of hospital financing and the steering of capacities in the in-patient sector, which took place in 1997 and which was already mentioned in this paper, may act as an instrument to strengthen priority setting on a federal and regional level, although several important steps have to be made.

In Austria there are currently no explicit models of rationing and setting priorities like those realised in the USA (Oregon), those suggested in the Netherlands and those discussed in Germany. But the financial bottleneck of the individual social health insurance bodies has triggered a process of reforming the set of service targets (see, for example, the amendments to the General Social Security Law) and the set of remuneration targets which is probably best described as a process of 'muddling through'. Thus, this process has the advantage of detailed knowledge, but will probably face the dilemma of creating social hardship and failing to set the important course for health care. The reform of the set of service targets mainly concerns the health care sector outside hospitals, where the existing form of remuneration of the doctors needs a defined catalogue of services, which are paid by the social insurance system.

Budgets in the Austrian Health Care systems are set in very different ways. These is no clear system of financial prioritising at the national level, nor are there clear explicit rules to divide the budgets between the different kinds of activities and localities. To a high degree, the allocation of funds is retrospective and subject to political decisions. Several cost containment initiatives have been undertaken:

1. The market for pharmaceuticals is highly regulated. Cost containment measures for pharmaceuticals therefore are a matter for negotiation between the representatives of the pharmaceutical industry and the social insurance system. By cutting the trade margin and by introducing positive lists, substantial savings have been achieved.

2. The increase in the costs for physicians working outside the hospitals were modest in the past. The increase is fixed in negotiations between the social health insurance system and the doctors' representatives. It is not a global budget, but there are several features in the mechanisms for paying the doctors which work in this direction.

3. Hospital costs increased very sharply in the past and this increase was a major reason for changing the hospital financing.[5] Since 1997, all hospitals get some kind of global budget, with the revenues of single hospitals determined by the number of Diagnosis Related Groups (DRG) points.

Regional integration of health care and the role of local initiatives in health care policy

The assignment of authority according to the Austrian Federal Constitution provides the framework for regional initiatives in health care and social welfare. A number of social tasks (for example, caring for old and handicapped people) that are a near substitute for or complement to health care fall within the competence of the provinces. In addition, each province may, within the framework of private enterprise administration, act independently of the barriers to authority imposed by sovereignty administration. Finally, municipalities, according to the principle of subsidiarity, are authorised and politically obliged to fulfil tasks which are exclusively and mainly in the interest of the municipalities and within the boundaries of a local community. This task fulfilment is limited, on the one hand, by political priorities at regional and municipal levels and, on the other hand, by the delegation of financial resources to the provinces and municipalities with financial resources. The very restricted possibility of an autonomous utilisation of municipal tax sources, the high burden of local infrastructure services on municipalities, and the high burden of financing and co-financing hospitals on provinces and municipalities presently leave only limited scope for the fulfilment of new health care aims. Additional income can be generated only if additional fees are introduced. Increased activities are also politically aggravated by the fact that other public households benefit from the financial yields (for example, long-term savings through increased preventive medicine activities), due to the strong division of authority and financial structure.

This general analysis should not lead to the conclusion that there are no local or regional initiatives. These initiatives, though, are characterised by the very heterogenous nature of the chosen objectives and foci of activities, of the quality of the services offered, of the achievement level of these facilities, of the historical traditions and the organisational starting points, of the types of organisation and financing chosen, of the incorporation of registered doctors, of the evaluation of services performed, etc. In many provinces WHO programmes have been initiated and tested (for example, Healthy Municipality, Healthy Cities).

In the following paragraph the exemplary activities of the Province of Vorarlberg will be described in more detail. As early as 1965 the Province of Vorarlberg established a working group for preventive and social medicine. In the course of this programme early disease recognition programmes were carried out in close cooperation with registered doctors. Simultaneously, the concept of a social administrative district came into being as a way of improving social structures at regional levels, as an instrument for coordinating social services and for the purpose of activating neighbourhood social welfare organisation. In 1983 a general concept of comprehensive health and social work at the local level was worked out for the first time and called 'Healthy Living Space'. In 1985 this concept led to a programme called 'Healthy Living Space Vorarlberg', which sees itself as a framework concept for a comprehensive social, health and environment policy and comprises a vast field of activities. This model is characterised by a linking of state-offered and private enterprise-offered services, the strong local establishment of programmes and the strong integration of registered doctors in the programmes. Moreover, (through cooperation with WHO) it is accompanied by a high level of national and international evaluation research concerning the quality of structure, procedure and results.

Currently, some forms of more strongly integrated health and social care are taking shape in all the provinces. In the interest of a comprehensive health care policy, it should probably be pointed out that the degree of integration intended is relatively low. In order to achieve a substantial shift in service structures, it would be necessary to include to a larger extent the area of registered doctors and in-patient health care. In the last few years the federal government has developed an 'Integrated Health and Social Administrative Districts' model, which provides a high degree of regional interlinking. However, the provinces will be responsible for the implementation of the concept. The restructuring of hospital financing in Austria described earlier includes important incentives for increasing regional integration and for promoting activities beneficial to health.

Conclusions

The following selection and evaluation is, of course, subjective and need not necessarily coincide with assessment by politically responsible institutions. From a public health point of perspective, the following conclusions can be drawn:

The basic structure of the Austrian health care system, in particular the distribution of political authority, is certainly a hindrance to quick and systematic implementation of public health concepts and priority setting. On the other hand, it should be pointed out that the federal structure creates information that is not available at such reasonable cost in centralised states. This is because the costs of gathering information about local particularities, the costs of the decision-making process, and the costs of wrong decisions may be lower in decentralised states. The federalist structure can also be utilised to test new initiatives. Therefore, the ways of implementing public health ideas in NHS-type health care systems are not applicable to Austria. Although there are tight financial restrictions at regional and provincial level many public health initiatives exist. These initiatives need more coordination on a federal level. The role of preventive services and health promotion within the social insurance system at the moment is low. But several initiatives exist to strengthen this role.

Public Health has a long tradition in Austria dating back to the initiatives of the Austrian-Hungarian Monarchy and based on the population policy of mercantilism. It is, however, the tradition of a hierarchical health policy. It is problematic to entrust to institutions and organisations which work for health protection the tasks of health promotion as provided for by the public health concept. From this point of view, a reform of the administrative area of 'public health' is urgently required.

Today the view that health-relevant information is particularly important for a public health concept is widely accepted. For decades, Austria has kept data on the health care system and the population's state of health. This information is mainly compiled and interpreted in the Federal Statistical Office, in the Federal Ministry for Labour, Health and Social Affairs and in the Main Association of Social Health Insurance Bodies. To use this data within the framework of public health concepts and the setting of national priorities, it would be necessary to pool data relevant for the health care system and its regulation, to improve the data's comparability, to have a functional rather than institutional orientation, to regionalise and coordinate data at various output/input levels of the health care system e.g. state of health, effects on health, services performed, capacities provided, health expenditures.

Based on improved health reports, it would be necessary to intensify evaluation research in health care at structural, procedural and result levels. In this respect, centralisation on a federal level would be absolutely necessary due to the existing cost structure.

Joining the European Union has not had a substantial impact on public health policy when we look at the initiatives which were undertaken over the last two years. But the strengthening of international contacts is encouraging new ways of thinking about public health policy.

References

1. Beirat für Wirtschafts- und Sozialfragen. *Neue Wege im Gesundheitswesen – Kurzfassung.* Wien, 1996.

2. OECD. *The Reform of Health Care Systems – A review of Seventeen OECD Countries.* Paris: OECD, 1994.

3. Federal Ministry of Labour, Health and Social Affairs. *Public Health in Austria.* Wien, 1998.

4. Meise U et al. *Die Versorgung Psychisch Kranker in Österreich.* Wien, 1991.

5. Theurl E. *Überleben die Krankenhäuser?* Thaur: Kulturverlag, 1991.

Additional Reading

Bundesministerin für Gesundheit, Sport und Konsumentenschutz. *Gesundheitsbericht an den Nationalrat 1994.* Wien, 1994.

Österreichisches *Bundesinstitut für Gesundheitswesen. Amtsarzt – Tätigkeitsbereich und Ausbildung.* Wien, 1991.

Österreichisches Bundesinstitut für Gesundheitswesen. *Österreichischer Krankenanstalten-plan.* Wien, 1994.

VAMED. *Österreichisches Krankenhauswesen bis 2010.* Wien, 1988.

14

Public Health and Health Care in Portugal

Victor Ramos

Introduction

Portugal is one of the oldest states in Europe having been a nation since 1143. It became a republic in 1910 and since the peaceful revolution in 1974 has established democracy. Portugal became a member of the European Union in 1986.

The land area of the country is 89,000 km^2 with a population of approximately 10 million. As in other European countries, the Portuguese population is ageing. Those over 65 now account for 14 per cent of the total population. During the last three decades, the fertility and birth rates have decreased and life expectancy at birth has increased. The average life expectancy in 1996 was 74.9 years (71.3 years for men and 78.6 for women).[1]

In 1997, income per capita was US$ 10,970, the annual inflation rate was 2.2 per cent and the unemployment rate 6.7 per cent.[1,2] The employment structure in 1997 was:

• Agriculture, forestry and fishery	14 per cent.
• Industry, construction, energy and water	31 per cent.
• Services	55 per cent.

The illiteracy rate is 11 per cent. School is compulsory to the age of fourteen, and since 1988 it has been extended to the 9th year after entry.

The Portuguese health care system

The Constitution of the Portuguese Republic gives every citizen the right and the responsibility to safeguard his or her health and such a right is assured through a

National Health Service (NHS). The NHS was created in 1979. Its main principles are: universal coverage, provision of comprehensive care and freedom from user charges (in general). Patients' rights are explicitly stated in the law and the health care services must inform citizens and patients of their rights. A Charter of Rights and Duties of the Patient was published in 1997.

The NHS is managed by the Ministry of Health, which covers the financing, administration and provision of all types of health care (primary, secondary and tertiary). There is currently a trend to decentralise the NHS through five Regional Health Administrations (Figure 1).

The NHS employs the large majority of health personnel. Only a few professionals work exclusively in the private sector. However, most doctors and a great number of other professionals work in both sectors simultaneously. Doctors and nurses are organised into public professional careers that are established by law. The medical career has three branches (Decree-Law 73/90): *public health*, *general practice* and *hospital medicine*. Public health medicine is a medical speciality and a professional career with equal status to any other medical speciality within the NHS. The nursing career offers three options (Decree-Law 437/91): *direct care* (hospitals or health centres), *management/ administration* and *teaching*.

For public health purposes the NHS covers the entire population and, in principle, is available to all through community or local health centres and public hospitals. In personal and family primary care, 80 per cent of people are registered with general practitioners/family doctors in the local health centres of the NHS. GPs have patient lists of 1,500 people, on average.

Access to secondary and tertiary care in the NHS requires a referral from a GP. However, in private practice and for some specific sub-groups (such as civil servants and military personnel) patients go directly to specialists. The NHS's total 103 hospitals (general and specialised, including mental health) have a total of approximately 28,000 beds. Portugal's 89 private hospitals have approximately 8,800 beds.[1]

Health care financing

There are three sources of health care financing. The NHS is financed predominantly from taxes through the State Budget. There are also some specific sub-systems (civil service, military, bank, large private companies) that provide access to health care through insurance or insurance-like schemes. A few people (less than 2 per cent) also have their own private health insurance. There is some redundancy in these schemes as everyone is entitled to benefit from the NHS.

The NHS is universal and aims to provide comprehensive care, or to assure that this care is provided by other institutions under contract with the NHS. The NHS believes that all citizens should have equal access to health care. Services are provided free of charge but there are very small moderating fees for the use of some care (consultations, tests, some

Figure 1
The organisational structural of the Portuguese National Service

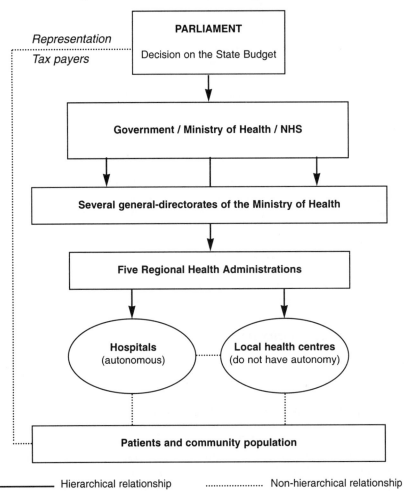

——————— Hierarchical relationship   .... Non-hierarchical relationship

treatments). Moderating fees were introduced as a way of rationalising demand but they represent a very small source of financing for the NHS. A proportion of the population (children, pregnant women, patients with certain chronic diseases, the elderly and some deprived people) are exempt from paying the moderating fee. This exemption is intended to deliver care to those in greatest need. There are also some co-payments for pharmaceuticals, these are less for people on low incomes (limits are defined by law).

The Government annually presents the proposed NHS budget to Parliament. The size of this budget is calculated retrospectively, based on the previous year's expenses.

The allocation of resources in the NHS is made centrally. The distribution of the budget to hospitals, primary care services and other institutions follows the pattern of their past expenditures and internal structure. There is currently a move to introduce prospective budgets negotiated with the institutions through five regional contracting agencies.

The NHS hospitals have administrative and financial autonomy and receive a yearly-defined budget. Primary care health centres do not have autonomy and their 'budgets' are administered by regional and sub-regional boards. Management and financial autonomy for primary care centres is expected to begin in 1999. Hospital doctors, GP/family doctors, nurses and other personnel receive fixed salaries. Until 1998 there was no specific budget for prevention and health promotion. Changes in professional remuneration and specific contracts for prevention and health promotion are currently being introduced.

The pharmaceutical industry and pharmacies are powerful interest groups that indirectly influence the components of the health budget. Rising and uncontrolled expenditures related to new medical technology have aggravated the imbalance between primary and secondary/tertiary care.

Total expenditure in health care accounted for 8.2 per cent of the gross domestic product (GDP) in 1997. Public expenditure on health care amounted to 60 per cent of the total expenditure (4.9 per cent of GDP). Citizens directly support 40.2 per cent of total health expenditure. However, these expenses are tax deductible.[3]

Health policy and priority setting

In 1990, the Parliament approved a new General Health Care Law, which was aimed at changing the health care system to a more decentralised and 'market-oriented' model. Several additional laws were introduced in the following years which led to organisational restructuring within the central and regional bodies of the Ministry of Health. However at local level health centres and hospitals, where health care is provided to citizens, there were no innovations.[4,5] Old problems and complaints about low accessibility, dissatisfaction of patients and professionals remained almost unchanged. In 1996, the new government defined a *'Health Strategy for Portugal 1998–2002'*, with the participation of several national organisations and partners. During this period the discussion of priorities in public health and methodologies for establishing those priorities took place at national and regional level. This explicit health policy has been patient-centred and oriented, with the goal of defined health gains or health outcomes for the population in specific and quantified terms.[6]

Inequalities and priority setting

Although in theory the NHS must ensure universal access to health care, many people have been adversely affected by hidden perverse mechanisms, such as waiting lists for consultations and surgical interventions. These mechanisms are frequently unrelated to the health status or health care needs of individuals and their families. The conflicting interests of professionals working simultaneously in the NHS and in private practice, together with the absence of penalties for the low productivity of the NHS institutions, are some of the main sources of this problem.

As explicit priorities within the NHS were undefined, there has been negative discrimination towards those in greater need, measured by waiting lists and avoidable deaths. The elderly, poor, illiterate and those living in inner rural areas are deprived of both preventive care and therapeutic and rehabilitative care.[7,8,9]

Inequalities within Portugal exist along dimensions such as: age, gender, social class/socioeconomic status, region and ethnicity. Most of these inequalities are unjust and unfair and can be minimised through appropriate health policy decisions and public health interventions. The debate about inequality in health and health care was introduced by researchers who have addressed this subject in Portugal.[10–13] These authors have studied the differences in health status/mortality, self-reported morbidity, determinant factors of health, accessibility and health care utilisation in the country. Striking inequities were found among social groups and among regions, confirming once again the 'inverse care law'.[14] The '*Health Strategy for Portugal 1998–2002*' addresses equity as an indispensable precondition to secure further health improvement.

Public health, prevention and health promotion

Demographic changes, changes in morbidity and mortality patterns, unemployment, social exclusion, increasing population mobility and rising public demands and expectations, are all present in Portugal. The challenges and problems facing Portuguese public health are in some ways identical to those present in the rest of the European Union, but to varying degrees.

During the last 20 years, some health status indicators of the Portuguese population have improved steadily. Infant, neonatal and perinatal mortality rates have decreased notably and are now closer to the European Union, compared to ten years earlier. Changes in life expectancy at birth have also been favourable. In several specific categories of mortality (for causes of death) the gap between Portugal and other European countries has narrowed, with some exceptions:

Cerebrovascular disease	238.1 / 100,000 (1996)
Diabetes	30.2 / 100,000 (1996)
Motor vehicle accident	22.2 / 100,000 (1996)

Accidents (traffic and workplace) represent the most important cause of potential years of life lost. Chronic liver diseases and cirrhosis are among the ten leading causes of death (26.7/100,000 in 1996) and also one of the most common causes of years of life lost. Incidence of tuberculosis was 38.5/100,000 in 1996 and this situation is closely related to the health conditions of immigrant groups and to the increase of HIV/AIDS.

The incidence of AIDS is increasing each year (38.1 per million, in 1996). Tobacco consumption is a growing trend in contrast with other European countries.[1,15]

As a general comment, those indicators sensitive to the improvement of global socio-economic conditions and to the development of maternal and child health care services showed a marked improvement. However, those that are more related to lifestyle, behaviour, civic and health education continue to pose serious public health problems.

The main public health problems can be considered both in terms of risk factors and diseases. Tobacco and alcohol consumption (with their related health problems and consequences), traffic accidents, hazards in the workplace, drug abuse and its links to HIV/AIDS infection, cerebrovascular disease, some forms of cancer, mental health problems (including suicide and self-inflicted injury) are now the main challenges for Portuguese public health.

The Portuguese infrastructure of public health – some historical notes

The recent history of the Portuguese public health infrastructure (although risking some oversimplification) encompasses two periods:

1. 1971 to mid-1980s: an expansion period; and

2. Mid-1980s to mid-1990s: a crisis period.

It is expected that the present and the near future will be a period of rebirth for public health.

The expansion period

In the sixties and early seventies Portugal had a marked maldistribution of doctors. The majority of doctors were specialists in urban hospitals, with part-time appointments in the ambulatory clinics of the then existing social insurance system. Rural and deprived areas were almost without medical assistance. Community approaches to health and the preventive philosophy were almost non-existent.

In 1971 a reform of the health system took place under the leadership of a few public health doctors. This reform was aimed at creating a well-organised and comprehensive infrastructure of public health services, including primary health care access for the entire population. Public health became a well established medical professional career and most of the principles of the primary health care concept stated at the 1978 WHO/UNICEF Conference held in Alma Ata were included in this reform.[16] A network of local health centres was established to cover the whole country with essential medical care and promote public health activities. The shortage of medical doctors and nurses, combined with several political and organisational obstacles, prevented full implementation of this reform.[17]

The new public health medical career attracted some enthusiastic doctors (around 30 across the country) who became the pioneers and leaders of a generation of public health doctors with an entirely new education, perspective and vision.

After the revolution of 1974, health became a political and social priority. Debates on a future National Health Service began. In 1975, an initiative was launched to address the problem of the maldistribution of doctors in the country. As a result, each young doctor was required to serve in rural and deprived areas for one year, if he/she wanted to work in the future National Health Service. This 'civic' medical service for young doctors created some favourable conditions for the implementation of the Portuguese National Health Service (NHS) in 1979.[18]

The 'civic' medical service of young doctors provided nationwide medical coverage from 1975 to 1982, with an emphasis on peripheral and deprived areas. The participating doctors gave the necessary medical support to health centres already established in the reform of 1971. Some of these doctors (around 300) decided to follow public health careers and a larger group (around 4,000) entered the new career of general practice/family medicine, created in 1982. At the creation of this new career of general practice within the health centres of the NHS, the 'civic' medical service was discontinued.

In 1983 the ambulatory clinics of the social insurance scheme were integrated in the first network of health centres that had been established in 1971. A new generation of local health centres arose, combining the 'curative' tradition of the old social insurance ambulatory clinics with the 'preventive' tradition of the previous health centres.

After 1983, the NHS primary health care infrastructure included around 2,200 primary health care local clinics attached to a network of 380 health centres which covered the whole country and were available to the entire population. Each health centre is devoted to a well-defined geographical area and population. The staff of health centres include: general practitioners/family doctors, public health doctors, general nurses, public health or community nurses, administrative staff, environmental health professionals, social workers and other professionals according to need.

The mission of the local NHS health centres is to increase the health status of the overall population through interventions at three levels: the individual, the family and the community (including the environment). The aim is to combine personal with community care and to integrate preventive and 'curative' activities.[19] The idea of the health centres is for general practice/family medicine and public health to collaborate closely to achieve their common goals.

A structured network of professionals and institutions of public health was developed in this period, including a well-established hierarchical career for public health doctors. These doctors possess delegated power from the State to act as public health authorities who can operate at central, regional and local levels all over the country. Historically, this structure had its roots in the beginning of the century ('sanitary police') and had the power to intervene in matters concerning the environment, housing, food commerce, control of transmissible diseases and threats to public health. The importance of public health authorities was markedly renewed and reinforced by the reform of 1971, which suggested that they should assume responsibility for the administration of community health, in order to achieve the best health gains for the population. Today, public health doctors and their multiprofessional teams (public health nurses, environmental health experts, social workers) cooperate frequently with a wide range of sectors such as environment, employment and work, agriculture, industry, commerce, education, social services and social insurance, non-governmental organisations, etc.

The most important institution for training and research in public health is the National School of Public Health (ENSP) in Lisbon. The School received a new identity and structure in 1971, moved into modern premises in 1976 and became a WHO collaborating centre for primary health care in the early 1980s. ENSP offers three core courses (public health, occupational medicine and hospital administration) in addition to seminars and several short courses.[20]

The National Institute of Health (INSA) created in 1971 is also a notable public health institution. Many departments of INSA have developed a great deal with regard to the epidemiological surveillance of transmissible diseases, environmental health control, nutrition and genetics. INSA is also the national public health reference centre.

The crisis period

From the mid-1980s to mid-1990s public health issues almost disappeared from the health policy agenda, in spite of public declarations to the contrary. 'Deregulation', 'market principles' and 'privatisation' were the keywords that influenced the policy decision-makers of that period. Public health doctors progressively lost their prestige and leadership in the NHS.

ENSP, the most prestigious centre for postgraduate training and research in public health, was in danger of closure in the early 1990s. Fortunately this situation was recently reversed and the School was integrated into the New University of Lisbon.

Public health seems to have regained political support after the political changes that occurred at the end of 1995. Portuguese public health experts and leaders face a huge task today, as public health resources, initiatives and efforts had been substantially disconnected and fragmented. There were, and still are, too many vertical national committees, commissions and councils established without effective coordination among them. The national infrastructure of public health had been running separately from those commissions and committees. The reactive principle that caused this situation seemed to have been the response: 'if there is a problem, a commission must be created'.

The present situation of public health

A new phase for public health and health promotion is beginning in Portugal. The current situation has strengths and weaknesses to take into account.

Some strengths

The universality of the National Health Service, together with the local primary care health centres already in place all over the country are major strengths of the system. This network of community-oriented health centres, with favourable conditions for multiprofessional and intersectoral cooperation, hand in hand with community participation at local levels, have great potential for future developments in supporting health promotion strategies in the country.

There are already important experiences of intersectoral cooperation in some 'Healthy Cities' projects, school health programmes relating to the control and prevention of drug addiction, and diverse initiatives for cancer and cardiovascular prevention.

The relatively long tradition of training and research in public health, the existence of well defined professional careers (public health; general practice/family medicine; hospital medicine; general nursing; public health nursing; etc.) and the reasonable standards of care in many services are also important potentialities to be explored and developed in the future.

In short, two major sources of strength must be highlighted: the network of local health centres and the system for training public health doctors.

Network of the health centres

The network of local health centres spans the country and is available to the entire population. The concept of a health centre is functional. Each health centre can integrate several buildings and primary care services. The size of each centre is linked to the demographics of the areas served. As a result, there is a wide range in sizes.

These centres have around 6,000 general practitioners/family doctors working in multiprofessional teams. Each person can choose his/her personal family doctor within the NHS. Family registration, the suggested method, is done by most people. Family doctors maintain patient lists, with an average size of 1,500 patients per list. Most of the lists are organised by family.

Services offered include: general practice/family medicine; PHC personalised nursing; home care and community nursing; family planning; maternal and child health; school health; dental health; occupational health (only in a few health centres); and environmental health. Some health centres also have clinical and/or public health laboratories and radiological services. A few health centres have physiotherapy services.

Some health centres, actually small community hospitals, have beds that were mostly inherited from the old local hospitals. This happens mainly in rural areas.

Some health centres also provide specialist consultations (paediatrics, gynaecology, obstetrics, cardiology, pneumology, dermatology, etc.) because they inherited such manpower from the old health insurance ambulatory clinics. Currently, under the

'Health Strategy for Portugal 1998–2002' specialists of hospitals cooperate with health centres as local consultants.

According to the intentions of the NHS, health promotion, prevention, treatment and some rehabilitation should be offered in a balanced way. However, treatment tends to get the most important share in time, attention and costs.

Until now health centres had neither managerial nor financial autonomy. This is expected to change in 1999, when health centres will begin to be responsible for running and controlling a prospective budget related to their population needs, expected institutional performance, outputs and some outcomes.

Training in public health medicine

One must complete a three year long post-graduate residency/vocational training programme in order to practice as a public health specialist doctor. The accreditation and certification of public health doctors is done by a joint committee (Government and College of Public Health of the Portuguese Medical Association). The residential training programme is based on the functions, activities and tasks of the Portuguese public health doctor. The first and the third year of training are rooted in apprenticeship and supervised practice of public health medicine in a health centre. During the second year the trainee attends the one-year post-graduate course in public health at the National School of Public Health. The trainers are selected among public health doctors working in health centres. Currently, there are around 500 public health specialist doctors in the country.

Some weaknesses

There are marked inequalities in health and in the use of health services. The fragmentation and the lack of coordination of resources, initiatives and efforts to address public health problems has caused many redundancies and inefficiencies.

One of the main problems of the health care system has been the accumulation of functions within the National Health Service: it is the provider, the purchaser and undertakes the regulatory functions. This means that the Ministry of Health and their central, regional and local institutions constitute a vertical, bureaucratic and hierarchical structure of command and control that distributes resources and provides care, simultaneously. Patients, citizens and taxpayers have not had appropriate influence in decision-making concerning allocation of resources, investment or management of health care services. Community participation still is weak on all levels.

The lack of incentives to provide efficiency or quality in the public health care services (NHS) and the perverse relationship between the public and the private sector has created severe problems of access to primary and secondary care, with inappropriate overuse of emergency departments as access points where it is possible for patients to obtain some immediate answers to common health care problems.

A current trend is decentralisation through five Regional Health Administrations that already have considerable decision-making capacity, but have been burdened with considerable interference of too many central departments of the Ministry of Health. Norms and standards are settled at the central/national level but assessment of performance (efficiency and effectiveness) and follow up are relatively new activities to be learnt at all levels.

For many years, all NHS institutions received a fixed budget and all professionals received a fixed salary, without any incentives to achieve effective outcomes. Management indicators were mainly of inputs. Outputs were rarely related to the inputs. Effectiveness and final outcomes of provision or utilisation of health care are still weakly addressed.

To promote community participation, the law has established formal consultative community councils for health centres and hospitals, but they have not been very effective. Nevertheless, there are notable and impressive examples of formal and informal interrelationships between some health centres and their communities. The same can be said about intersectoral cooperation. This depends mainly on individual energy and the motivation of some exceptional leaders.

Prevention, health promotion and the health care reform

An explicit health policy is presently stated in the '*Health Strategy for Portugal 1998–2002*'.[6] The main elements of the current health policy and health care reform are:

(a) The citizens and the population as the central focus of the strategy;

(b) Priority setting for prevention, health promotion and defined health gains to be achieved;

(c) Development of 'local health systems' (population-based and health gains oriented) as a level of planning and coordination of health care and public health interventions – each 'local health system' involves several health centres, hospital care, other public and private health care institutions and partners for health in a defined geodemographic area;

(d) Development of five regional agencies for contracting/commissioning on a prospective basis, with hospitals, health centres and other health care institutions, taking into account the above and including community participation;

(e) Experimental models for organisation and remuneration of GPs and of other health care providers;

(f) New organisation and internal management for hospitals ('integrated responsibility centres') promoting internal commissioning between the managers of the hospital as a whole and the leaders of the operational clinical departments;

(g) Management and financial autonomy of community health centres in order to make them responsible and accountable to the contracting regional agencies.

Among the main tasks of the regional contracting agencies is one of identifying and meeting the health needs of communities. One of the potential expected benefits of these developments is to put health before health care and to introduce greater flexibility and adaptability into public sector management. A greater responsiveness to patients and to citizens' expectations and preferences is also expected to balance the traditional predominance of professional interests and influence.

An increasing number of governmental bodies and non-governmental organisations are devoting efforts and resources to address the main health problems. Some of the plans, programmes or projects are clearly intersectoral. The media are now devoting increasing attention to health matters because it has become a mainstream issue.

Several international health intervention programmes have representatives and activities in Portugal. The Healthy Cities programme is well established in Amadora (a city close to Lisbon) and eight more cities are working, in cooperation with their local health services, to follow the framework of this international project. The CINDI (Countrywide Integrated Noncommunicable Diseases Intervention) programme also inspired preventive activities in Setúbal and Lisbon. At national level 'DiabCare' is a good example of an integrated disease management programme aiming at improving health outcomes for the diabetic patients. New projects for health promotion and disease management contracting at regional and local levels are currently under study, namely for a new vaccination plan, lifestyle issues, asthma and stroke and ischaemic coronary disease, among others.

Recently, the EU legislation has had a considerable influence on the national legislation and initiatives in health.

There are a great number of 'health intervention areas', with national coordinating bodies and variable levels of development and implementation at the local level.[21] They can be organised in four groups:

Lifecycle phase and family health The national plan for immunisations at different ages; family planning; maternal and child health; health of the elderly; minorities and deprived groups;

Health determinants Promotion of active life; food and nutrition; tobacco; alcohol; drugs);

Specific health problems Tuberculosis; HIV/AIDS and other transmissible diseases; mental health problems; diabetes mellitus; cardiovascular diseases; cancer; disabilities, accidents;

Environment Healthy city projects; environmental health; occupational health and work safety; school health and the network of health promoting schools.

Several health-related projects and activities involve different ministries, in close cooperation with the Ministry of Health (Figure 2).

Figure 2

Examples of health-related shared responsibilities between different ministries

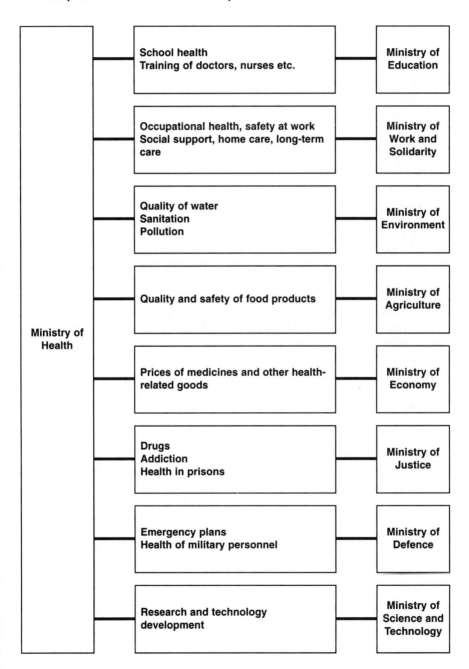

Occupational health is mainly the responsibility of companies. Each company must organise its own services or buy occupational health care from the private or the public sector. Small companies can request the support of the NHS local health centres to accomplish their occupational health obligations. However, there is a shortage of occupational health professionals, both in the NHS as well as in the private sector, to meet the legal requirements.

There have been some actions, both by the State and NGOs, to address social and health care needs of migrants and ethnic minorities, namely people from Africa and East Timor. There is not yet a global comprehensive policy to address this problem.

A new type of migrant population consists of people from northern European countries, some of them retired, who move on a temporary or permanent basis to the southern regions of Portugal.

Data and information

Most data and information are collected at local level, by doctors (obligatory notifications in some cases) and other health care professionals of the NHS, in the local health centres and hospitals. Apart from this routine data collection, there are multiple and separate initiatives collecting information on morbidity and use of health services. HIV/AIDS has a voluntary/confidential notification system. There is a National Inquiry on Health for self-reported morbidity, utilisation and family expenses in health care.[22] A GP Sentinel Network and the Regional Cancer Registers are examples of those initiatives.[23-26] In 1998 a National Observatory for Health (ONSA) was implemented to permanently monitor the Portuguese population's health status and its main determinants.

Trends and conclusion

Work is being done to achieve, through participatory measures, more explicit health policies and public health strategies at national and regional levels. At the same time there is an emphasis on the development of coordinating mechanisms concerning public health, health promotion interventions and activities in order to counteract the extreme fragmentation and absence of coordination of resources in the past. The goal is to put into practice the health policies and public health strategies previously defined.

The Ministry of Health is presently committed to substantially increasing accessibility to primary and secondary care and to developing a 'citizen-centred' culture in the NHS, by improving communication and encouraging new organisation of the services of GPs/family doctors.

Decentralization is also a main trend in the Portuguese health care system. The implementation of administrative and financial autonomy and responsibility at the local level in primary health care centres and the development of the role of purchaser/agency of citizens as a separate function of the health administration within the NHS, go hand in hand with the development of new methods of financing health services based on the needs of defined populations. The purchaser/agencies are beginning to be responsible for the allocation of resources to the different NHS institutions (hospitals and health centres) based on the institutions' explicit achievements in productivity, efficiency and quality. Performance based assessments will follow, focused on outputs and results.

Based on experience since the reform of 1971, and considering the present situation in Portugal and the EU, some perspectives seem to be emerging for the future, such as the development of patient-centred approaches with a permanent focus on changing health problems, health care needs and expectations of the population. This will necessitate the development of partnership with patients – directly at local level – as well as through consumers and other similar organisations. The involvement of local communities and participation of the population must be considered as a key for partnership for health.

In a context of new social challenges and limited resources, the expression of concrete health policies conductive to a broad national consensus for responsibility and action for health in the country requires appropriate priority setting practices, including efforts to identify causes and possible strategies to reduce inequities in health.

The implementation of cost-containment policies through several measures, including new organisational and financial arrangements, combined with decentralisation leading to financial and administrative autonomy of primary health care, must accompany the concern with outcomes management and technology assessment. The above measures shall profit from exchanges with other EU countries, especially concerning evidence of effectiveness of specific interventions (preventive, health promotion, therapeutic, etc.).

References

1. Ministério da Saúde – DGS. *Portugal – Saúde 1996*. Lisboa: Direcção-Geral da Saúde, 1998.

2. INE (Instituto Nacional de Estatística). *Statistical Yearbook of Portugal*. Lisboa: INE, 1998.

3. OECD. *Portugal 1997–1998 – Special Features: Health Reform; Creating Employment*. Paris: OECD Economic Surveys, 1998 and *OECD Health Data 1998*. (CD Rom) Paris: OECD, 1998.

4. Ferrera M. *EC Citizens and Social Protection: Main Results from a Eurobarometer Survey*. Brussels: Commission of the European Communities, 1993.

5. Ramos V. O que deveria ser melhorado nos serviços públicos de saúde – Estudo de opinião, de base populacional, na Freguesia do Lumiar (Lisboa). *Arquivos do Instituto Nacional de Saúde* 1994/95;20–21:5–14.

6. Ministério da Saúde. *Saúde em Portugal – Uma Estratégia para o Virar do Século 1988–2002*. Lisboa: IGIF, 1998.

7. Pereira J. *Inequality in Health Care in Portugal: Evidence from the National Health Interview Survey.* York: University of York, 1988 (mimeo).

8. Pereira J, Giraldes R, Campos, AC. *Desigualdade e Saúde em Portugal.* Lisboa: IED, Caderno 19, 1991.

9. Giraldes M R. *Desigualdades Socioeconómicas e Seu Impacto na Saúde.* Lisboa: Editorial Estampa, 1996.

10. Pereira J. Horizontal equity in the delivery of health care in Portugal. *Revista Portuguesa de Saúde Pública* 1992;10(3):35–46.

11. Vaz AM, Simões JA, Costa RJ, Santana P. Desenvolvimento de um modelo de avaliação do estado de saúde das populações. *Revista Portuguesa de Saúde Pública* 1994;12(2):5–24.

12. Dias JA. Évora e Beja: vizinhos, mas ... diferentes! – gradientes na morbi-mortalidade e determinantes de risco a nível distrital. *Revista Portuguesa de Saúde Pública* 1994;13(3):33–48.

13. Giraldes MR, Ribeiro AC. Desigualdades sócio-económicas na mortalidade em Portugal no período 1980/1982 – 1990/1992. *Revista Portuguesa de Saúde Pública* 1995;13(4):5–28.

14. Hart JT. The inverse care law. *The Lancet* 1971;February 27;405–11.

15. World Health Organization. *WHO Global Health-for-All database.* Geneva, 1996.

16. Ferreira FG. *Política de Saúde em Portugal – Uma Experiência de Definição Legislativa e de Organização de Serviços de Saúde.* Lisboa, 1972.

17. Sampaio A, Campos AC. Serviços de saúde em Portugal – uma reflexão crítica. *O Médico* 1980;96(1517),489–502.

18. Gomes DS, Dias JL. *O Serviço Nacional de Saúde – Descrição Sumária do seu Desenvolvimento.* Lisboa: Direcção-Geral dos Cuidados de Saúde Primários, 1987.

19. Sakellarides C. Centros de saúde integrados: nova espécie de estereótipos ou instrumentos de desenvolvimento? *Revista Portuguesa de Clínica Geral* 1984;1:12–5.

20. Ferreira C. O Professor Arnaldo Sampaio e a Escola Nacional de Saúde Pública. Alguns momentos de história. In: *Livro de Homenagem ao Professor Arnaldo Sampaio*, pp. 15–19, Lisboa, 1980.

21. Ministério da Saúde – DGS. *A Saúde dos Portugueses.* Lisboa: Direcção-Geral da Saúde, 1997.

22. Ministério da Saúde – DEPS. *Inquérito Nacional de Saúde – 1995/96.* Lisboa: Departamento de Estudos e Planeamento da Saúde, 1997.

23. Miranda AC. *Incidência e Mortalidade – Registo Oncológico Regional Sul.* Lisboa: Centro de Lisboa do Instituto Português de Oncologia de Francisco Gentil, 1991.

24. Dias JA, Miranda AC. Tumores malignos das principais localizações em Portugal. *Revista Portuguesa de Saúde Pública* 1993;11(3):15–31.

25. Falcão JM. 'Médicos-Sentinela' – aplicações de um instrumento de medida de saúde. *Revista Portuguesa de Saúde Pública* 1993;11(3):45–58.

26. Coelho AM. A importância da vigilância epidemiológica no controle das doenças transmissíveis. *Revista Portuguesa de Saúde Pública* 1994;12(3):5–14.

15

Finnish Public Health Policy and Health Care in Transition

Arpo Aromaa

Introduction

In the late 1960s, international comparisons revealed that, despite high mortality and high perceived morbidity, the utilisation rates of ambulatory health care were low in Finland.[1] The high perceived morbidity coincided with low utilisation in the East and North, in remote areas and in lower socioeconomic groups.[2] Since then, a central aim has been to strengthen the provision for health care, which has increased considerably, and the population's health has greatly improved. After a period of centralised administration, Finnish health policy and health care have now entered a phase of decentralisation.

Country, population and government

The 5.1 million inhabitants live in a large country with many sparsely populated areas and small local communities. Finland is economically and socially highly developed. Employment in agriculture and forestry has declined from over 30 per cent to 7 per cent of the workforce, and employment in public services has increased to one third. The economic recession of the 1990s led to a high level of unemployment, which still in 1996 was around 16–17 per cent of the workforce, but by 1998 had declined to 10–12 per cent. The economy is improving but the recession has forced some reduction in the budget of social security and public services.

Owing to the ageing of the population, the need for health and social services is increasing. In 1995, 14.3 per cent of the population was aged 65 and over; the number of aged people increased by 44 per cent between 1975 and 1995 and a further 42 per cent increase is expected to occur during the next 20 years.

Finland has a tradition of local municipal self-government, which has been strengthened in recent years. It is the task of municipalities to provide services to their inhabitants. Central government formulates policies, prepares legislation and takes part in financing. The population size of the 455 municipalities varies by a factor of 100 and the smallest have about one thousand inhabitants. Their ability to provide services differs. However, all residents have similar rights to publicly provided services and benefits, and the duties of all municipalities are the same. A system of state subsidies reduces differences between municipalities' resources.

The state administrative structures are the elected President, Parliament, central government with its ministries, and the provinces. There used to be 12 provinces but the number was reduced to five in September 1997 following a complete reorganisation of state regional administration. Municipal administration is based on elected councils, which in turn elect the municipal government and committees such as the Social and Health Committee. Joint municipal activities are organised by regional administrative structures such as hospital districts.

For social security, additional central structures are in place. Much of the national social insurance is implemented by the Social Insurance Institution, for the Parliament is administratively responsible. Other obligatory parts of social security such as the earnings-related pension schemes are administered mostly by private insurance companies.

Public services are financed from income from general state taxes and municipal taxes. Both the state and the local municipalities levy taxes on income. There are separate additional payments by employees, the self-employed, employers and, lately, also by pensioners towards social security and social insurance.

Health in Finland

The following summary is based on recent analyses of the population's health.[3,4]

In the 1960s, Finland was known as a country with healthy children but very ill adults. Child health continues to be among the best in Europe and this has been attributed to free preventive care and health education offered to all expectant mothers and children. The single most important change over the past 25 years has been a considerable decline in mortality of the middle-aged and older population resulting mainly from a reduction of cardiovascular disease. For example, the decline in coronary heart disease mortality since the 1970s has been about 60 per cent. The life expectancy of Finnish men (72.1 years in 1993 and 72.8 years in 1994) is approaching the Nordic level and that of women (79.6 years in 1993 and 80.2 years in 1994) has reached it and is already above the European average.[5,6] Improved health has been ascribed to health promotion and disease prevention strategies as well as to improved access to medical care. Traffic accidents have been decreasing: the number of fatal road traffic accidents has decreased from 1,086 in 1973 to 484 in 1993. Smoking has declined in men. Food habits have improved. Intake of dairy fat and salt has decreased and consumption of vegetables and fruits has grown. Leisured physical activity has been increasing. Coverage of hypertension treatment has also been much improved. Infectious diseases have been very well controlled by childhood vaccinations, and by good hygiene. AIDS remains rare, which has partly been attributed to a control strategy based on health education.

On the other hand, cardiovascular diseases remain important public health problems. Musculo-skeletal disorders and mental problems are not declining. Allergic conditions and asthma are becoming more prevalent. Oral health of children has improved considerably but that of adults remains poor. The good dental health of children and young adults is in part attributable to free preventive dental care, and the poor dental health of older adults partly to under-utilisation of dental care. The continuing rather high prevalence of smoking among teenagers and smoking among middle-aged women remains a threat to future health. Obesity has been increasing in the 1980s. Alcohol-related mortality has been growing with increasing consumption since the 1970s. The changes in availability of alcohol brought about by Finland joining the European Union may result in further increases in consumption and endanger the health of teenagers and adults (see below). Drug abuse may become a more serious problem. Infectious diseases may spread with increasing travel. Many infectious diseases, almost non-existent in Finland, are prevalent in neighbouring Russia.

Although the overall level of health has improved, relative variations in health between regions and socio-economic groups have not diminished. The high level of unemployment is a new threat to public health. The main determinant of an increasing need for health services and social security is the ageing of the population.

Health care

A recent English language description of Finnish health care can be found in brochures published by the Ministry of Social Affairs and Health.[7] Health care provision and financing involve a combination of central direction and local self-government, and an interplay of public and private services. In the 1990s, a change of the planning and state subsidy system is leading to more decentralisation of planning and management of public services. Resources are being redirected from the hospital sector to community care, and there is a strong movement towards combining the administration and financing of health services and social services in the municipalities.

Health care provision, administration, and financing

All inhabitants are entitled to publicly provided health care, which is either free or subject to modest patient charges. All employed people are entitled to free occupational health care. Costs of medication and of private health care are covered in part by national sickness insurance. Most primary health care and almost all hospital care is provided by local municipalities (and their federations), occupational health care is provided by employers, and private health care by private doctors and medical institutions, of which a few have specialist level hospitals. About 72 per cent of ambulatory physician visits are to health centre doctors and the remainder are to doctors who are either in occupational care or in the private sector.

The public health care system provides non-specialist services in the community and specialist services mainly in regional and central hospitals, and the most specialised services in the five university central hospitals. In the private sector both non-specialist and specialist services are available. The patient has freedom of choice, but his out-of-pocket costs will be higher than in the public sector.

An overview of health care administration is presented in Figure 1, and health care providers and their tasks in Figure 2. The financing of health care and selected health-related obligatory insurance schemes are presented in Figures 3 and 4.

Publicly provided health care At the central government level, this is provided by the Ministry of Social Affairs and Health and several central agencies and research institutions. At the regional level, provincial governments participate in planning and supervise public and private health care. Specialist regional and central hospital services are provided by 21 hospital districts, which are federations of local municipalities. In local municipalities, administration consists of elected municipal councils, municipal government and social and health committees. The director of health care (now often of social and health care), and various medical directors are key persons. Municipal health care is financed by local taxes, by state subsidies from state tax revenue, and relatively modest co-payments by patients.

Occupational health care Employers are obliged to provide occupational health services, both preventive and curative, to their employees. Large employers have their own health services, but other employers buy these services from municipal health centres or from private medical institutions unless several employers run a joint facility. Employers pay the cost and receive a refund of 50 per cent of approved costs from the Social Insurance Institution (see below). Estimated coverage is about 90 per cent of employees.

Private health care Private doctors and medical institutions provide services and part of the cost is reimbursed to patients by sickness insurance.

Dental care Dental care for children (under 19 years of age) is provided by dentists employed in municipal health centres. Young adults (born 1956 or later) may obtain dental care from health centres or from the private sector and older adults from the private sector. Sickness insurance coverage is available only for young adults.

Pharmaceuticals Pharmaceuticals are sold by licensed private pharmacies and part of the cost of medication is reimbursed to the patient by sickness insurance.

Sickness insurance Sickness insurance covers the whole population.[8] It is financed by contributions from both employed and self-employed persons, pensioners and employers. The benefits include daily allowances and reimbursement of part of the following costs: costs of physician-prescribed medications, approved costs of occupational health

Figure 1
Central administration of health care in Finland

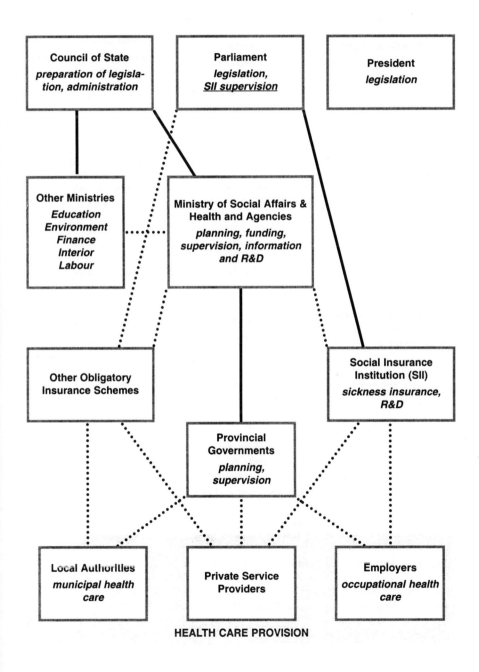

Figure 2
Health care providers and their tasks in Finland, 1996

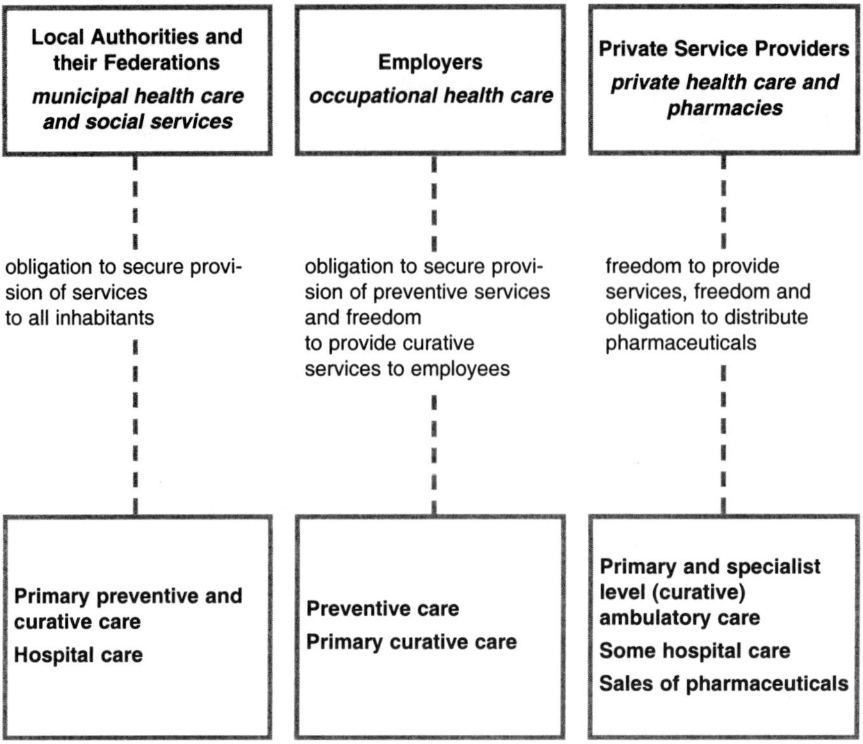

Local Authorities and their Federations *municipal health care and social services*	Employers *occupational health care*	Private Service Providers *private health care and pharmacies*
obligation to secure provision of services to all inhabitants	obligation to secure provision of preventive services and freedom to provide curative services to employees	freedom to provide services, freedom and obligation to distribute pharmaceuticals
Primary preventive and curative care **Hospital care**	**Preventive care** **Primary curative care**	**Primary and specialist level (curative) ambulatory care** **Some hospital care** **Sales of pharmaceuticals**

care to employers, travel costs incurred because of medical care, and costs for private doctor visits, examinations and treatments as well as the costs of private dental care for 'young adults' born in 1956 or later. Reimbursements for private care are calculated according to a scale of maximum fees proposed by the Social Insurance Institution and decided by the Ministry of Social Affairs and Health. There is co-payment by the patient, which for private medical care is high, i.e. about 65 per cent. It is lower for dental care, for laboratory examinations and for prescribed medicines.

Health care developments until the early 1990s

From the 1950s to the late 1980s the goal of health policy was to improve provision of and access to health care, and health care expanded. The numbers of health care personnel of working age increased sharply. As an example there were 5,583 doctors in 1973 and 9,793 in 1983.[9] Central government had strong directive powers with regard to

Figure 3
Financing of health care and related compensations schemes, 1998

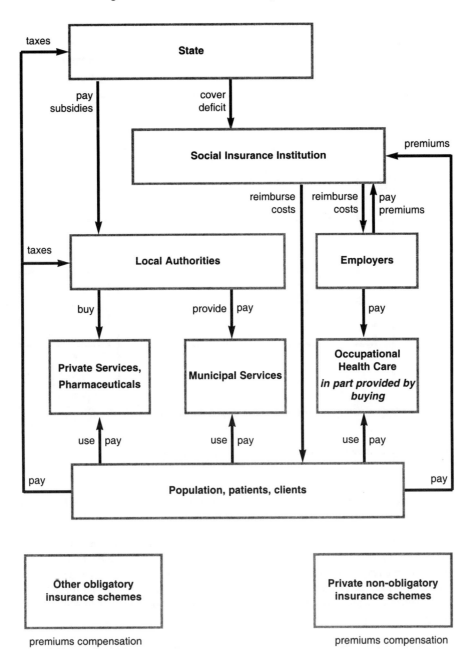

Figure 4

Obligatory insurance schemes compensating for health care costs, for income lost due to disability or for other losses in Finland, 1996

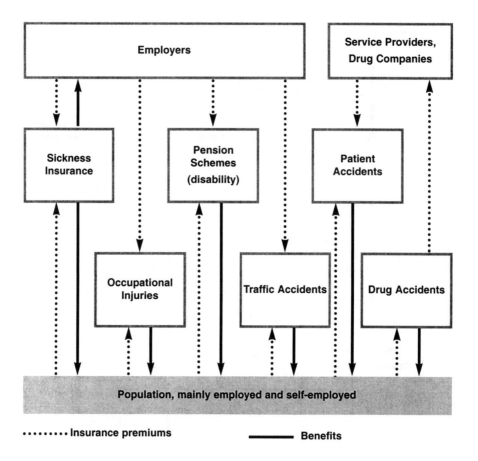

health care. The state subsidy was a percentage of approved costs and ranged from 30 to 70 per cent depending on the wealth of the municipality.

The specialist district and regional hospital system was set up to cover the whole country in the 1950s and 1960s. Federations of local municipalities, known as Hospital Districts, are responsible for operating these hospitals. There were separate institutions and districts for mental care, for the care of the mentally handicapped and for tuberculosis, but both mental care and tuberculosis care have since been integrated with general hospitals.

The sickness insurance scheme introduced in 1964[10] was intended to facilitate use of ambulatory health care by reducing the patient's costs – initially both in the private and public sectors. However, there was a lack of accessible ambulatory care in medical services.[2,11] Local primary care services expanded fast following the Public Health Act,[12] which took effect in 1972 and stipulated that municipalities had to provide primary care free of charge to their inhabitants. New health centres were built and new personnel employed giving preference to the more remote areas.

The introduction of occupational health care to all employees in 1979 and of sickness insurance coverage for dental care for young adults in 1986 led to further expansion.

Health care developments in the 1990s

The economic recession of the 1990s has necessitated savings at all levels. Co-payments have been increased and improvements which would create new costs have been postponed.

Restructuring and functional changes are in progress. The marked reduction in the number of hospital beds had already begun in the 1980s (Table 1). The relative share of community care has continued to grow and ambulatory care costs have increased to 30 per cent of total health care costs. Primary care in health centres has been evolving towards a more personalised care system, and in 1995 over 70 per cent of the population lived in municipalities where each inhabitant had been assigned his/her own doctor. However, in psychiatric care and in the care of the elderly, institutional care seems to have been reduced too fast, and corresponding community care has not yet been sufficiently developed.

Table 1
THE NUMBER OF HOSPITAL BEDS BY TYPE OF HOSPITAL

	1973	1983	1994
General hospitals	24,766	21,564	19,183
Health centre hospitals [a]	5,745	17,689	22,923
Psychiatric hospitals	19,671	18,533	7,708 [b]
Tuberculosis hospitals [c]	3,105	2,102	
Total	53,287	59,888	49,814

Notes:
a. the majority are nonspecialist longstay beds
b. contains in 1994 all psychiatric hospital beds regardless of type of hospital
c. annexed to general hospitals in 1987

Source: Health care registers of STAKES. Previously published in this form in Aromaa et al 1996.

In specialist hospitals, efficiency has been increasing as shown by a higher turnover and shorter stays. From 1988 to 1994 the number of treated patients increased by 6.6 per cent, the number of in-patient days was reduced by 19 per cent and the mean stay was shortened from 6.8 days to 5 days.[4,9] Short-stay surgery and day surgery have helped to bring about increased efficiency. Despite this, waiting lists have recently become longer for some operations indicating a relative shortage.

If the increasing needs for health service are to be met, restructuring must continue. This may mean further reduction in the provision of hospital in-patient services although the ageing population requires more care. There is a pressing need to improve home care and intermediate forms of care. The care processes within hospitals and between community and hospital need to be optimised, and municipalities should buy more services from each other and from private service providers. The reduction in the number of hospital beds is likely to continue. Finnish health care is in the middle of rapid changes and the outcome is not yet clear.

Health policy, preventive policies and actions

Health policy: aims and strategies

Central aims have been to improve provision of services and to ensure equal access to them. This was the background for the construction of the regional and central hospital network in the early 1960s, for the introduction of sickness insurance in 1964, and for the creation after 1972 of the network of local municipal health centres to provide free primary health care. Prevention of the major chronic diseases, in particular of coronary heart disease, has had a high priority since the 1970s. Alcohol abuse, smoking and other unhealthy habits were combated by health education and control mechanisms. Nation-wide screening for cervical cancer was carried out. Medical care programmes and guide-lines were prepared to control common public health problems.

The emphasis on equal access to care, on primary care and prevention were already part of the Finnish tradition when WHO introduced its 'Health for All' (HFA) programme. Its aims were well received and the HFA policy contained many of the principles which had been applied. Finland prepared an HFA programme of its own.[13] There has been criticism, however, that the HFA programme had little influence on local health care and little impact on any other health sector. An international evaluation of the progress toward HFA goals,[14] while applauding many of its aims was not without criticism.

Current health policy emphasises the HFA goals and a new version called the HFA cooperation programme has been developed.[15] It stresses the need to reduce health differences between socio-economic groups to improve the population's functional abil-ity, to improve services, to improve prevention and health promotion and to give prior-ity to primary care and community care over institutional care. It also calls for better participation of the population, for better health care management, for better education of personnel and for intersectoral cooperation.

The last central government five-year Plan for Municipal Social and Health Care reflects the above mentioned priority areas.[16] Health promotion and preventive social and health policy are important aims and so is equal access to high-quality care for all. Other goals are intersectoral cooperation, healthy housing and living environment, promoting the healthy development and growth of children and adolescents, promoting healthy living habits, and enhancing working ability and rehabilitation. Structural changes in the services are seen as essential prerequisites, which enable the care system to respond to growing needs. The plan has a target of at least 90 per cent of the population aged 75 or over living at home with support from organised community care. As of 1998, a new national health programme was under development.

The latest health specific document is the Government's Report on Public Health to the Parliament.[17] It was orginally planned that this document would be prepared every two years and it was expected to help focus discussion in Government and in Parliament on health and health policy. It was also intended to provide information for and to provoke discussion among various interest groups. The last report contains an analysis of health and health developments, which is based on reports on health[4] and health care.[18] It also contains chapters describing what various ministries have done and plan to do to promote health and to prevent health problems. It ends with a concluding chapter outlining future priority areas for health policy. It calls for support for local municipalities by using national expertise and improved health information systems.

Goals include equity in health and in access to health care, health promotion particularly in young age groups (teenagers, young adults), alleviation of the consequences of unemployment, combating alcohol and drug dependence, strengthening of health education, and improving the ageing population's functional ability.

By December 1996, the report was discussed in Parliament, particularly in the social and health committee. After this process a new decision was taken to produce an integrated social and health report at two-year intervals.

Prevention policies and actions

Preventive services are offered to the whole population free of charge. Participation rates for specific prevention programmes have always been high. Although the central government's powers to direct the actions of local municipalities reduced greatly after the 1980s (see below), equal provision can be ensured by legislation and by the five-year plans. Such tools have been used for example, to control tobacco smoking and to ensure that cancer screening is provided.

The following gives examples of some specific preventive actions. A more detailed account of many of the following has been recently published.[4]

Immunisations. Immunisations in childhood are provided free of charge by local health centres against diphtheria, whooping cough, tetanus, polio, measles, mumps, rubella, tuberculosis and haemophilus influenzae B. The national immunisation rates vary between 98 and 99 per cent for all of these.

Antenatal services. These are provided free of charge by local health centres, and mothers are expected to visit antenatal clinics early enough in pregnancy to be entitled to all maternity benefits. Attendance rates approach 100 per cent.

Breast cancer and cervical cancer screening. Regular free of charge screening by mammography is offered to all women aged 50 to 59 and cervical cancer screening for all aged 30 to 59. Participation exceeds 75 per cent. These screening programmes are financed by the local municipality which organises them in cooperation with the hospital district and with the Finnish Cancer Society.

Smoking. Health education, 'quit smoking' classes, high prices (taxation) and strict anti-smoking legislation are cornerstones for combating smoking. Advertising is prohibited. The legislation first introduced in 1976[19] was updated in 1995. It severely limits smoking both at work and indoors in public places, and also prohibits the sale of tobacco to under 18 year olds. For all practical purposes smoking indoors has disappeared other than in homes and restaurants.

Alcohol and drug abuse. Health education and control of availability, high prices (taxation) on alcohol and banning advertising have been cornerstones of the policy. Alcohol production and distribution were a State monopoly. The situation changed after Finland joined the European Union in 1995. Alcohol advertising is allowed, prices are falling, and availability is increasing. Finland has retained the State distribution monopoly and wants to continue to limit private imports and to maintain a high price policy, but within a few years availability and prices of alcohol are likely to approach the general European Union level. It is likely that alcohol use and the consequent health problems will increase but there is no defined new strategy for combating these problems.

There are also early signs of a worsening narcotics problem. It is likely that stricter control measures to limit illegal imports and distribution will be introduced.

Diet. The main activities have been recommendations by the National Food and Nutrition Council, health education and preventive programmes concerning for example, coronary heart disease and hypertension. The production of low fat and low salt products has been encouraged, and requirements for the declaration of contents on packages have been introduced. Large scale catering services, mostly those providing school meals, meals at the work place and in institutions, covering 75 per cent of the population are subject to national dietary recommendations.

Chronic disease control. National strategies for hypertension control were developed in the 1970s (last up-dated in the 1990s), and for coronary heart disease control in the 1980s. Recommendations have also been issued for lipid lowering, for asthma control, and for the control of musculo-skeletal disorders. The strategies and guidelines have been developed by expert groups or committees, which have been appointed by the Ministry of Social Affairs and Health, by one of its agencies, by a large patient organisation, or by professional organisations. It is likely that this problem-centred approach, which was strong in the 1970s, will regain popularity.

AIDS. AIDS control has relied heavily on comprehensive health education, which starts early in schools, and on free anonymous HIV testing. The AIDS situation is much better than in most countries in Europe. Between 1980 and 1995 there have only been 725 AIDS cases.[20]

Road traffic accidents. The strategy has been developed by Parliamentary traffic committees. Actions have included structural measures (roads, separating heavy and light traffic, speed limits etc.), obligatory safety equipment (seat belts, helmets), better education and traffic regulations with strict control of adherence as well as strict control of drunk driving. In the past 20 years the number of fatal accidents has been reduced by half and is now (under 500 deaths in 1993) at roughly the Nordic level.

Environment. A national programme for environmental health is currently being prepared jointly by the Ministries of Environment and Social Affairs and Health. The need remains for continuous control of the spread of infectious diseases through food and water by hygienic measures as well as to ensure safety of food and water. Other important environmental health problems stem from the quality of indoor air, the effects of traffic and energy production on outdoor air, and the pollution of water in some areas. Mould due to moisture in buildings is a widespread problem. Lead pollution has practically disappeared, since only unleaded petrol is available.

Inequality. There is a growing concern about health inequalities between regions and between socio-economic groups. These relative differences have not been reduced although the general level of health has greatly improved. With the exception of service provision, there is a lack of practical measures which could be adopted to reduce health differences. Although discussion is concerned with health inequalities, health policy continues to stress equal access to health care. A research-based programme has been launched with the final goal of determining new ways to reduce these differences. In the spring of 1996, the Academy of Finland supported by the Ministry of Social Affairs and Health set up a working group to prepare an action programme for research on differences between population groups in health and well being. Special earmarked research funding has been made available for the years 1998 to 2000.

Planning, administration, finance and budgeting

The planning processes in the public sector differ from those in occupational health care and the private sector and are changing. Some structures related to planning and decision-making at the central level are presented in Figure 5 overleaf and comparable schematic information for the local (and regional) level is provided by Figure 6.

During the period of expansion of health care provision, legislation and direction from central government were important tools, backed by detailed resource allocation. Investments, the numbers and categories of personnel and the total yearly costs were centrally controlled. The effective levers were the rotating five-year plans and the state subsidy system, whereby only accepted functions and investments qualified for state

Figure 5

Planning and decision-making in health and health care in Finland, national level

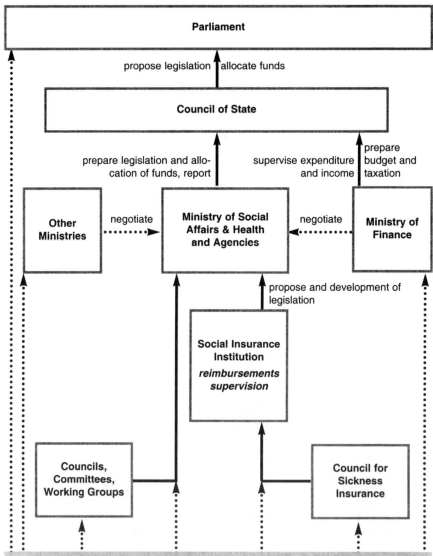

Figure 6
Planning and decision-making in municipal health and health care at regional and local levels in Finland, 1998

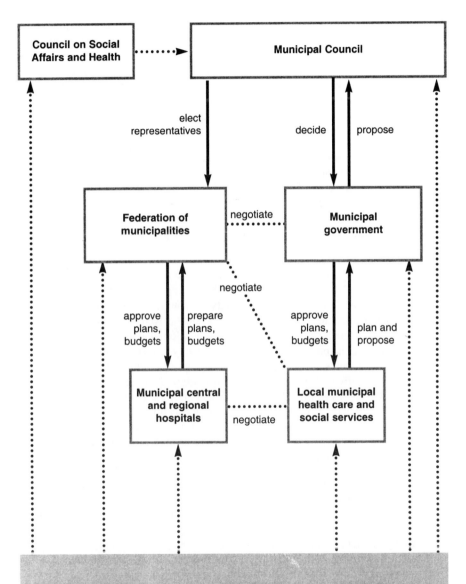

subsidy. The central health agency, the National Board of Health, also issued directives concerning the contents of services.

During the 1990s, the roles of local municipalities and the central government have changed. New legislation concerning planning of social and health care and state subsidies took effect in 1993.[21] The autonomy of local municipalities in deciding their priorities and services has been greatly strengthened. The central government's remaining methods for influencing health policy and service provision are setting general goals, controlling large investments, the total amount of state subsidies and, if need be, using legislation to prescribe that certain tasks and programmes be carried out all over the country. The Public Health Act[12] is a good example. It defines the duties of municipalities as providing preventive services and necessary (basic) non-specialist and specialist medical care to all inhabitants.

The central government-prepared five-year plans deal with both social and health services. They set priorities and list 'large' approved investment projects (over FIM 25 million or approximately EUR 4,205,000), which entitle the local municipality to receive a state subsidy. Smaller (FIM 2–25 million or approximately EUR 336,365–4,205,000) investment projects are approved after preparation by the provincial government. The separate subsidies for investments cover 25 per cent to 50 per cent of their total cost.

The state subsidy system for running costs has been changed from reimbursing a proportion (30 per cent to 70 per cent) of the incurred costs to a system of block grants, which are based on estimated need. The block grants are now for social and health services, and may soon include the state subsidy for education as well. The amount of the state subsidy for health care is separately calculated using a formula, which takes into account the size of the population, the area of the municipality, age structure and mortality. In 1996, the basic amounts per person in different age groups were the following: age 0–6 years FIM 1,163/EUR 196, 7–64 years FIM 1,097/EUR 185, 65–74 years FIM 2,724/EUR 458 and 75+ FIM 4,374/EUR 736, and these are adjusted by using the other factors of the formula.[15] However, the municipality may divide the block grant funds to social and health care as it chooses as long as it fulfils its service provision duties. At the same time, the administration and the budgets of municipal social and health services are being merged.

Owing to the big deficit of the State economy, there is a trend towards reducing the total amount of state subsidies to local communities. The budgetary process involves preparation by the Ministry of Social Affairs and Health and negotiations with the Ministry of Exchequer followed by an agreement on the budget proposal by Government and approval by Parliament. Other decisive detailed planning and budgetary processes take place in the local municipality (community care) and in the interplay of municipalities with the hospital districts (specialist-level hospital care). Some big municipalities run their own specialist-level hospital services and the allocation of resources (and patients) between their own hospital(s) and the district hospital creates continuous tension. Decision-making is a two-stage process with negotiation and proposals by the municipal government and approval by the elected council. Negotiation in hospital districts concerns the hospital's functions and budget, which are approved by municipal representatives and are dependent on the budgets and plans of their respective local municipalities which pick up the bill.

The role of health professionals, mostly municipal medical directors, is central at the local level. This situation may be changing towards health administrators (with a background in social services) particularly with the ongoing change to joint social and health care administrations. In the provincial governments public health matters are handled by health professionals (such as 'province doctors'). In hospital districts management powers rest with the directors of the hospital districts, often medical doctors, and medical directors of the hospitals.

The local municipalities (and their health professionals) are seen as purchasers of services on behalf of patients. In most parts of the country their main supplier is the central hospital but the municipality is free to buy elsewhere (such as other hospitals or the private sector). However, it is not easy to introduce a market model to a health care system, which is based on regionalisation and public provision of services.

Occupational health care. The need for approval by the Social Insurance Institution, which pays the 50 per cent refund for occupational health care, has been used to create guidelines, which give much weight to prevention and early rehabilitation. Actual planning and budgeting is handled by the employers, who are constrained by legal and refunding requirements and their own financial resources. Trade unions and employers' organisations negotiate agreements which influence the content of occupational health care.

Private sector. The private sector operates on market principles, and planning and budgeting follow corresponding rules. The central government and the Social Insurance Institutions influence private sector services and pricing mainly through the reimbursement scheme i.e. by setting the level of reimbursable fees and by including services (and pharmaceuticals) in the reimbursement scheme or excluding them from it. Only the costs of medically sound examinations and treatments of illness are reimbursable, and this principle is reflected in guidelines.

Health policy decisions and setting of priorities

Policy

Health policy decisions at the central level are made mainly by central government and influenced by the other parties involved. Among them are the municipalities' central organisation, provincial governments, the large patient organisations and other interest groups, professional organisations, employers' organisations and trade unions, and the Social Insurance Institution. Evidence based evaluation of health policy and health outcomes plays an important part in the process.

Interest groups such as patient organisations do not have any official role in formulating health policy and priorities. However, they function as pressure groups and are important channels e.g. of health education and service provision. Interest groups have often been involved in programme planning and current health strategy documents stress the need to cooperate with them. Examples of influential patient organisations include the Heart Association, the Cancer Society, the Diabetes Association and the Mental Health Society. A plan has been established which sets up a Public Health Council with representation from interest groups.

In specialist-level hospital care, policy is influenced by hospital district administrations and by the larger more influential member municipalities of the district. At the local level, the health professionals and other management of social and health care influence policy and decision-making in the preparatory phase, but final decision-making is in the hands of local government, the elected social and health committee and the elected council.

Priorities

Priorities at the national level are determined during the planning processes and incorporated into strategies and the five-year plans. Service priorities are set locally and at the district level but the central government may give guidance and, as a last resort, issue directives (legislation) and sometimes separate funding. This has resulted in the high priority given to health promotion, prevention and equitable access to health care. The only population group which has been given preference over others is armed forces veterans, who have special arrangements for rehabilitation and reimbursable dental care.

Priorities for individual patients are decided by their doctors. However, mainly owing to the expenditure involved, local municipalities have recently become much more interested in controlling, for example, referral to hospitals and hospital use. So far, all doctors can refer their patients, although in many municipalities referrals by health centre doctors are controlled by a chief medical officer.

Prompted by the economic recession and international examples of priority setting, an advisory working group has been set up to make recommendations concerning priority setting.[22] Its report deals with the process of making choices and the values affecting them. The report also presents ethical, economic and administrative issues related to making choices. However, it does not offer lists for prioritising diseases, treatments, individuals or groups. Thus, there has not been and is no official priority listing. In both the public sector and in the reimbursements of sickness insurance, priority is given to medically sound examinations and treatments, which are necessary because of illness.

The reason for excluding services or for allowing waiting lists is based mainly on lack of resources to cater for all possible demands and on rational use of the existing resources. However, until now it has been possible to meet practically all medically sound care needs. Unfortunately, waiting lists for some types of operative care have grown recently. Cosmetic surgery is not available in the public sector and not reimbursable in the private sector. Alternative medicine is another example. *In vitro* fertilisation has been available to a limited extent in the public sector and is available and reimbursable in the private sector. Some types of elective surgery are only available in the public sector from a waiting list and may be obtained more quickly privately, but reimbursement is quite low. Dental care for older adults is only available in the private sector but not reimbursed. The same goes for expensive dental prosthetic treatments and for dental treatments which are deemed cosmetic. Major surgical procedures such as hip prostheses or coronary by-pass surgery are available both in the public and in the private sector.

Use of public services is somewhat limited by public resources and that of private services by the relatively low level of reimbursement of user charges. However, currently, virtually all of the need for major surgery is being met. Examination of the effects of the savings and cuts of the 1990s has led many to conclude that these have hit hardest psychiatric patients, those with alcohol-related problems and mentally handicapped patients, but scientifically valid evaluations have not been carried out. In the future, shortage of funds may create new pressures for deciding about priorities politically and some media-led discussion about the need for explicit priority setting has taken place recently.

Patients' rights

All inhabitants are entitled to necessary care, but within the limits of resources available. The Act on the Status and Rights of the Patient[23] provides that the patient's agreement must be obtained for treatment and that all relevant information must be given to the patient. It also provides for submission of complaints. Obligatory insurance for patient injuries and injuries caused by medicines provides for financial compensation regardless of any error, negligence or carelessness, and is an important safeguard for patients.

Role of public health, health information and research

At the central level and in provincial governments there are doctors and other health professionals specialising in administration and public health matters. Monitoring and evaluation is carried out by public health professionals in the central agencies and research institutes. However, at the local level, public health is integrated into service provision. The local municipalities' health professionals, generally doctors but also nurses, have a central responsibility for the planning and administration of public health activities. Preventive services and immunisation, health education and screening are all integrated parts of primary health care and its clinical services. In practice, much of the responsibility lies with the medical director of each health centre, although in larger cities several doctors and nurses may concentrate on public health and administration. Some of the medical directors of health centres may be public health specialists, but the rule is that they are general practice specialists. Public health has little direct influence on clinical services and its role is essentially limited to hospital services. The regional responsibilities of hospitals are carried out by hospital districts and the key profession-

als are their directors and medical directors. Generally they are not public health specialists. In December 1996, public health as a medical specialty was threatened by a
proposal from a Ministry of Education working group to harmonise medical specialties
with those adopted in the European Union and to reduce their number. However, following joint efforts by University Departments of Public Health, the Public Health Doctors'
Association and the Ministry for Social Affairs and Health, the specialty now remains.

Health information

The back-up for local planning of preventive services is central support. For infectious
disease control this is provided by the National Public Health Institute (KTL). KTL also
attempts to improve national health monitoring and offers advice on prevention with
regard to chronic non-communicable diseases. The Institute of Occupational Health has
a corresponding role in occupational health. National monitoring of health care is
provided by the National Research and Development Centre for Welfare and Health
(STAKES), which also runs an online database containing municipality level health and
health care data. The Social Insurance Institution monitors especially the private sector
and occupational health care.

Efforts are being made to improve analysis, presentation and interpretation of existing
statistical and survey data on health as well as on a long-term plan to create a comprehensive system of health monitoring. Despite a good statistical basis, there is currently
a lack of information on, for example, musculo-skeletal disorders, mental disorders and
functional limitations. The development process has been initiated by publishing the
first comprehensive report on the population's health,[4] which is intended to become a
regular publication timed to coincide with the Government's Public Health Report to
Parliament. The other background document for the Government's report is the report
on health care[17] first published in 1995.

Public health research

Public health research to support decision-making is being carried out by Agencies and
Research Institutes, some of which are subordinate to the Ministry of Social Affairs and
Health. Important institutions are KTL, STAKES, the Institute of Occupational Health
(IOH), and the Social Insurance Institution's Research and Development Unit as well as
specialised institutions such as the Cancer Registry. Other institutions carrying out
public health research are university departments of public health and of social sciences.

Conclusions

Many principles applied in Finnish health policy are in line with those of the WHO's
'Health for All' policy. For a long time, emphasis has been put on increasing the provision of health care, especially on primary care, and on enabling equal access to health
care. Preventive activities including the prevention of major chronic conditions have
also been important. The centrally directed policies of the 1960s, 1970s and 1980s have
been successful when judged on the basis of increased and more equitable utilisation of

health care. Moreover, health improved considerably. The 1980s and 1990s have led to some shifts in health policy. Key issues now are restructuring and improved efficiency of services, development of community care, a combination of specific prevention and more general health promotion, and an increase in intersectoral cooperation. The economic recession of the 1990s has forced changes which have increased the efficiency of health care. The need for services is increasing because of the ageing of the population. There are some negative health developments and some emerging threats. There are also indications that the savings on health care have caused some negative effects, including overburdening of health care personnel. It is essential to continue a health policy, which gives high priority to health promotion and prevention as well as to the provision of accessible community care.

Future needs cannot be met unless restructuring of the health services continues. This may also require additional resources which can probably be made available only if economic growth continues. Finnish health care is undergoing major changes and the planning and budgeting mechanisms have shifted from central direction to decentralised local planning and decision-making. It is not yet clear what the long term effects of decentralisation will be. What is clear, however, is that future developments can only be directed by better information. Therefore, central agencies must give more emphasis to national evaluation and planning based on high quality health information and public health research, and to the provision of information and expertise in support of local health policy and planning.

References

1. Kohn R, White KLM, (eds.) *Health Care, an International Study.* London: Oxford University Press, 1976.

2. Purola T, Kalimo E, Nyman K. *Health Services Use and Health Status under National Sickness Insurance.* Helsinki: Publications of the Social Insurance Institution, Finland, A:11, 1974.

3. Aromaa A. Finn's health and health care seen in a European perspective. *Finnish Medical Journal* 1994; Special Edition No. 3:1623–38 (Original Finnish language version: Suom Laakaril 1994;49:1623–38).

4. Aromaa A, Koskinen S, Huttunen J (eds.) *Suomalaisten Terveys 1996.* Kansanterveyslaitos, Sosiaali ja terveysministerio, Helsinki, 1996. (*Health in Finland 1996,* in Finnish, to be published in English as an updated vesion in 1998).

5. WHO. *World Health Statistics Annual 1993.* Geneva; WHO, 1994.

6. WHO. *World Health Statistics Annual 1994.* Geneva: WHO, 1995.

7   Ministry of Social Affairs and Health. *Health Care in Finland.* (Brochures 1996:1) Helsinki, 1996.

8. *Statistical yearbook of the Social Insurance Institution, Finland, 1994.* Helsinki,1995.

9. STAKES. *The central register of health care personnel* (published and unpublished data). Helsinki, 1996.

10. Sairausvakuutuslaki 4.7. 1963/364, sairausvakuutusasetus 1.11.1963/473 (Sickness Insurance Act).

11. Aromaa A. Health surveys in the planning and implementation of sickness insurance in Finland. In: *The Role of Research in Social Security. Studies and Research No. 25.* Geneva: International Social Security Association,1988:65–84.

12. Kansanterveyslaki 28.1.1972/66 (Public Health Act).

13. Ministry of Social Affairs and Health. *Health for All by the Year 2000. The Finnish National Strategy.* Helsinki, 1987.

14. WHO. *Terveytta kaikille ohjelma Suomessa.* WHO:n terveyspolitiikan arviointi. Maailman terveysjarjesto, Euroopan aluetoimisto, Koopenhamina 1991 (Evaluation of the Health for All programme in Finland, in Finnish).

15. Ministry of Social Affairs and Health. *Terveytta kaikille vuoteen 2000.* Uudistettu yhteistyoohjelma. Sosiaali ja terveysministerion julkaisuja 1993:2, Helsinki, 1993. (The updated Health for All programme).

16. Kunnallisen sosiaali ja terveydenhuollon tavoitteet ja toimintaperiaatteet. *Valtakunnallinen suunnitelma sosiaali ja terveydenhuollon jarjestamisesta vuosina 1996–1999.* Helsinki, 1995. (*The Finnish Government's plan for social and health care for the years 1996–1999,* in Finnish).

17. The Council of State of Finland. *Public Health Report.* Finland. Helsinki, 1996.

18. Uusitalo H, Konttinen M, Staff M (eds.) Sosiaali ja terveydenhuollon palvelukatsaus. STAKES, Raportteja 173, Jyvaskyla 1995 (A review of the situation in the social and health services 1995, in Finnish).

19. Laki toimenpiteista tupakoinnin vahentamiseksi 13.8.1976/693 (Antismoking Act, last updated 1995).

20. KTL (The National Public Health Institute). *National Infectious Disease Register and Surveillance System,* 1996. (published and unpublished data).

21. Laki sosiaali ja terveydenhuollon suunnittelusta ja valtionosuudesta 3.8.1992/733 (Act on Planning and State Subsidies in Social and Health Care).

22. National Research and Development Centre for Welfare and Health (STAKES). *From Values to Choices. Report of the working group on health care prioritisation.* Helsinki, 1995.

23. Laki potilaan asemasta ja oikeuksista 17.8.1992/785 (Act on the Status and Rights of Patients).

16

Public Health and Priority Setting in Sweden

Johan Calltorp

The structure and characteristics of the health services system

One of the most important characteristics of the Swedish health care system is that it is overwhelmingly public in regard to financing, ownership of health care facilities, policy planning and control.[1] Among the five Nordic countries, with great similarities between them, Sweden has the most public provision (around 90 per cent in all areas).[2] The main units responsible for both financing and delivery of health services are the county councils that cover defined geographical areas with local elected political boards. By law, they have a responsibility to plan and provide health services for the entire population along the whole spectrum from preventive to curative services. Successive changes of the health law during recent decades have put a stronger emphasis on integrated approaches between the different activities to enhance and restore health. The present law is radical in adopting WHO's 'Health for All' aims in giving a 'right to citizens' to be able to achieve a healthy life.[3] The county councils are responsible for putting this ideology into practice. A strong emphasis in general policies is also placed on intersectoral cooperation and planning at different levels in society. This is enhanced by the relatively large public sector within Swedish society – a circumstance that from another perspective, that of economic integration in Europe, is seen as a problem.

Financing of the health services system is closely linked to the county councils' right to levy taxes. At the moment around 80 per cent of health financing comes through this mechanism. Except for a relatively insignificant amount from patient fees (around 1.5 per cent) the rest of the financing is derived from Government contributions allocated to the county councils mainly according to a per capita formula.[1] Tax raising powers give the Swedish county councils a stronger and more independent position towards the central Government than seems to be the case for example with the local health authorities in Britain.

The Government contributions to the county councils have both decreased in relative size over time and have also changed in character. Twenty years ago they were typically directed towards different sectors of the health services system. Some were linked to development of primary care initiatives, some were directed towards out-patients and specific sectors, e.g. psychiatry etc. Much of the Government financing was directed towards health policies to achieve innovation and change within the sector and to introduce preventive measures into public health. The development towards block allocations was part of a process where the roles of central Government and county councils became more clear-cut. The county councils now plan and provide health services, and they do it with an integrated population perspective. The national Government has the role of setting overall rules and giving guidance, supervision and control, emphasising the character of a national health care system with divergence within acceptable limits.

Previously, the Government actually ran parts of the system; psychiatric care (until 1968) and the primary care system with district doctors (*'provinsialläkare'*) and nurses (until 1972). The Government also financed and administered two teaching hospitals (Karolinska Hospital in Stockholm and Uppsala Academic Hospital until 1980). The same was the case for some rehabilitation and tuberculosis hospitals.

The health service facilities are structured and planned throughout the country in a very comprehensive and remarkably similar way. It is typically a four-level system with primary care facilities at the base (primary care physicians, district nurses and some specialist out-patient services in one organisation). Smaller hospitals (around five different medical specialities and some hundred beds) form the basis of in-patient services within each county council area. In each county council a multi-specialism hospital (15–20 medical specialities and up to 800 beds) takes the role as the main hospital.

An important element in the system is the regional structure for planning and delivery of highly specialised services. This idea arrived quite early in Sweden compared with other European countries. As early as the late 1950s, a master plan was adopted dividing Sweden into a number of so-called medical regions for the most specialised services.[4] A national law requires the county councils to cooperate in this way (typically four to five county councils jointly form a region). Joint financial agreements govern how a tertiary care (regional) hospital is financed. The regional hospitals are thus the most highly specialised units in the country covering all established medical specialties. This cooperation between the county councils to maintain and finance highly specialised care has gradually evolved to include many aspects. In the most advanced regions, the cooperation between the county councils is broken down into planning and work division within each medical specialty and linked to protocols for care and professional agreements regarding what type of patients and conditions should be treated at the different functional levels. Rotation schemes for doctors under training is another example of planning and cooperation activities linked to the regional structure. The six medical faculties in Sweden are linked to the regional hospitals in respective cities and form centres of excellence and nuclei for future development.

Until now, the Swedish health care system has been very comprehensive and the system components have been developed and linked to each other in a similar way all over the 26 county councils. This is remarkable given the great formal freedom that is inherent in a decentralised system where the county councils by law are given the obligation to plan and provide all health services. They have the power of tax collectors and there are local elected health politicians (these are the two major differences to the system in the United Kingdom which in other aspects has very similar structural features). There are two main explanations for this paradoxical homogeneity. One is the long-term national planning tradition that has been guiding health policies during the whole post-war era. Another is the tradition of consensus politics.[5] Although the county councils have had their formal freedom, they have been linked to a national planning system that has created this homogeneity.

National health insurance was introduced by law in 1955 and replaced the earlier voluntary insurance arrangements. The national compulsory insurance gives the legal right to health care for residents in Sweden, and the responsibility to plan and deliver the services according to both individual and population needs is given to the county councils. Some quite distinct phases can be distinguished in the development after the mid 1950s.[6] During the 1960s, there was a big hospital and facilities construction period. The Swedish economy was remarkably strong in that phase, the health and social sectors were prioritised and became centrepieces in the construction of the strong welfare society (the concept 'welfare society' – in Swedish '*folkhem*' – had already been coined in the mid 1930s). During this period the Swedish health system developed its emphasis on in-patient services and on hospital beds and there was a relative decline in the earlier quite strong primary care system. The strong economy, the idea of the welfare society and a general belief in biomedical and technical solutions to create welfare helped produce the basic characteristics of the system as we still see it today. Although technocratic, in its basic approaches, the system also had an early emphasis on intersectoral cooperation and an understanding of how health is produced by a combination of individual, social and medical factors.

The 1970s became the big planning era when functional levels in the system became imprinted in the structure. The regional structure was consolidated. A medical manpower planning system[7] was developed with the overall aim of balancing supply and demand of manpower, but also with ambitious attempts to direct the physicians both geographically and in the different medical specialties according to long-range plans (towards a 'planning horizon'). This machinery where national authorities both cooperated with and tried to direct the county councils could be described as perhaps the best example of the cooperative forces or 'consensus politics' that have been so important in shaping the Swedish system.[8] An important condition for this far-reaching planning was that physicians had been working on a totally salaried basis since 1970 (the so called '7-crown reform') with defined working hours. This is still the case but what has happened inbetween is a development of a relatively generous compensation scheme in free time for physicians' working hours on call and at night. This has somewhat distorted manpower planning and projections and considerably delayed the creation of a physician's surplus which did not emerge until the early 1990s.

In terms of health planning, the 1980s could best be described as a structural consolidation period when the major expansion was over. An interest and focus was placed on how different parts of the system were interacting and a population and public health perspective was emphasised in the different national health plans.[9] Ambitious wide ranging plans were drawn up for totally transferring psychiatric and geriatric services to out-patient care and a steady policy emphasis was put on strengthening primary care. Gradually, primary care regained some of its earlier position and status, and that was possible since the health economy was still increasing. Cost containment has actually shaped health policy since the early 1980s, although Sweden tried to escape the harsh realities longer than other countries and to avoid strong constraints.

Recent health policy developments

Table 1 below provides a survey of the major trends in health reforms in the Swedish system in recent years.

Table 1
Phases of cost containment measures since 1982:

Less capital investment, general saving campaigns, wage freezes (during 1980s)
Personnel reductions (1990 onwards)
Transfer of long-term geriatric care to municipalities (1992)
Transfer of parts of psychiatric services to municipalities (1994)

Purchaser provider split 1991–1994
Approximately half the county councils adopted this strategy, no uniform arrangements. Continuation and development of the system in some county councils at present.

Hospital mergers, fusion and integration processes from 1995 onwards
A wave of mergers and integration processes started in 1995. They are not uniform over the whole country, they include two or more hospitals or whole health care areas. The macro structural changes are followed by micro organisational change.

Until the beginning of the 1980s, Sweden allocated a steadily increasing proportion of its GDP to health care services; 1982 marked the top year in this respect with 9.7 per cent of GDP spent on health services.[1] Since 1982, there has been a steady decrease, with at present around 7.5 per cent devoted to health services. These official OECD-statistics do not however tell the whole story and somewhat exaggerate the constraints achieved. Some major reforms have transferred parts of what was earlier defined as medical care to the social sector. In 1982, a reform transferred what was defined as non-medical geriatric and long-term care from county councils to municipalities, and in 1994 parts of the psychiatric care and care for the mentally handicapped was moved in the same way. Money was reallocated in relation to the activities, and this accounts for about 1.5 per cent of the decrease of the GDP-percentage between 1982 and 1995. But even after this is taken into account, there has been a decrease of resources in real terms and Sweden seems, jointly with Ireland, to have one of the most pronounced and successful cost containment programmes at the system level among the European countries.[10]

This strong economic pressure has resulted in successive waves of containment policies – first, during the 1980s general savings campaigns, wage freezes and decreased budgets for investment in equipment and buildings.[11] Around 1990, pressure had accumulated in the system partly because no major structural reforms had been undertaken during the first cost containment phases in the 1980s. Relative over-capacity of hospital beds and imbalances between different segments of the system had emerged. The search for new organisational methods and the need for a more flexible and responsive health care system led to a rapid introduction of the purchaser-provider split in some of the county councils around 1990.[11] This was also stimulated by the emergence of this method in the UK and the general interest in market solutions at that time in several European countries. The purchaser-provider split was not introduced all over the system in a uniform way as in the UK. It may be typical for the quite decentralised structure of Swedish health care that different county councils organised the internal market in their own way. The movement among the county councils during the beginning of the 1990s to come up with their own 'model' (the 'Stockholm model', the 'Bohus model', the 'Dala model') for the internal market underlines a further move towards decentralised authority. The growing relative proportion of the health budget financed through county council taxation enhances this.

In the mid- and late 1990s the health policy picture is dominated by resource problems for the health sector, following on the cost containment policies, and the urgent need to adjust the delivery structure to the resources available. This has started off a wave of rapid structural changes of mainly horizontal integration in the system.[11] Decisions about hospital mergers have been taken in many county councils, mainly bilateral arrangements between two hospitals but in some cases formations of county council-wide new structures covering in one organisation all in-patient services for a whole county council population (200 – 500,000 population). In two regions of Sweden (south and west) the different county councils are in the process of abandoning the old borders and forming a new structure covering the whole region (around 1.5 million population). Many actors see the future development of the health services area in the greater economic units and the concept of 'regions' within the European Community.

To summarise, a rapid organisational restructuring is going on in the health sector as a direct result of economic pressure. Other pressures like demographic trends and the rapid spread of new medical technology innovations also play a role in speeding up the need for change.

An interesting aspect of these changes is that the traditional homogeneity within the country is in some ways breaking up. The main new initiatives for structural changes and innovation are taken at the county council level and they are taken in different ways in different parts of the country. Local conditions, traditions and circumstances play a new and more important role for the development of the health system than before. By tradition, Sweden has generally been a centrally governed country and this tradition strongly shaped the system during the big expansion phase between 1950 and 1980.[5,8] Structural planning, hospital building and manpower planning were performed according to national plans and central policy principles. The centre was strong, had many policy planning tools and could effectively balance the county councils' strength based on local taxation power and locally elected health politicians. The development of forceful local innovation and structural changes that go in different directions thus seems to be creating a diversity which is a new tradition within the Swedish health sector and in society as a whole.

During recent years, this development has been striking and quite rapid. Centralising efforts now appear in the health system as a reaction towards the new local innovative power and it seems unclear where and when a stable balance point will emerge. The rapid phase of structural change is new for the health sector as such and this has created turmoil that makes it difficult to predict how and when power within the system will stabilise.

Public health functions

During the first half of the 20th Century public health had its base in the function of the district physician (*'provinsialläkare'*). They were assigned to defined geographical areas all over the country and were employed by the Government according to a tradition several hundred years old.[12] Their task was to treat the sick in the traditional role as primary care doctors but they also had surveillance functions regarding general public health and hygiene. They wrote annual public health reports. These reports give today's readers an illuminating picture of the health situation and general living conditions. This function and documentation is the traditional base for the development of modern public health in Sweden. Here are also found some of the roots of mechanisms that have been important for forming the welfare society in integrating medical and social perspectives at the local level as well as linkages to population records.[13]

The system of district physicians declined in the 1960s and the specialised part of the health care system became predominant (hospitals and medical specialists). This change in the structure is an interesting and still somewhat puzzling aspect of Swedish health politics.[8] After the second world war, the economic conditions were present to give the means rapidly to construct the public and tax financed welfare society planned in the 1930s. Health care became a centrepiece in this, and a blend of ideas regarding technocratic planning, belief in progress through specialisation and biomedical development seem to have been guiding forces. The local political power within the county councils also provided motives for the building of many hospitals and the structure thus shifted rapidly from an out-patient public health dominated system to a system where hospitals and specialists became dominant. Still today Sweden is different from many countries in Europe in that the primary care functions are weaker than the hospital specialist system.[14]

Parallel to this decline in the public health functions of the district physicians, specialised public health functions started to emerge in each county council and munic- ipality. This was first seen through an establishment of medical officers (*'länsläkare'*), one within each county council, with the task of collecting public health statistics and with some supervision tasks. Then followed development of central departments of public health within the county councils (*'samhällsmedicinska enheter'*). They do not have a uniform staffing or function throughout the country but generally they are staffed by physicians with a specialisation in social medicine or public health as well as epidemiologists and social science trained health workers. These have, at present, the major task in trying to link epidemiological data to planning of services within the county council machinery and trying to influence policy towards preventive aspects.

A key tool in these activities are public health reports (*'folkhälsorapporter'*) that are made mostly locally by collecting epidemiological data, household surveys and other data from registries that describe the population's health, as well as social conditions. There are also national public health reports issued by the National Board of Health and Social Welfare every third year. The first national report was published in 1987[15] following a decision by Parliament in the middle 1980s to collect more comprehensive data on the development of the population's health. The reports contain in principle the following parts:

- description of health resources and their distribution
- overview of activities performed
- living conditions
- health risks
- disease and illness patterns

This series of public health reports could be described as a revival of the old reports on the population's health by the district physicians. They mark a clear ambition by the Government (all parts of the political spectrum) to make public health aspects central in policy. During the last ten years, several governmental documents have dealt with public health policy and underlined the goals regarding equity, intersectional cooperation and successive shifts towards preventive strategies. Sweden early on endorsed the WHO 'Health for All' programme. Through the relatively strong epidemiological research undertaken both at county council and national levels helped by the long tradition of registries and personal identification numbers, a constant watch is kept on health trends and improvements in health (especially length of life).

Regarding the distribution of health and illness between the social classes, there was steady progress towards a more equitable pattern until around 1990, and after that a standstill but no significant move backwards. There are differences among the Nordic countries: Denmark, with an earlier economic recession than Sweden, has experienced widening health gaps and a less favourable health development overall.

Within the six university hospitals and medical schools (all combined with regional tertiary care hospitals) public health capacity is brought together in university departments of community medicine (or social medicine which is the term for the university discipline). The traditional focus in these departments is on epidemiological research, health services distribution according to needs, social class and other social aspects. Gradually, a broadening into general health services research (including health economics, medical sociology and management) is taking place within the university departments.

The number of physicians in public health medicine is relatively small, not more than around 100 (social medicine-trained). However, one should also include some physicians with primary care training and occupational medicine carrying out mainly traditional public health functions (in total around 300).

Nationally, the functions of planning and supervision in public health in Sweden lie with the National Board of Health and Welfare. Extensive data collection forms a backbone in the activities of the board. Public health policies are mainly formed within this agency.

Previously, the National Board of Health and Welfare had several specialised functions in respect of drug issues, health promotion and other specific public health areas. In 1992, a new national agency – the National Institute for Public Health ('*Folkhälsoinstitutet*') – was formed with the specific task of dealing at the national level with health promotion of all kinds. Resources for this were transferred from the National Board of Health and Welfare and from some sectoral organisations. There are also other sectoral research bodies like the National Environmental Institute and the National Psychosocial Worklife Institute. This decision-making structure is illustrated in Figure 1.

Targeted public health functions and programmes

There is a long tradition in Sweden of specific targeted programmes for prevention of important diseases and conditions within the health sector. The first of these were the early programmes for antenatal/maternity and child health preventive services. They were mainly linked to the obstetric/gynaecology departments and paediatric departments of hospitals and were staffed by specially trained nurses under the supervision of physicians. These programmes have generally been regarded as important for assuring early and good child health records besides support of mothers and young families.

An important aspect of these, and all social programmes and benefits in Sweden, is their universal character, covering the whole population with few or no barriers, such as fees. An important principle has also been that benefits in this area should be delivered uniformly to everybody concerned. There is no income level requirement for child benefits for example. In the present tight economic situation, discussions have also now begun about these principles and their practical application. For example, the routine child health examinations for all children at the age of four is being questioned with regard to value and resource use. This has led to heated debates because these

Figure 1
Decision-making process in the Swedish public health system

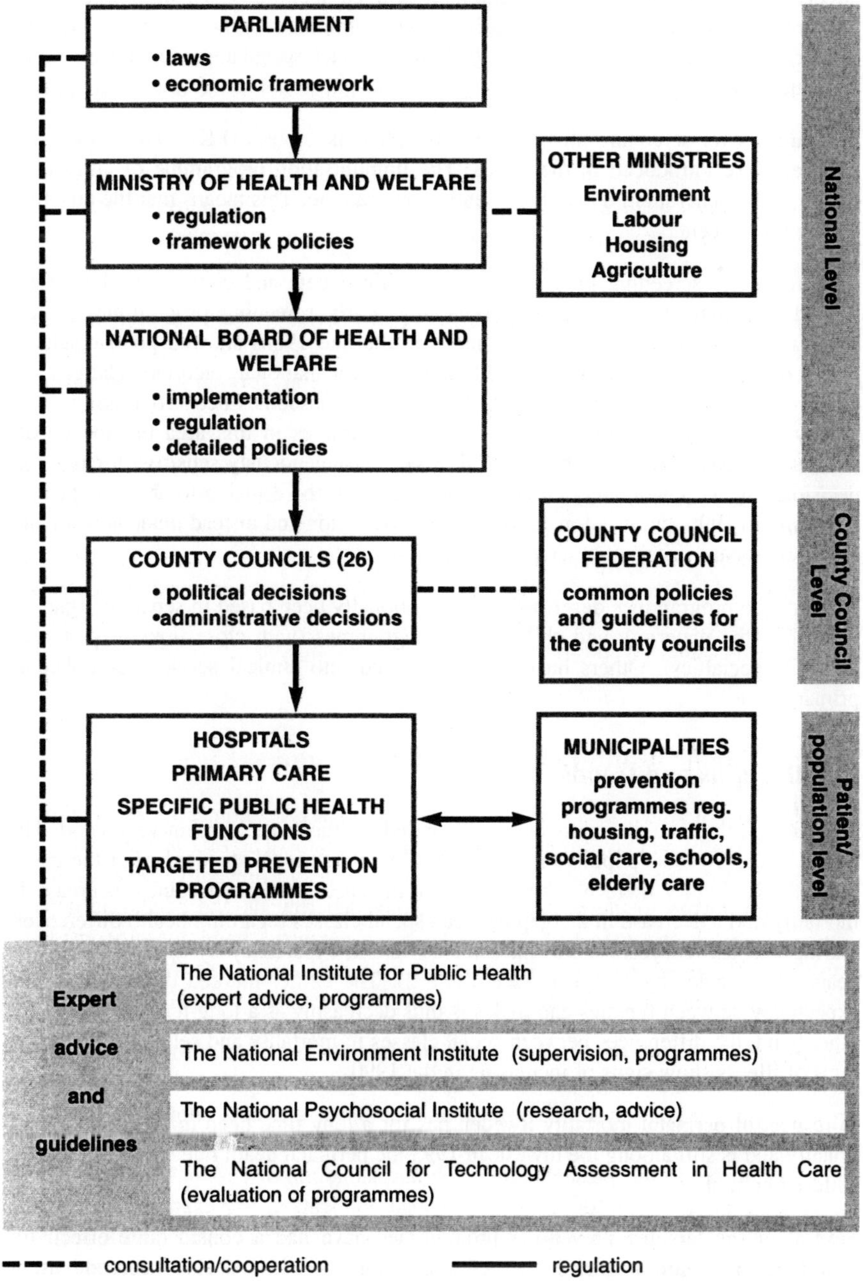

PARLIAMENT		
• laws		
• economic framework		

National Level

MINISTRY OF HEALTH AND WELFARE		OTHER MINISTRIES
• regulation		Environment
• framework policies		Labour
		Housing
		Agriculture

NATIONAL BOARD OF HEALTH AND WELFARE		
• implementation		
• regulation		
• detailed policies		

COUNTY COUNCILS (26)		COUNTY COUNCIL FEDERATION
• political decisions		common policies
•administrative decisions		and guidelines for
		the county councils

County Council Level

HOSPITALS PRIMARY CARE SPECIFIC PUBLIC HEALTH FUNCTIONS TARGETED PREVENTION PROGRAMMES		MUNICIPALITIES prevention programmes reg. housing, traffic, social care, schools, elderly care

Patient/ population level

Expert advice and guidelines

The National Institute for Public Health (expert advice, programmes)

The National Environment Institute (supervision, programmes)

The National Psychosocial Institute (research, advice)

The National Council for Technology Assessment in Health Care (evaluation of programmes)

— — — consultation/cooperation ———— regulation

programmes in a way symbolise the welfare state – both its large scale, uniformity and universality. The approach taken at the moment is to try to evaluate scientifically the effects of the different programmes and their detailed operations. Arguments have been put forward that resources could be redistributed within the programmes with somewhat less frequent general examinations of all children and a targeted approach towards those at greater risk.

Programmes for screening all new-borns for phenylketonuria (PKU) and some other diseases were introduced in the 1980s. The immunisation programme of children is linked to the general child health preventive programme. This means that the coverage is over 95 per cent.

With regard to screening programmes, a specific debate and controversy has arisen around radiological mammography screening. Early screening programmes with a scientific approach in two county councils in the late 1980s showed good results in terms of lives saved. This triggered demands for national recommendations for mammography screening, and a lively debate on this issue has been continuing. Most county councils have introduced screening programmes in this area but the debate has become more and more heated. This issue is tremendously sensitive for political decision-makers. One county council, Älvsborg, took the decision to abandon general screening in 1996, but was forced to cancel this decision and instead made adjustments to age-limits and criteria for screening selection.

Some of the programmes described have traditionally been based in separate organisations, like the maternity and child health programmes (with close links to particular medical specialties). Others have been integrated into clinical services or linked to primary care.

Health status and trends

Statistically, the overall results of the integrated welfare society seem very good. The health of the Swedish population is excellent by international standards. For the major part of this century there has been a steady increase in life expectancy, decrease in mortality and a decrease in the gap between social classes regarding health differences. During the last ten years males have increased life expectancy by approximately 2.5 years and females by 1.5 years (see Table 2). The earlier marked difference in life expectancy between females and males is thus decreasing as a long-term trend. On the other hand, the differences between social classes in mortality and self-reported symptoms of illness show signs of increasing in the 1990s.

In respect of perinatal mortality Sweden has for a long time been in the lead internationally and is still among the lowest. In 1993 the perinatal death rate was 4.8 per 1000 children born alive.

Several of the targeted prevention programmes have had a considerable effect, for example, with regard to smoking in the last ten years. Sweden has also recorded reason-

Table 2
Life expectancy at birth, at 50 years of age and at 65 years of age (1982–1997)

Year	At birth		At 50 years		At 65 years	
	Male	*Female*	*Male*	*Female*	*Male*	*Female*
1982	73.4	79.4	26.4	31.3	14.6	18.3
1985	73.8	79.7	26.6	31.6	14.7	18.5
1990	74.8	80.4	27.5	32.2	15.3	19.0
1992	75.4	80.8	27.8	32.4	15.6	19.3
1994	76.0	81.4	28.4	32.9	16.0	19.8
1996	76.5	81.5	28.6	33.0	16.1	19.7
1997	76.7	81.8	28.8	33.2	16.3	19.9

Source: National Statistical Bureau, SCB

ably low numbers of cases of HIV which might be attributed to control of drug abuse, a generally high level of education and the relatively small part of the population outside the reach of health information campaigns.

So far, no link has been found between the strongly enforced cost containment measures taken since the mid-1980s and unfavourable changes in health. Health indices still show a favourable development. There are signs that the steady decrease in health differences related to social class stopped at the beginning of the 1990s. However, this appears to be linked primarily to general economic and social policies and not to changes in the health systems, although since the mid-1990s there has been a growing debate about social barriers in the health system linked to increased co-payments. There is still no clear evidence of this point but it demonstrates important trends and issues to watch in future.

A very important aspect of the general social changes during the 1990s is the increasing level of unemployment (currently 8 per cent). By traditional Swedish standards this is perhaps the most important social change that will threaten the health of parts of the population.

Health policy decisions and priorities

The Swedish health care system has a public character in its tax financing, with political decision-making at county council level and the traditionally strong influence from national planning and supervising agencies. Despite this – or maybe linked to this –

there has also been a strong tradition of clinical freedom in decision-making about individual patients that is surprisingly only restricted to a small degree. Clinical freedom has been present to almost the same extent as for example in the UK, and over recent years to a considerably greater extent than in the United States. Decision-making has been guided by broad policy programmes either specific on diseases and conditions or for whole services. Guiding programmes are issued by the National Board of Health and Social Welfare, by medical specialists associations or by the supervising pharmaceutical agency. However, there has always been strong resistance towards letting national guiding programmes directly influence local clinical decision-making. An emphasis has therefore been put on developing local programmes and guidelines on the basis of national recommendations.

At present, this tradition of great clinical autonomy and independence in decision-making is slowly being circumscribed. The main factors behind this are the economic constraints described earlier, the general need for a health care system that is as rational as possible and efforts following from this to streamline medical practice through new management techniques. The harsh economic realities have provoked great interest in this area of new medical and administrative management. One of the key roles in running the system has been the function of the heads of clinics ('*Chefsöverläkare*'), normally a physician having a combined medical, economic and administrative responsibility for a clinic or a primary care centre. This post has been in place for about eight years and builds on a long tradition of physicians taking management responsibility. At present, with extensive cuts in the clinical budgets the inherent conflicts in these roles of having to take account both of economic interests and the medical interests of a population or a service have become more and more pronounced. These roles will evidently become increasingly controversial and it may be not so easy to recruit strong clinicians to these posts. Thus a new law from 1 January 1997 changed the mandatory requirement for a physician to take this combined post.

The whole area of clinical autonomy and independence will also become more and more problematic and there will presumably be a gradual development towards more guided medical practice. These developments follow international trends with the introduction of strong management and feed-back techniques in the clinical setting.[16] The separation of purchaser-provider in some county councils described earlier is an example of this. They have generally enhanced the search for new and more specific management methods in the clinical setting.

All priority decisions above the level of individual patients (services, specialties, structure within a county council) are taken by the county council political boards. The professional management within the county council has an important role in the decision-making process. At the regional level there are similar processes going on with both political and administrative as well as medical input from the respective county councils to facilitate cooperation. In the political decision-making process within the county councils an important consideration is to balance the system – that is both to prioritise between medical specialties and services as well as handle the geographical distribution of health resources. Politicians especially have to pay attention to how the use of services as well as the health level or sickness pattern is distributed in the population. Issues regarding population minorities and deprived groups are constantly on the political agenda.

An important input into the discussions on priorities and policy building in the whole health sector in recent years has been the reports from the Parliamentary Commission on Choices in Health Care. After several waves of public and media discussions about the resource needs for health services in the late 1980s, the Government appointed a commission for this task in the spring of 1992. The commission was composed of seven Members of Parliament representing the main political parties with nine expert advisers from areas of clinical medicine, health economics, health administration, law and ethics. The commission finished its work in March 1995 with a report entitled 'Priorities in health care – ethics, economy, implementation'.[17] The full text is available in English as well as the discussion document the commission presented in November 1993 with the title 'No easy choices'.[18]

In many ways this Swedish report on choices covers similar material to the national reports put forward in Norway (1987), The Netherlands (1992) and Finland (1994). The general outlook for health services with the gap between available resources and increasing demands is discussed in detail, as well as the interaction between the factors that will make the problem more acute in the years ahead.

Of special importance is the discussion in the report of the traditional goal of the health services system in Sweden to maintain and enhance an equitable society. The report emphasises that to maintain equity in access and outcome requires a balanced health system. The search for equitable allocation of resources and efficiency in methods used are key strategies in this direction.

The two most concrete proposals in the commission's report are the description of a so-called 'ethical platform', that is, key principles that should guide detailed decision-making in all parts of the system, and the description of priorities. The ethical platform contains the principle of human dignity, the principle of need and solidarity and the principle of cost-efficiency. The principles are described in this rank order and are supposed to override each other.

With regard to concrete advice to the health community to guide decision-making in more detail, the commission developed two lists of priorities. One is directed towards political and administrative areas (decisions on the aggregate level and for anonymous groups). The other is directed towards guiding clinical decision-making. The lists – which are quite similar in construction and content – define in broad terms different diagnostic and treatment conditions. The clinical list is as follows:

IA   Treatment of life-threatening acute diseases. Treatment of diseases which, if left untreated, will lead to permanent disability or premature death.

IB   Treatment of severe chronic diseases. Palliative terminal care. Care of persons with reduced autonomy.

II   Individualised prevention during contacts with medical services. Habilitation/reha-
bilitation etc. as defined in the Health and Medical Services Act.

III   Treatment of less severe acute and chronic diseases.

IV   Borderline cases.

V   Care for reasons other than disease or injury.

The commission's idea is that the lists should guide decision-makers in general terms, and be used in general discussions and deliberations within the health system. It gives its own judgement that group IB above receives insufficient resources by comparison with groups II and III. In annexes to the report, the commission discusses, in more detail, concrete examples and tries to place them in the grouping scheme. With regard to specific public health aspects, the commission explicitly places 'prevention having a documented effect' in group II on the list for political/administrative prioritisation. It underlines in discussion that prevention is a goal of long-term national health policy, but stresses that the preventive activities have to have documented benefit in order to be priorities. Preventive programmes have to be looked at individually in this respect.

The commission's report has been well received in Sweden and has been widely discussed. It has been regarded as a plea for a fair health system and an instrument in the fight to maintain the traditional values of equity and humanity in the Swedish 'model'. It has also been criticised for being too vague and general and there will presumably be calls for national decisions on a number of detailed issues where policies now tend to diverge between different county councils (for example regarding access to services such as in vitro fertilisation). It is too early to judge what concrete impact a general discussion and symbolic document like this can have.

Moreover, of great importance for judging the scene and discussion in Sweden is the fact that parallel to the national commission's work, there have been several local working groups on prioritisation in individual county councils. They have taken similar approaches to that of the national committee, but often their conclusions are more concrete and therefore easier to implement. In this context the national commission has mainly served the purpose of advocating general principles and values in the national debate and at the county level.

In late December 1996, after public consultation, the Government put forward a proposal to Parliament based on the Priorities Commission report.[19] It was proposed that the principles described in the report should be further underlined by Parliament as guiding health care decision-making. A formal strengthening of the health care law regarding distribution of resources according to need was proposed as well as a more pronounced respect for the equity and dignity of the individual patient. The concrete guiding principles for prioritising were adopted by the Government and approved by Parliament in spring 1997. The Government brought together the two different prioritising lists (for clinical and for administrative/political decision-making) into one, with four levels instead of the proposed five (level IV 'Borderline cases' was deleted). The

Government strongly underlined the need for research, follow-up and public discussion on how priorities are made in a more constrained health care situation. It proposed a special national committee for this task. A decision based on the proposal was approved by Parliament in spring 1997.

The new national government committee for priorities began its work in Spring 1998. It is composed of Members of Parliament, experts in the field and representatives of unions and patients' organisations. It has a three-year mandate, with the basic tasks of informing the public on parliamentary decisions concerning priorities, monitoring implementation of policies within county councils and making proposals for national action that is required.

Background data for policies and decisions

The Priorities Commission in Sweden and the associated debate has had the effect of underlining the need for reliable data to guide policy-making at both national and local levels as well as in clinical decision-making. It points out in a similar way as, for example, the Dutch priorities report[20] that data on effectiveness and efficiency of clinical interventions are the key to more rational decisions and policies. It is of equal importance to have reliable data at the population level regarding health, well-being and distribution of disease. The health services system needs these data to be able to plan activities and monitor the system's performance. The trend to separate the system into purchasers and providers has rapidly enhanced this need for data both on the population and technological levels. This search is worldwide and to an increasing extent international cooperation to share technology assessment information is developing effectively.[21]

In some important aspects Sweden has a solid tradition in this area. There is a long tradition of population records (since the 18th Century) and medical records that have been stored and maintained through the years. The use of personal identification numbers has helped epidemiology as well as clinical research. A system has been developed to collect clinical data in each county council and report to the regional and national level.

Several national registries of specific diseases and treatments have been built mainly through initiatives of medical specialties during the last ten years (for example the registry of hip replacements, all operations performed since 1979). There are 30 registries, and they are used to an increasing extent for technology assessment purposes as well as for local feed back for clinical quality assurance programmes. Interesting possibilities to use the excellent population records and link them more actively to planning of services and technology assessments are being explored for the future.

Conclusion

The Swedish health services system – in many ways a centrepiece and symbol for the welfare society – is in a situation of tension, as are all health systems in Europe. Cost containment has been especially stressed since the beginning of the 1980s because Sweden has had to adjust the size of the system to present economic conditions. This means both a decrease in real terms and a shifting of health resources for long-term care to the municipalities. Resulting from the economic pressure, the system has moved into a phase of rapid structural and organisational change. Awareness of the danger in this situation of increasing social inequities and differences both in access to health services and in actual outcome of the services is high.

The national Priorities Commission has put forward a document that underlines the importance of safeguarding the achievements regarding equity and solidarity that form a strong value base in Swedish society. The commission has also underlined the need to maintain a balanced system regarding prevention and treatment services in an economically tight situation. The Government has endorsed the commission's view and proposed that Parliament takes a decision based on the document's principles and a slightly modified version of the practical directives.

These directives are general, not detailed or binding for health practitioners and managers. Although the health community has a strong desire for concrete practical guidelines on priorities – the commission's report and governmental proposals based on it have been favourably received, which may reflect a need for general guidelines when a health system is undergoing change. Besides the national work of this kind, several county councils have developed their own more concrete and practical guidelines for priorities. These add to a new and interesting dimension of growing diversity in the Swedish health care and public health system.

The Swedish health system is in considerable and growing tension. It and the whole welfare society is confronting great challenges. The obvious challenge is to maintain as much as possible of universal and equitable provision when public resources are shrinking. Several technological and population trends are forcing the health system and society in general to move towards more diversity and individualism. Sweden has to strike a balance here and find workable definitions of equity in the new more open European situation and context. The openness to and influence of the European Community will affect all sectors of the society. At first glance health care and public health may not be affected much, but the indirect effect of policies in other areas could be considerable. This has already been seen, for example, in the traditional public health area of alcohol taxation and policy, where Sweden has fought for, and partly succeeded in, maintaining a restrictive policy. More areas will cause tensions like this in the future. A final important issue for further consideration is how Sweden can contribute to intersectoral practice and thinking.

References

1.   Calltorp J. The Swedish model under pressure – how to maintain equity and develop quality? *Assurance Health Care* 1989;1:13–22.
2.   Rohde T, Garpenby P, Häkkinen U, Mabeck CE, Vohlonen I. *Privat och offentlig insats*

i Nordens helsevesen (Private and public components in Nordic health care). Oslo: Gruppe for helsetjenesteforskning, Statens Institutt for folkehelse 1986 (Rapport 3/1986).

3. Swedish Governmental Proposal. Om hälso-och sjukvuardslag (Swedish health care law) Stockholm: 1981/82:97.

4. Swedish Governmental Proposal. Förslag till riktlinjer för regionsjukvärdens utbyggnad (Proposal to development of the regional health care system) Stockholm: 1960:159.

5. Anderson OW. *Health care: Can there be equity? The United States, Sweden and England*. New York: Wiley, 1972.

6. Calltorp J. *Priority setting and the decision-making process in health care. Some postwar characteristics of health policy in Sweden*. Uppsala: Department of Social Medicine, 1989 (thesis).

7. Calltorp J. Physician manpower politics in Sweden. *Health Policy* 1990;15:105–18.

8. Heidenheimer AJ, Elvander N (eds.) *The shaping of the Swedish health care system*. London: Croom Helm, 1980.

9. Swedish Committee report: *Hälso- och sjukvärd inför 90-talet (Health services towards the 1990s)*. Stockholm: Department of Health. SOU. 1984:39.

10. OECD Health data base. Paris: OECD, 1996.

11. Calltorp J. Swedish Experience with Fixed Regional Budgets. In: Schwartz FW, Glennerster H, Saltman RB (eds.) *Fixing Health Budgets; Experience from Europe and North America*. Chichester: Wiley, 1996.

12. Gustafsson RÅ. *Traditionernas ok Den svenska sjukvårdens organisering i historie-sociologiskt perspektiv (The burden of traditions. Swedish health care organisation in a historical sociological perspective)*. *Stockholm:* Esselte, 1987 (Ph.D. thesis).

13. Diderichsen F. Health sector reform and sustainability of the welfare state. *Health Policy*. 1995;32:141–53.

14. Culyer AJ. *Health Care and Health Care Finance in Sweden: The crisis that never was; the tensions that ever will be*. Stockholm: Studieförbundet Näringsliv och Samhälle, SNS. Occasional paper 33, 1991.

15. *Folkhälsorapport (National public health report)*. Stockholm: Socialstyrelsen redovisar, National Board of Health 1987:15.

16. Iglehart JK. The Struggle between Managed Care and Fee for Service Practice. *New England Journal of Medicine* 1994;331:63–7.

17. The Swedish Parliamentary Priorities Commission (final report). *Priorities in health care. Ethics, economy, implementation*. Stockholm: Department of Health. SOU. 1995:5.

18. The Swedish Parliamentary Priorities Commission (interim report). *No easy choices.* Stockholm: Department of Health. SOU. 1993:93.

19. Swedish Governmental Proposal. *Prioriteringar inom hälso- och sjukvärden (Priorities*

within health care). Stockholm: Department of Health. Prop 1996/97:60.

20. Government Committee on Choices in Healthcare. Ministry of Health, Welfare and Cultural Affairs. The Netherlands: Rijswijk, 1992.

21. Orleans M. The Cochrane Collaboration. Lessons for public health practice and evaluation. *Public Health Report* 1995;110:633–4.

17

Setting Public Health Priorities in the UK

Michael O'Brien

Introduction

This chapter uses the definition applied to public health by the report of the Committee of Inquiry into the future development of the Public Health function in England in 1988.[1] The report wrote of, 'the science and art of preventing disease, prolonging life and promoting health through organised efforts of society'. In 1957 a joint committee of the International Labour Office and the World Health Organisation crystallised a description of industrial health which can be paraphrased to develop the above definition of public health. Using this description as a basis it is suggested that Public Health should aim at:

- the promotion and maintenance of the highest degree of physical, mental and social functioning for all;

- the prevention among populations of departures from health caused by their circumstances;

- the protection of populations from risks resulting from factors in their environments adverse to health;

- the maintenance of populations in circumstances adapted to their physiological and psychological abilities;

- the restoration to health, where possible, and the maintenance of residual function in others, when there is ill health; and to summarise

- the adaptation of life to people and people to their lives.

This is a sophisticated expansion of the traditional triad of needs to protect the health of the public, namely security from disease, starvation and violence. It reflects the complexity of life in Europe at the end of the twentieth century.

Background

Social and economic changes in the British Isles prior to the eighteenth century created a situation ripe for industrial development. New sources of power, mechanisation and new methods of transport all combined to provide new health problems for the population. The effects of the new industrial life gradually led to organised attempts at easing the burden. Writing later about industrial conditions in the nineteenth century Hunter[2] stated that by 1850 the principle of interference by the legislature for the good of the population had been established.

Legislative contribution to the public health now extends to virtually every aspect of life. Most Departments of State are involved in some way and there is legislation which deals with the health aspects of recreation, education, occupation, housing, transport and the environment.

Public Health policy is considered here under the three broad headings of structure, process and outcome.

The political and managerial structures affecting the public health

National structures

(i) Government departments

Most Departments of State are involved in some aspects of public health policy although the lead position is held by the Department of Health (DH). DH is responsible for all health policy in England, including public health, and not simply for the National Health Service (NHS). The responsible elected government minister is the Secretary of State for Health. There are additional Ministers of State in support of the Secretary of State. Each carries a portfolio of work which contributes to the overall policy on health matters. The government which was elected in 1997 appointed a Minister with specific responsibility for Public Health. This was the first time that such an appointment has been made in the UK.

Civil service support to the Secretary of State includes a Chief Medical Officer (CMO) responsible for the coordination and provision of all professional health related advice to government. The CMO, although employed in DH is nevertheless the chief medical adviser to other government departments. Similar responsibilities are discharged by the Scottish, Welsh, and Northern Ireland Offices for their respective territories. Each has its own Minister of State and its own Chief Medical Officer. Figure 1 shows in schematic form the structure governing the health and social services in England. The typical health structure in a territorial government department is similar, except that they do not have Regional Offices. It is normal practice for the four government departments

Figure 1
Schematic structure of public health services in the UK, 1998

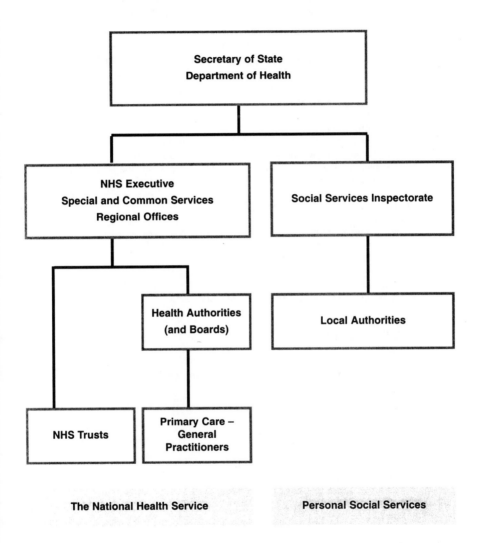

to act in harmony over matters of public health policy, and for DH to take the lead in international discussions on health policy. These arrangements might vary after the year 2000 when devolution of some governmental responsibilities to a Scottish Parliament and a Welsh Assembly take place.

Major components of health policy impinge on the work of other Departments of State. Their responsibilities are shown in Table 1. Evolving policy about the interaction of the environment and health is shared between six government departments in England and the three territorial Offices of State for Scotland, Wales and Northern Ireland.

Table 1

Allocation of responsibilities for public and environmental health between government departments

Department of Health (DH)
Public health
Health promotion
Health care services (The National Health Service)
Health effects of environmental microbiology and toxicology
Microbiological and toxicological safety of food, water and the environment
Communicable disease control

Department of the Environment (DoE)
Housing
Waste management
Environmental protection, air pollution and noise control
Water, sewage and sewage disposal
Building regulation
Health and safety at work
Effects of working practices on the general public

Department of Transport (DT)
Traffic-related pollution
Traffic accidents

Ministry of Agriculture, Fisheries and Food (MAFF)
Food composition, standards and labelling
Food science research
Pesticide and veterinary product safety
Control of products of animal origin
Animal health and welfare

Department of Trade and Industry (DTI)
Consumer protection

Home Office
Bylaws
Licensing
Administration of justice
Controlled drugs

Department for Education and Employment (DfEE)
Health of children and young people in primary, secondary and higher education

---

Adapted from: Department of the Environment and Department of Health. UK Environmental Health Action Plan: Consultation Draft. London, HMSO, 1995

The long tradition of cabinet collective responsibility means that there is an established method of ensuring coordination of policy across all these government departments. There is a Ministerial sub-committee on health strategy which brings together representatives of all government departments to discuss and coordinate views on policies affecting the public health which extend beyond the individual remit of any one department. It is advised by the CMO.

(ii) The National Health Service (NHS).

Within the DH there is the NHS Executive (NHSE) which has the specific responsibility for policy formulation, priority setting and oversight of the NHS. Civil service support to the NHS includes a Medical Director, who is one of the two Deputies to the Chief Medical Officer. The NHSE has a central office and eight regional offices through which its responsibilities are discharged. The National Health Service has major implications for both individual and community public health.

Details of expenditure in the UK, under a selection of headings which are relevant to public health, are set out in Table 2. Illustrative expenditure figures for England are set out in more detail in Table 3.

Table 2					
Government expenditure on public health related services, 1996–97 (£ million)					
Service	*England*	*Scotland*	*Wales*	*N. Ireland*	*Total*
Health and social services	40872	5225	2833	1603	50533
Housing	2944	575	300	248	4067
Other environmental services	7623	1222	708	358	9911
Social security	78288	9142	5478	3203	96111

Source: Public Expenditure: Statistical Analyses 1998–99. London, HM Treasury, 1998.

Table 3	
National Health and Personal Social Services Expenditure in England, 1996–97	
Service	*£ million (approx)*
Hospital and Community Health Services	23,877
Family Health Services	8,192
Centrally Managed Health Services	614
Department of Health Administration	292
Personal Social Services (provisional)	8,131
TOTAL	41.106

Source: Department of Health. The Government's Expenditure Plans 1998–99. London: HMSO, 1998.

81.5 per cent of the total NHS and Personal Social Services expenditure comes from general taxation. The balance is made up of a mixture of charges, capital receipts and a proportion of National Insurance.

The only clearly identified public health expenditure is £325 million of the centrally managed health services expenditure which supports the development of health strategy and some health promotional and allied activities.[3] The rest of public health expenditure is subsumed in the other budgets. Health Authority administration represents approximately 4 per cent of total hospital and community health services expenditure, of which Public Health expenditure is a fraction. Community Health services which represent the clinical component of public health activity take 15 per cent of total hospital and community health services expenditure.

(iii) Special and common services

Special Health Authorities and Boards have been established within the NHS. Each one has a nation-wide remit for a single aspect of the overall health services. Examples include the Health Education Authority (HEA) in England and the Health Education Board for Scotland (HEBS). The National Blood Authority deals with the collection and processing of blood for transfusion and the manufacture of blood products for therapeutic purposes in England.

Although not officially designated as a Special Health Authority, the Public Health Laboratory Service (PHLS) and its associated Communicable Diseases Surveillance Centre (CDSC), plays a vital role in the central coordination of the detection and control outbreaks of infection in England and Wales. The Scottish Centre for Infection and Environmental Health (SCIEH) plays a similar role in Scotland.

A recent development has been the establishment of the Environment Agency.[4] This is a national body set up, as part of the UK government response to the Second European Conference on Environment and Health, to take over and coordinate the responsibilities of several formerly separate organisations each of which dealt with a segment of environmental health and regulation. It is responsible for the enforcement of standards in the areas of water resources, pollution control, waste disposal and radiation.

It is proposed to establish a Food Standards Agency (FSA).[5] Legislative time has yet to be found so it unlikely that the FSA will be operational before 1999 at the earliest. Its purpose will be to separate responsibilities for consumer concerns from those of the producers to avoid the conflict of interest which is perceived to exist while both are managed by MAFF. It is expected to have a role in the control of outbreaks of foodborne infection. This means that the relationships between the FSA and health authorities, local government and the PHLS/CDSC will have to be carefully managed to avoid confusion and potential conflict.

(iv) Other bodies influencing public health policy at a national level

There are many other statutory and non-governmental bodies whose activities influence the public health. These include organisations representing the interests of health profes-sionals. Some are standing organisations statutorily established to advise government. The Standing Medical Advisory Committee and The Standing Nursing and Midwifery Committees are examples.

There are also Trade Unions (The British Medical Association) and charitable bodies (the Medical Royal Colleges and their Faculties) which seek to influence both policies and priorities.

Voluntary organisations, especially those which represent single issue lobbies, devote a considerable part of their efforts to affecting policy to favour their issues. There are prominent examples concerned with mental health matters, individual clinical condi-tions and with various aspects of disability.

The media frequently take up the themes of many of the lobby movements and apply pressure for policy change. Examples include sudden infant death syndrome and BSE. Media coverage of health and public health matters can have undesirable effects, for example reductions in vaccine uptake when unsubstantiated 'scare' stories are published.

Sub-national structures

(i) Health Authorities and Boards

Management of the NHS, including planning, priority setting and purchase of health and health care services is the responsibility of District Health Authorities (DHAs) (known as Health Boards (HBs) in Scotland (see Figure 1). The structure in Northern Ireland varies from the rest of the UK to the extent that Health and Personal Social Services are managed together in combined Health and Social Services Boards (HSSBs). There are approximately 120 DHAs and Boards in the UK.

DHA/Board members are divided into non-executive and executive directors. People are chosen for non executive positions to bring to NHS management a range of expertise from industry, commerce and public and voluntary services. The executives include a Director of Public Health (DPH) who is the chief professional adviser to the DHA.

Each Director of Public Health has a department which includes supporting staff. Departments vary in size but a typical example would have a Director plus three Consultants in Public Health Medicine, technical and administrative staff. The training of the Directors and Consultants in Public Health Medicine, which is similar in form to that of hospital specialists, takes four to five years and concentrates on the public health aspects of medical practice. The range of duties that they perform for the Health Authorities includes: health promotion, surveillance, needs assessment, planning, evaluation, disease control, teaching and research. Public Health Consultants make up most of the doctors employed by the Health Authorities. Former general practitioners are employed to assist with the development of primary care. All other NHS doctors are either employed in specialist roles by the NHS Trusts or are in general practice.

The major providers of health and health care services are general practitioners and NHS Trust Hospitals dealing with acute, community and mental health services. Minor providers include private sector hospitals and nursing homes.

(ii) Local authorities

Elected local government carries large scale responsibilities for services which have an impact on public health. Housing, education, many aspects of food hygiene, infection control, consumer protection, health and safety at work, environmental health and public health engineering are delegated to local authorities by the government departments mentioned above. Local authorities discharge their policy responsibilities through a committee system. Most authorities have environmental health committees, made up of elected councillors, to undertake the delegated tasks. The committees are supported by professional staff, including Environmental Health Officers, who play vital roles. Some of their responsibilities are shared with consumer protection control officials. Although, in theory, they have health promotional responsibilities there are so few of them that most of their time has to be devoted to enforcement duties. A complicating factor is that legal requirements vary between the four countries of the UK. For example the laws governing communicable disease control differ between England and Wales on the one hand and Scotland on the other. Both sets of legislation are out of date.

(iii) Other bodies affecting public health policy at a local level

Within the NHS the DH has set up Community Health Councils (CHCs). There is at least one for the area of each DHA. Their membership is drawn from representatives of local government, (one third) voluntary organisations (one half) and the balance from names submitted to the Secretary of State by NHSE Regional Offices. The remit of the CHCs is to comment on NHS services on behalf of the public and especially to represent local opinion when contentious policy matters are being discussed.

Processes affecting public health policy

National strategy

Public Health data are published annually, allowing both levels of and trends in mortality, avoidable deaths and life expectancy to be seen nationally and regionally.[6] In common with many other developed nations one of the matters of concern has been the growth in population, especially the increasing proportion of old people. It has been stated recently, however, that available evidence on population growth does not indicate unmanageable growth in demand on services.[7] By the late 1980s there was increasing concern about the funding and direction of public health policy and of the NHS. One of the most significant contributions to the public debate was about levels of health.[8] The government responded to the concern by starting a public consultation process in 1991.[9] Wide debate took place and comments on policy were received from many interested political and professional groups and from individual members of the public. At the conclusion of the process in 1992 the *Health of the Nation*[10] policy document was published. Although health in England is at its best ever levels, it is conceded that there is still room for improvement. For some time after its publication the *Health of the Nation* was the main source of public health policy and the driving force for action both in and out of the NHS. It set a range of targets for improvement in health and related measures to be achieved by the early years of the 21st century.

Similar Public Health policy statements were issued by each of the territorial offices of state representing Scotland, Wales and Northern Ireland. Each statement was broadly similar in content to the Health of the Nation, although there were differences to cater for local needs.

Early in 1998 the government published a consultation paper entitled *Our Healthier Nation*.[11] This is a forerunner to a new White Paper which will replace *The Health of the Nation* as the definitive health policy statement for England over the next few years. Once again similar Green Papers have been issued for Scotland, Wales and Northern Ireland. There is an intention to shift the balance within the NHS from hospital domination to a more evenly balanced provision of care. Behind every aspect of policy is a drive for increased efficiency so that more can be provided within the available resources. From time to time there are new policies to deal with emerging single issues, for example the government White Paper on drug misuse.[12]

Although the *Health of the Nation* has been the main driving force for improvements in the public health, other government policies contribute. For example Care in the Community has, for some years, been the preferred means of securing care for those with mental illness. Recently it has been called a failure and the government is now calling for improvements to the mental health services.[13] Continuing care for those who are old, demented or suffering the long term after effects of illness or accidents is shared between the NHS and local authority social services.

National tactics

DH has published aims and objectives.[14] These are:

- to reduce avoidable illness, disease and injury;
- to treat people in need quickly, effectively and on the basis of need alone;
- to enable people who are unable to perform essential activities of daily living to lead as full and normal lives as possible; and
- to maximise the social development of children within stable family settings.

NHSE has a Business Plan which is a set of ten priorities[15] to enable it to contribute to the fulfilment of the DH aims and objectives. These are:

- to promote implementation of the *Health of the Nation*;
- to improve the quality and responsiveness of services to patients;

- to maximise the NHS contribution to community care;
- to improve the effectiveness of mental health services;
- to develop a primary care led NHS;
- to secure cost effective prescribing;
- to encourage good employment practice;
- to strengthen the science and information base of the NHS;
- to strengthen the central management of the NHS; and
- to increase public understanding of the NHS.

NHSE sets annual priorities and planning guidance for DHAs.[16] Each issue of the priorities and planning guidance rehearses the policy context and points out the current priorities as seen from the centre. Criteria of success for each of the priority areas are suggested. They are taken into consideration in the corporate contract negotiations between DHAs and NHSE Regional Offices.

Local strategy

Within the framework of central policies and guidance DHAs create their own local strategic plans. A typical method is that followed by Northumberland Health; the northernmost authority in England. In June 1994 Northumberland Health issued a consultation draft policy.[17] Every household in the county, covering some 300,000 people, received a summary of the draft and an invitation to take part in the consultation process. The consultation document described the state of health in the locality, the resources available to deal with health problems and a set of actions designed to improve the situation. Comments were invited from individual members of the public, from the health professions, MPs, local government and from special interest groups. Public meetings were held in strategic locations to explain the policy proposals and to listen to public reaction. After three months of consultation the plan was revised and finalised. In October 1994 a summary of the comments received as a result of the consultation process was published together with the final plan.[18,19]

Strategy in local authorities derives in part from guidance provided by the Departments of the Environment and Health and in part from the local democratic process which determines priorities in response to local expressions of need.

The Environment and Health Action Plan for Europe (EHAPE) which resulted from the Second European Conference called for states to prepare their own action plans by 1997. The UK consulted about its proposed plans and published *An Environmental Strategy for the Millennium and Beyond.*[20]

Local tactics

Once the Government has established its policies, both the NHS and other relevant bodies have to implement them, each adding its own variants to deal with particular local circumstances. Guided by the work of their DsPH, Health Authorities base their policy judgements on evidence about burdens of disease, avoidable deaths, effective interventions and available resources.

The market style of working adopted in the NHS in 1991 meant that the DHAs had to obtain services to meet the health and health care needs of their populations through a system of contracts with service providers. With the election of a new government in 1997 the competitive element of the market has been replaced by collaboration between commissioners (the DHAs) and providers. There is still an annual business cycle in which NHSE agrees corporate contracts with DHAs to achieve their local contribution to overall national policy. Within the strategic direction set nationally and in corporate contracts DHAs must negotiate service agreements with the providers of health care in the NHS. Health Authorities agree with their counterpart local authorities what levels of care can be provided in mental health, community and continuing care.[21]

The public is informed in official publications and through the media about what can be expected from the health and social services. Many policy documents are available on the Internet at http://www.open.gov.uk.

As a result of the changes to the structure of the NHS in England, announced by the new government in its White Paper *The new NHS: modern, dependable*,[22] the responsibility for the negotiation of service agreements will shift from DHAs to Primary Care Groups in the future. Primary Care Groups will be formed by aggregation of existing general practices into larger federal groups each serving a population of approximately 100,000 people. Annual health and health care plans will be replaced by longer term Health Improvement Programmes. During 1998 Health Action Zones have been designated. They are communities with defined public health problems. The purpose of the Zones is to ensure close working between health and local authorities, the commercial and voluntary sectors of society, concentrated on resolution of the problems.

Accountability

Government can be called to account for its actions through the system of Parliamentary Select Committees. These comprise groups of MPs drawn from all political parties. They can summon cabinet ministers, civil servants, managers of both public services and private businesses and question them about their policies and practices. There is a Select Committee for Health which can look at both management and clinical issues. There is also a Select Committee for Finance which can look into the way money is spent on health services.

All the directors of DHAs are required to abide by a code of conduct designed to ensure financial propriety, strict observance of relevant laws and political impartiality. They can be subject to the accountability process through the Parliamentary Select Committees. Similarly, local authority councillors and officers can be summoned to account by Parliamentary Select Committees.

DHAs are held to account for their performance, centrally, through their corporate contracts with the NHSE Regional Offices. At the start of each fiscal year DHAs agree with the Regional Offices how they are to meet the targets set in the annual planning and priorities guidance. The Regional Offices undertake quarterly monitoring of progress. There is an overall review at the year end to assess the degree to which the authorities met their targets. Together with the planning and priorities guidance the outcome of this process contributes to the next year's corporate contract.

Each DHA accounts to its local community by publishing an annual report which describes the activities of the authority and in particular explains how the funds have been used to achieve the national and local aims.

Accountability can be exercised through a process of Public Inquiries into specific events. It is also exercised through the courts if negligence is suspected.

Advisory contributions to priority setting

One of the means by which the CMO discharges his functions is through the publication of an Annual Report which comments upon the state of health of the nation, reports on progress in dealing with problems highlighted previously and indicates areas for future priority attention.[23] The CMO is assisted in this task by the Central Health Monitoring Unit which undertakes surveillance of the state of health of the population and enables the CMO to alert DsPH to changes in health.

Each of the territorial CMOs publishes an annual report dealing with similar issues to that published in England.

One of the important elements of the work of Directors of Public Health of the DHAs is the publication of Annual Reports on the states of health in the districts. These are local variants of the report published by the CMO. DsPH reports frequently echo some of the themes of the central report and add priority topics of local concern. The DsPH use the techniques of health needs assessment, surveillance and monitoring to inform the production of the report. In particular they explain the strategies to meet the needs, suggest priorities within the range of needs and inform the market process for the purchase of services.

In addition to locally conducted surveys there are central initiatives to help DHAs, and others, place their policies in a wider perspective and implement them. An example is the publication by the Health Education Authority and the Office of Population, Censuses and Surveys (now part of the National Statistical Office) of the results of a survey to find out what people know and believe about factors that contribute to some of the Health of the Nation targets and how they behave.[24]

The NHSE Information Management Group is developing a tool, described as Health Benefit Groups, to help purchasers to make better use of information about health care interventions.[25] Its purpose is to provide a common language for all involved in the health care contracting process.

Many professional and voluntary groups are developing guidelines of care to help bring evidence of effectiveness into the NHS. One example is the Scottish Inter-collegiate Guidelines Network (SIGN). The NHSE also plays a role in this respect, an example being guidelines for the management of patients with ischaemic heart disease published in the north of England.[26] A series of epidemiological overviews, including needs assessments was commissioned by the Department of Health during the approach to the NHS market. The needs assessment documents explain the various concepts of need, and the methods used for its assessment. They describe approaches to need for a range of topics; some of which are clinical conditions, some are care groups, some are clinical procedures.[27]

The changes outlined in *The New NHS: Modern, Dependable* include provision for the publication of National Service Frameworks[22] intended to be blueprints for cost effective services of the future.

An example of the efforts to influence central thinking is *Setting priorities in the NHS*, published by the Royal College of Physicians.[28] Its comments include reference to the tension between what is technically possible and what can be afforded in a publicly provided health care system. It also highlights the tension between process quality measures, such as waiting lists, beloved of politicians, and clinical outcome measures such as frequency of hospital admission for control of the complications of diabetes.

The work of a variety of government agencies and academic units contributes to a range of publications, such as reviews of effectiveness of interventions and the Public Health Common Data Set,[6] with collated national, regional and local data with comparators, intended to help Directors of Public Health assess the position of their own localities in relation to the rest of the country.

An initiative, aimed at keeping public health matters in focus, has been the publication of guidance for non-health agencies to enable them to assess the impact of their policies on health.[29] It gives guidance on identifying, quantifying and valuing health effects and upon quantifying uncertainty and risk.

A Research and Development policy is emerging intended to support identification of priorities and the establishment and delivery of health and public health policy based on sound information about the results of research.[30] A central Research and Development Committee was established in 1991 with a Director of Research and Development as its Chairman. Applications for central research funding are judged on scientific merit, study design, method and relevance and value to the NHS. The great majority of centrally approved and funded research is clinical. There are projects of public health significance which include studies of ethnic and social variation in cardiovascular disease, methods of assessing mental health needs of a population, studies of behaviour modification before pregnancy and childbirth, the causes of cancers and efficacy of screening.

Outcomes

Some positive progress

Current policy continues to follow the principles set out in the *Health of the Nation* and *Our Healthier Nation* and the associated territorial statements. *The Health of the Nation* identified five key areas, in which there was need for improvement and scope for its achievement. The decisions about key areas rested on the conditions being major causes of premature death or avoidable ill health. Secondly, there had to be effective interventions available which could give scope for improvement. Thirdly, for each key area objectives were established and targets were set so that progress could be charted. Central monitoring of progress has resulted in several publications on progress towards the targets. Although there are indications that progress is broadly in line with expectations, there is concern that issues such as obesity, smoking among teenagers, suicide in young men and lung cancer in women are not proceeding according to plan.[31]

Our Healthier Nation reduces the number to four key areas, all of which reinforce those previously published and revises the targets for improvement.

The original baseline date was 1990 with targets to be achieved by 2000. The new baseline is 1996 with targets to be achieved by 2010.

The key areas are:

• Coronary heart disease and stroke
• Cancers
• Mental illness
• Accidents

In broad terms the proposed targets are twofold. They are:

• to improve overall health by increasing length of life and number of years disease free; and
• to improve the health of the worst off members of society and narrow the gap between the best and worst.

The creation of the *Health of the Nation* policy (and its territorial counterparts) and its continuance through *Our Healthier Nation* has given both purpose and direction to Public Health in the UK that will survive well into the next century. As the dates for the attainment of targets approach the policy will be revised in light of prevailing circumstances.

The establishment of Health Improvement Programmes, coupled with performance review will enable those responsible for the delivery of policy to agree and measure intermediate targets. The framework, though bureaucratic, allows accountability for the pursuit of public health policy to be clear to everyone.

The *Health of the Nation* stimulated some authorities to develop health marketing programmes instead of traditional health education campaigns. Central initiatives in health education are intended only to stimulate and support more sustained and focused local action.

When the NHS market was created in 1991 the watchwords were 'steady state' and 'no surprises' to ensure smooth continuity of existing services. The system rapidly fell into disfavour with the health professions[32] and external pressure to improve the process was applied.[33] Despite the best efforts of many people in the NHS faults in the implementation of market policy remained. They were described in a report from one of the English Regional Offices of the NHSE.[34] The government recommended improvements so that contracts for health and health care services should be:

- comprehensive and based on clinical need;
- aiming to integrate primary, secondary and other levels of care;
- involving continuing dialogue between Health Authority staff and providers, including clinicians;
- using evidence of effectiveness and auditable outcomes of care.[35,36]

Now that market forces are being replaced by collaboration these principles remain relevant.

Even now most service agreements for health care are based on historical levels of activity rather than on comprehensive evidence based programmes which include primary prevention and are designed to achieve specified health outcomes. The Medical Royal Colleges anticipated the official advice about contracts and supported a pilot project to improve the system. The project started in 1993 with some financial assistance from NHSE. It involved local medical practitioners in the process and based service agreements on assessed needs for services for a specific named clinical condition. It succeeded in creating service agreements which dealt with the whole range from primary prevention to tertiary care, using evidence of effective interventions and including target outcomes.[37,38] Now that collaboration has replaced competition the principles developed in the Royal Colleges' project still hold good.

The development of a primary care led NHS is one of the basic tenets of current policy.[15,22] It requires a strategic shift of resources from hospital to primary care. Such a shift is in conflict with the expectations of the public for specialist services, with some of the standards specified in the Patient's Charter and with the demands of the Efficiency Index imposed by the Treasury. The Index, with its accent on acute, mainly hospital based activity, acts as a disincentive to the strategic shift. Many in the NHS acknowledge that the efficiency index needs amendment but there is no confidence that it will be revised appropriately.[39] The new NHS: modern, dependable proposes a broader set of performance measures to replace the efficiency index.

A major feature of the NHS market was the development of fundholding by general practitioners. This process allows GPs to undertake some of the purchasing of services.

There are several grades of fundholding. Some practitioners, usually those from the smaller practices, purchase community care services only. The majority purchase community care services and a limited range of elective acute services. The latest development is the 'Total Fund'. Practitioners involved in Total Fund pilot projects undertake to purchase the full range of health and health care services for their practice populations. A recent study has identified some improvements in communication between general practice fundholders and hospitals and in cost effective prescribing but the report is critical of the management and financial skills of the practitioners.[40]

One of the most significant effects of the development of fundholding is that money for the purchase of health care is being transferred from the statutorily appointed Health Authorities into general practices. Although progress in this direction is patchy it has made substantial differences in some quarters. For example, there are authorities with 70 per cent of the population covered by fundholding practices and half their revenue transferred to GPs. The consequence for the DHAs is that they become more strategic planning bodies and less involved with direct purchasing of services.

Naturally, individual practice budgets are very much smaller and less flexible than DHA budgets. They will be vulnerable to the incidence of the sporadic low volume high cost clinical problem. A tight check has been kept on the administrative overheads of DHAs in recent years. The proliferation of fundholding practices, each with its inevitable management costs, had created the possibility that proportionately more would be spent in aggregate on overheads and less on services. In future the scale of Primary Care Groups will mitigate against both these potential problems to some extent.

Changing the terms of service for general practitioners has stimulated some approaches to health promotion, both systematic and opportunist. Clinics have been established in which health educational and health promotional messages are given about behaviour; smoking; nutrition and obesity and about the benefits of the careful control of long term illnesses such as asthma and diabetes.

There has been improvement in the uptake of childhood immunisation and cervical cytology screening services. These successes have been rooted in the creation of relatively modest financial incentives. Extra payments to GPs are triggered by achievement of threshold percentages for practice population coverage of the relevant procedure. There are lower and higher percentages each of which attracts extra payment. The overall effects have been to increase uptake of the procedures to their highest overall levels ever.

Local Authorities play a large part in the provision of some services, particularly those for the elderly, disabled and mentally ill. Specific financial grants for some of these services allow NHS funds to be used to underpin local authority services. In other circumstances it is difficult to transfer funds from services within the sphere of one government department to those of another. Such a transfer would normally be ultra-vires.

Some NHS services and procedures are being rationed as the tension sharpens between demand and resource. Topics that require difficult policy decisions include cosmetic surgery and fertility services. It is being recognised that it is not satisfactory for rationing decisions to be taken at authority level only. In many places the public is being consulted and its views considered before the decisions are made. Consultation is undertaken both directly and using the assistance of Community Health Councils. Some service users and patient groups are helping authorities to make sensitive policy judgements. The involvement of the public in decisions on priorities is to be welcomed as it can enhance understanding of the complexities of providing a modern health service.

Priority response to worsening of the drug misuse culture has required the establishment of Drug Action Teams in all DHAs. The teams are joint, bringing together representatives of the law enforcement agencies, the health services and local authority social services. Each team has had to submit a plan of action to government to demonstrate the coordinated approach that it proposes to take with the problem of drug misuse.

Unfinished business

There is a lack of clearly identified responsibility for the systematic surveillance of the interaction of the environment with health. To the extent that DsPH must advise on all health matters in the area covered by their DHAs there is an implied expectation that the DPH will do the job. That responsibility is not made explicit and there is no cadre of trained individuals able to support such surveillance.

Lessons derived during two World Wars about dependence on other countries for food supplies have stimulated post-World War II governments to encourage domestic food production. They have been very successful. There have been some deleterious consequences, however, the most evident having been salmonella in eggs and BSE in cattle. Despite these problems the ready availability of convenience foods has meant that the main issues now are of overnutrition rather than undernutrition.

The last fifteen years has seen a large increase in crime recorded in the British Crime Survey although the rate of resolution has failed to keep pace. There is increasing pressure for vigilante solutions to the State's apparent inability to cope.[41] The development of a vigilante society is likely to militate against the successful conclusion of more overtly health and health related policies. Crime, particularly violent crime, derives from and leads to social psychopathology which harms the public health. When compared with the effects of tobacco smoking the death toll from violence is small. Nevertheless, violence contributes to avoidable premature mortality and to long term morbidity. It has prompted the new government to propose crime and disorder partnerships to tackle the problem.[42]

One of the achievements stemming from the *Health of the Nation* was the first government acknowledgement of inequalities in health, marked by the publication of *Variations in Health*.[43] Despite this achievement, the fact that official policy does not look for causes or solutions outside the health services makes it the subject of criticism.[44] The new government openly acknowledges both the inequalities and the fact that not all the problems can be tackled by the NHS. The non health service influences on health, in particular the effects of both social differences and environmental influences, need more attention. In its description of the 'New Public Health' approach the government includes the Welfare to Work programme aimed at reducing unemployment as a major contributor to health improvement outside the NHS. Attention is to be given in the R&D programme but it needs more emphasis.

Homelessness has been the subject of several reports in recent years. A comprehensive report stemming from a public health source[45] has made recommendations about investment in public and private housing, affordability of accommodation and temporary housing for those in need.

There is a marked shortage of information to support policy and priority decision-making.[46] Much of the currently available information is concerned with process measures and not with outcomes. Information to underpin policies with research evidence, epidemiological and other surveillance data, and outcome information is being developed gradually. Its development will be a significant move towards DHAs and local authorities making their policy and priority decisions on the basis of validated, agreed, common information. A set of proposed outcome indicators has been published on a consultation basis.[47] When finalised they are expected to be used in the NHS.

To sustain the delivery of the public health policies and priorities set out in the UK programme a considerable workforce needs to be recruited, trained and retained. There are signs that careers in the NHS are waning in attractiveness. The reasons need to be examined and remedies found. There is a particular need to recruit, train and retain a cadre of research staff. They need to be drawn from a variety of professional disciplines. They need to be trained and to undertake supervised research for two to three years before being capable of working independently. They need to have a career pathway clearly available to them in order to ensure their retention in the academic departments and authorities.[48]

Postscript - the influence of Europe?

Since November 1 1993 Article 129 of the Maastricht Treaty is supposed to have begun to influence EC and therefore UK approaches to public health issues.[49] The only perceptible impact in the UK has been confined to academic departments. Firstly, there has been concern about the draft Directive on Data Protection. Until its modification the effect of the draft Directive would have been to inhibit medical research.

Research and Development sponsored by the EC in the Fourth Framework Programme includes Public Health Research and Health Services Research in BIOMED 2. DH and the Medical Research Council represent UK on the EC management group for BIOMED 2. Calls for research proposals will generate interest in academic departments.

Outside academic departments the EC makes little noticeable contribution to either national or local public health policies. In particular it is doubtful whether anyone working in the NHS has noticed any effect at all arising from Article 129. The new article

129 agreed in Amsterdam (new Article 152 of the Amsterdam Treaty) is likely to have a greater impact in the UK.

By universal acclaim the biggest single contribution to health world wide would be a cessation of tobacco use. The European Commission ought to exert its influence for the good of the public health in respect of tobacco production. Cessation of subsidies for the production of tobacco would earn the Commission even greater credibility in the eyes of public health workers than its current rather weak proposal to agree a common position on tobacco advertising.

References

1. Department of Health. *Public Health in England: The Report of the Committee of Inquiry into the Future Development of the Public Health Function.* London: HMSO, 1988.

2. Hunter D. *Diseases of Occupations.* (3rd edition) London: EUP, 1962.

3. Department of Health. *The Government's Expenditure Plans 1998–1999.* London: HMSO, 1998.

4. Environment Agency. *Aims and Objectives.* Website, 1996.

5. The Food Standards Agency: *A Force for Change.* London: HMSO, 1998.

6. Department of Health. *Public Health Common Data Set 1997.* University of Surrey: National Institute of Epidemiology, 1997.

7. *The National Health Service: A Service with Ambitions.* London: HMSO, 1996.

8. *UK Levels of Health.* (Volumes 1 & 2) London: Faculty of Public Health Medicine, 1991/2.

9. *The Health of the Nation: A Consultative Document for Health in England.* London: HMSO, 1991.

10. *The Health of the Nation: A Strategy for Health in England.* London: HMSO, 1992.

11. *Our Healthier Nation: A Contract for Health. A Consultation Paper.* London: HMSO, 1998.

12. The Lord President's Office. *Tackling Drugs Together: A Consultation Document on a Strategy for England: 1995–98.* London: HMSO, 1994.

13. Department of Health. *Frank Dobson Outlines Third Way for Mental Health.* Press release 98/311, 29th July 1998.

14. Department of Health. *Aims and Objectives of the Department of Health.* London: Department of Health, 1998.

15. NHS Executive. *Aims and Objectives.* Leeds: NHS Executive, 1997.

16. NHS Executive. *Priorities and Planning Guidance for the NHS 1996/7.* EL(95)68. Leeds: NHS Executive, 1995.

17. Northumberland Health Authority. *Better Health in Northumberland: Discussion Document.* Morpeth: Northumberland Health Authority, 1994.

18. Northumberland Health Authority. *Better Health in Northumberland: Summary of Responses to Strategy Consultation.* Morpeth: Northumberland Health Authority, 1994.

19. Northumberland Health Authority. *Better Health in Northumberland: Implementation Plan.* Morpeth: Northumberland Health Authority, 1994.

20. The Environment Agency. *An Environmental Strategy for the Millennium and Beyond.* London: HMSO, 1997.

21. Northumberland Health Authority. *Meeting Continuing Health Care Needs: Policies and Eligibility Criteria.* Morpeth: Northumberland Health Authority, 1996.

22. *The New NHS: Modern, Dependable.* London: HMSO, 1997.

23. Department of Health. *On the State of the Public Health: The Annual Report of the Chief Medical Officer of the Department of Heath for the Year 1994.* London: HMSO, 1995.

24. *Health in England 1995: What People Know, What People Think, What People Do.* London: HEA/OPCS, 1996.

25. *Health Benefit Groups Development Project: Information Sheet.* Winchester: NHS Executive/IMG, 1996.

26. *Guidelines for the Management of Patients with Ischaemic Heart Disease.* Newcastle upon Tyne: NHS Executive (Northern & Yorkshire) 1996.

27. Stevens A. Raftery J. (eds.) *Health Care Needs Assessment: The Epidemiologically-based Needs Assessment Reviews.* Oxford: Radcliffe Medical Press, 1994.

28. *Setting Priorities in the NHS: A Framework for Decision Making.* London: Royal College of Physicians, 1995.

29. Department of Health. *Policy Appraisal and Health: A Guide from the Department of Health.* London: HMSO, 1995.

30. NHS Executive. *Research and Development: Towards an Evidence-based Health Service.* London: Department of Health, 1995.

31. Department of Health. *Fit for the Future: Second Progress Report on the Health of the Nation.* London: Department of Health, 1995.

32. Bury B. Letter to Mrs Bottomley. *British Medical Journal* 1993;306:702–3.

33. Audit Commission. *Their Health, Your Business: The role of the District Health Authority.* London: HMSO, 1993.

34. NHS Executive (Northern & Yorkshire Region). *Contracting Between Health Authorities and NHS Trusts: A Working Group Report.* Newcastle: NHS Executive Regional Office, 1995.

35. Mawhinney B, Nichol D. *Purchasing for Health: A Framework for Action.* Leeds: NHS Executive, 1993.

36. Purchasing Unit. *Managing Contracts: Further Good Practice and Innovation.* Leeds:

NHS Executive, 1994.

37. O'Brien M, Halpin J, Hicks N, Pearson S, Warren V, Holland WW. Health-care commissioning development project. *Journal of Epidemiology* 1996;6:S89–S92.

38. *Health Care Programmes in the NHS.* vols. 1-3. London, Academy of Medical Royal Colleges 1997.

39. Millar B. Wiping the flaws: the efficiency index is to be revamped. *The Health Service Journal* 1995;105(5473):13.

40. Audit Commission. *What the Doctor Ordered: A Study of General Practice Fundholding in England and Wales.* London: HMSO, 1996.

41. Rose D. *In the Name of the Law: The Collapse of Criminal Justice.* London: Jonathan Cape, 1996.

42. *Crime and Disorder Act: Introductory Guide.* London: Home Office, 1998.

43. *Variations in Health: What can the Departments of Health and the NHS do?* London: Department of Health, 1995.

44. Smith GD. Income inequalities and mortality: why are they related? *British Medical Journal* 1996;312:987–8.

45. *Housing or Homelessness: A Public Health Perspective.* (2nd edition). London: Faculty of Public Health Medicine, 1992.

46. Holland WW. *Achieving an Ethical Health Service: What Information do we Need?* The Queen Elizabeth the Queen Mother lecture, Faculty of Public Health Medicine, 28th February 1995.

47. *The New NHS Modern and Dependable: A National Framework for Assessing Performance – Consultation Document.* EL(98)4. NHS Executive, Leeds 1998.

48. Holland WW, Fitzsimmons B, O'Brien M. Back to the future – public health research into the next century. *Journal of Public Health Medicine* 1994;16:4-10.

49. Department of Health. *On the State of the Public Health: The Annual Report of the Chief Medical Officer of the Department of Health for the Year 1993.* London: HMSO 1994.

Index